La Leche League International
Leader's
HANDBOOK
Fourth Revised Edition—2003

CONTRIBUTORS

This revision is a result of work from the following LLL Leaders.

Beth Hilleke, South Carolina, USA

Carol Miranda, New Jersey, USA

Cindy Garrison, Pennsylvania, USA

Claire Eden, Georgia, USA

Diane Jeffer, New Jersey, USA

Edie Boxman, Heraliyah, Israel

Isobel Fanshawe, Chirstchurch, New Zealand

Juanita Watt, New Mexico, USA

Judy Torgus, Illinois, USA

Karen Butler, Coventry, Great Britain

Kristin Marshall, British Columbia, Canada

Nancy Spahr, Indiana, USA

Nikki Julien, Washington, USA

Sandra Tourret, Tortebesse, France

Shirley Phillips, Manitoba, Canada

Sue Ann Kendall, Texas, USA

Special thanks to Shirley Phillips, who coordinated the team of women who updated text and reorganized topics; and to Sue Ann Kendall, who provided editorial assistance in the production phase of the book.

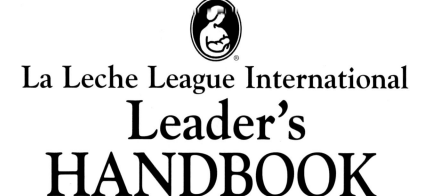

La Leche League International
Leader's
HANDBOOK
Fourth Revised Edition—2003

La Leche League International
Schaumburg, Illinois

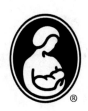

La Leche League International
957 North Plum Grove Road
P.O. Box 4079 Schaumburg IL 60168-4079 USA
847-519-7730
847-969-0460, fax
www.llli.org

Fourth edition, March 2003
    First printing, 6,000 copies
    Second printing, 250 copies

Third edition, March 1998

Second edition, Three printings, 1989, 1991, 1994

First edition, 1977

© 1997, 1989, 1998, 2003 La Leche League International, Inc.

All Rights Reserved

Printed in the United States of America

Cover and book design by Digital Concepts, LLC

Library of Congress Catalogue Card Number 2003103431

ISBN 978-0-912500-95-9

Photo Credits:
Cover photos and pages xiii, 29, 61,135,153, David Arendt; page 1, Paul Torgus;
page 81, Kaye Lowman; page 171, Kim Cavaliero; page 199, Judy Torgus

To the seven Founders, who started it all;

To the 40,000 Leaders so far, who have made

La Leche League what it is today; and

To the Leaders of the future, who will touch the lives of

mothers and babies in the 21st Century.

CONTENTS

CHAPTER 8—LLL SERVICES AND PROGRAMS   199

APPENDICES   211

INDEX   261

A HANDBOOK FOR LEADERS

The purpose of the LLLI LEADER'S HANDBOOK is to provide the basics you need to effectively perform your work as a La Leche League Leader by:

- Describing the Leader's role,
- Offering examples of ways to accomplish the work of an LLL Leader, and
- Suggesting resources.

You will find here the Leader-to-Leader encouragement and support you need to fulfill your job with confidence and pleasure. While this book is intended as a primary reference or resource for Leaders, it is designed to be supplemented and updated with information and ideas from other published and people resources within LLL.

The legal documents of La Leche League provide the framework within which we work as Leaders. Some of the LLLI or Affiliate policies and guidelines that directly apply to your work as a Leader are included in Appendix 1 of this handbook. LLL policies and guidelines are updated regularly. The most current versions of the LLLI Bylaws and *LLLI Policies and Standing Rules Notebook* are available on the LLLI Web site.

Information in this edition of the LEADER'S HANDBOOK is current at the time of printing. LLL is a dynamic organization that is constantly changing. New information is provided through your Leader support system, Leader publications, and on the LLLI Web site.

In 1998, the LLLI Board of Directors outlined activities basic to LLL leadership. In 2001, it updated the definition of an active Leader. The new definition reflects the awareness that, while the basic responsibilities remain central, Leaders can be active and work to fulfill the mission of LLLI in a variety of ways.

Support for Leaders in their work is fundamental to La Leche League. The position titles of those providing this support and the structure within which this support is provided vary throughout LLL. Throughout this handbook, a Leader who provides support for other Leaders—District Advisor, District Coordinator, Assistant Area Coordinator of Leaders or Area Coordinator of Leaders (DA/DC/AACL/ACL)—is referred to as a *support Leader*. A Leader who provides specialized support and information for other Leaders—Coordinator of Leader Accreditation, Professional Liaison Leader, Communication Skills or Human Relations Enrichment Facilitator/Instructor, Area Financial Coordinator, Area Leaders' Letter Editor or Publications Administrator, Area Conference Supervisor or Area Coordinator of Events—is referred to as a *resource Leader*.

In addition to NEW BEGINNINGS and LEAVEN, which are published by LLLI, many La Leche League entities around the world also publish member and Leader newsletters or magazines. The phrase *member publication* or *Leader publication* is used throughout this handbook when reference is made to these publications.

The generic term *LLL Office* is used throughout this handbook, since the Affiliates and many Areas in the International Division have offices to provide local services to Leaders and members in addition to or in place of services provided by the LLLI Office in Schaumburg, Illinois, USA.

INTRODUCTION

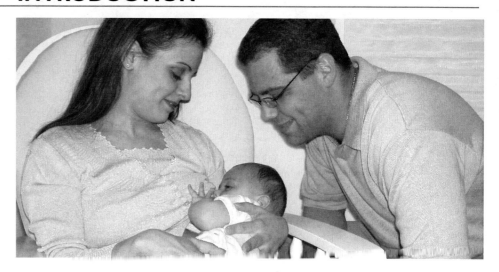

WHY WE ARE LA LECHE LEAGUE LEADERS

Most of us started our relationship with La Leche League with a need for reassurance and accurate breastfeeding information. A Leader—another mother—answered our questions and offered support.

We attended LLL meetings, and as our babies grew older we realized that our personal experience could be important to other new mothers with similar concerns. We wanted to help, to pass on what we ourselves had received. This desire to help other mothers and babies, as well as the satisfaction we receive from doing so, is why we are La Leche League Leaders.

When the problems facing today's world seem overwhelming, it may be hard to believe that one person can make much of a difference. Yet the children of the world are its future. And so, by helping just one other woman establish that special breastfeeding bond with her child, we touch and help shape the future of the world.

As LLL Leaders, we convey values, as much through example as through words: the importance of the family and the value of being a mother, respect for children and their needs, appreciation of nature's wisdom.

We develop and improve skills that we can apply in all the roles we fill in our lives. Active listening helps us respond more effectively to mothers who contact us with questions and problems. Refining our communication skills can enhance our relationships with others, from breastfeeding mothers to family, friends, and co-workers in La Leche League or elsewhere.

We also learn problem-solving techniques. As we gain experience helping women breastfeed, we soon learn that the first question asked may not be the real concern and that finding workable solutions for complex situations requires creativity, patience, and determination. Careful inquiry and creative thinking are useful anywhere we direct our energies.

Assuming responsibility for an LLL Group—organizing materials, keeping financial records, writing reports, and effectively overseeing Group management—helps us gain or increase marketable skills and develop insight into working cooperatively with others in many situations.

We can apply our experience leading Group discussions in many contexts. Learning to offer information and express our thoughts clearly and with conviction, while communicating caring and respect, can be invaluable whether we are speaking with our children, our children's friends, or groups of adults.

As we continue our involvement in LLL, we encounter many opportunities to expand our parenting skills. Through workshops, conferences, books, and personal interaction with other parents, we can improve our ability to meet challenges throughout all the stages of our children's development.

For many, a compelling benefit of our commitment to LLL is the support and companionship of the network of mothers who share our philosophy. LLL work offers us the opportunity to further personal growth and to attain important goals while maintaining our dedication to our families. We can adapt our degree of involvement as our families' needs change. Every individual Leader is vital. LLL is built on the knowledge gained from each personal experience and the unique contribution of time and talent from each of us.

BALANCING FAMILY NEEDS AND LLL COMMITMENTS

La Leche League was founded by women with growing families, and continues to depend on mothers to carry on its work.

How do you balance the needs of your family with your commitment to represent La Leche League?

Setting goals and establishing priorities are keys to achieving this balance. Meeting your baby's needs always comes first. And a baby's needs are perhaps the easiest to combine with LLL work. You can breastfeed the baby while talking to a mother on the telephone. You can take the baby along when leading Series Meetings—the best visual aid possible! Many Leaders have spoken at Area Conferences or childbirth classes with a baby snuggled up in a carrier or sling.

Sometimes a Leader may need to modify her responsibilities for a time. For example, if you are pregnant, you may prefer not to be responsible for leading a meeting near your due date, because you might have to cancel the meeting. Perhaps you'll want to avoid lengthy telephone calls for a while, because your toddler will need extra attention as he adjusts to his new sibling.

At other times in your life, you may welcome new challenges. Perhaps you no longer have a breastfeeding baby and wonder if there is still a place for you in La Leche League. It may be reassuring to know that there are many dedicated Leaders who have been active for ten years or more; many have been involved for more than twenty-five years. The seven women who founded LLL have themselves all continued to be actively involved in the organization for more than forty-five years.

La Leche League offers various avenues of commitment and opportunities for self-expression to fit all the stages of a Leader's life. Leaders may focus on the basic responsibilities, or they may take on support responsibilities, concentrate on reaching populations that haven't traditionally had access to LLL information, or develop new and creative ways to fulfill the LLLI mission.

As your children get older, it may become more difficult to fit LLL activities into family life. Still, Leaders who continue in LLL find a great deal of personal satisfaction in being able to help new mothers enjoy breastfeeding their babies. In evaluating their commitment to La Leche League, some Leaders have commented that there are many who can act as volunteers in their children's school or other activities, but only a limited number of women are able to help mothers breastfeed. La Leche League work is something very special.

You may find, as so many Leaders have, that your parenting values are reinforced by continuing a close association with others who believe in being sensitive to children's needs and feelings. As you remind new mothers to trust their parenting instincts and place people before things, you strengthen your own ability to do the same.

The Balancing Act

Some tips that may help you fit LLL work into your busy life:

- Decide what's important to you, set reasonable goals, and allow plenty of time to achieve those goals.
- Make lists and mark your calendar to help budget your time. The less you carry in your head, the freer your mind may be for creative thinking.
- Know your own limits and learn to say *no* when you reach them. Saying *no* is more responsible than saying *yes* and not following through.
- Use your most productive time most effectively by setting priorities. Don't do an unimportant job during your highest energy/most creative time.
- Find and use hidden time. For example, keep reading material in the car for times that you are waiting to pick up children. Make telephone calls or listen to tapes while cleaning up the kitchen.
- Make good use of spare minutes. A few minutes is enough time to do a quick follow-up telephone call, read a short article, dash off a postcard or note, or address the envelope for a leaflet and add a short note.
- Emphasize the positive. Don't dwell on the negative: guilt over yesterday's things undone, worry over tomorrow's things yet to do. The magic word is *start*.
- Be kind to yourself. Eat right, exercise, take care of your appearance, and find time to relax.
- Let your partner and family know how much LLL work means to you. Communicate your needs and listen to theirs.
- Make time for people and activities important to you. Be flexible when family needs arise. Enjoy life.
- Reward yourself.
- Remember the powerful message we send others when we respond to our children's needs at a meeting or while talking on the telephone.

LA LECHE LEAGUE INTERNATIONAL PURPOSE, PHILOSOPHY, AND MISSION

La Leche League was founded to give information and encouragement, mainly through one-to-one helping, to all mothers who want to breastfeed their babies. LLL recognizes the unique importance of one mother helping another to understand the needs of her children and to explore the most appropriate ways for her to fulfill those needs.

LLLI Bylaws
Section 1. General Purpose

The purpose for which the corporation is formed is charitable and educational and solely in furtherance thereof:

To help the mother learn to breastfeed her baby;

To encourage good mothering through breastfeeding thereby stimulating the optimal physical and emotional growth of the child and the development of close family relationships;

To promote a better understanding of the values of breastfeeding, parenting, childbirth, and related subjects;

To offer discussion meetings and conduct lectures on the purposes stated above and on related subjects for such educational purposes as are herein expressed.

LLLI Purpose and Philosophy

LLLI believes that breastfeeding with its many important physical and psychological advantages is best for baby and mother and is the ideal way to initiate good parent-child relationships. The loving help and support of the father enables the mother to focus on mothering so that together the parents develop close family relationships which strengthen the family and thus the whole fabric of society.

LLLI further believes that mothering through breastfeeding deepens a mother's understanding and acceptance of the responsibilities and rewards of her special role in the family. As a woman grows in mothering she grows as a human being and every other role she may fill in her lifetime is enriched by the insights and humanity she brings to it from her experiences as a mother.

The purpose of LLLI is distinct. The purpose as stated in the Bylaws does not prevent interaction with other organizations with compatible purposes but La Leche League will carefully guard against allying itself with another cause, however worthwhile that cause might be.

The basic philosophy of LLLI as expressed in THE WOMANLY ART OF BREASTFEEDING is summarized in the following concepts:

- Mothering through breastfeeding is the most natural and effective way of understanding and satisfying the needs of the baby.
- Mother and baby need to be together early and often to establish a satisfying relationship and an adequate milk supply.
- In the early years, the baby has an intense need to be with his mother which is as basic as his need for food.
- Breast milk is the superior infant food.
- For the healthy, full-term baby, breast milk is the only food necessary until the baby shows signs of needing solids, about the middle of the first year after birth.
- Ideally the breastfeeding relationship will continue until the baby outgrows the need.

- Alert and active participation by the mother in childbirth is a help in getting breastfeeding off to a good start.
- Breastfeeding is enhanced and the nursing couple sustained by the loving support, help, and companionship of the baby's father. A father's unique relationship with his baby is an important element in the child's development from early infancy.
- Good nutrition means eating a well-balanced and varied diet of foods in as close to their natural state as possible. *From infancy on, children need loving guidance which reflects acceptance of their capabilities and sensitivity to their feelings. (LLLI Policies and Standing Rules Notebook, Appendix 1, rev Feb 98)

Mission Statement

Our Mission is to help mothers worldwide to breastfeed through mother-to-mother support, encouragement, information, and education, and to promote a better understanding of breast-feeding as an important element in the healthy development of the baby and mother.

(LLLI Policies and Standing Rules Notebook, May 89; rev Apr 93)

Leader Roles and Responsibilities

The basic responsibilities of leadership (refer to Appendix 1) are:

- Helping mothers one-to-one by telephone or in person.
- Planning and leading monthly Series Meetings.
- Supervising the management of the LLL Group.
- Keeping up-to-date on breastfeeding information.
- Helping other mothers find out about leadership and prepare to become LLL Leaders.

Leader responsibilities can be shared when there is more that one Leader in a Group. Most Leaders have found it beneficial to concentrate on the basic responsibilities for a period of time before considering expanding or changing their service to LLL.

When thinking about changing your LLL involvement, you may find it helpful to take time to evaluate what you are already doing, set priorities and goals, assess your personal interests, and discuss plans with co-Leaders, support and resource Leaders. By choosing carefully among options, you can find activities to revitalize and strengthen your LLL commitment. In any activity in which you are representing La Leche League as a Leader, it is important to remember that how you fulfill your responsibilities reflects on the organization as a whole-you are the visible face of LLL to your community.

Whatever your priorities, there are many LLL resources available to help you. La Leche League wants you to enjoy and find fulfillment in your work.

Definition of Active Leader

An active LLL Leader pursues the La Leche League mission through basic Leader responsibilities as defined in the Policies and Standing Rules Notebook and/or other service to LLL. An active Leader's fees are current, she keeps up to date with Leader education, and she communicates regularly with the organization.

(LLLI Policies and Standing Rules Notebook, Oct 91, Mar 01)

A BRIEF HISTORY OF LA LECHE LEAGUE

An Idea Is Born

Never underestimate the power of a woman. In the case of La Leche League, never underestimate the power of seven determined women. What started in 1956 as a "nice little local group of mothers" has turned into an international organization that has been helping thousands of mothers and babies all over the world for more than 45 years.

LLL members are fond of saying the group began at a picnic, and, in a way, it did. Two of the Founders, Mary White and Marian Tompson, were sitting under a tree nursing their babies during a church picnic. They were astonished by the number of women who approached them, saying, "I had wanted to nurse my baby, but . . ." They realized the problems these women had faced in trying to nurse their babies were not unusual. They were convinced each of these mothers could have nursed her baby if her questions had been answered.

Mary and Marian consulted Mary's husband, Dr. Gregory White, who was supportive of breastfeeding, although he had little practical advice to offer. They searched through his medical books for what little scientific information was available and recalled their own breastfeeding experiences. They decided that the secrets of successful breastfeeding were information, encouragement, and support.

The two women had no formal plans, but they agreed to meet at Mary's house and invite some friends to discuss breastfeeding. Marian called Edwina Froehlich, who in turn invited Viola Lennon. Mary contacted Mary Ann Kerwin, her sister-in-law, and Mary Ann Cahill, who thought of Betty Wagner. These seven met several times during the summer and early autumn to make plans for their breastfeeding group.

It seemed clear that two main worries for new mothers were having enough milk and whether their milk was right for their babies. Mother-to-mother help had been an important source of encouragement for each Founder when she was learning how to breastfeed. Each Founder contributed her own background, experiences, and special talents to the fledgling organization.

The first official meeting was held on October 17, 1956 in Franklin Park, Illinois, USA. The seven Founders and five of their pregnant friends attended. However, the group did not stay small and intimate. To the surprise of the Founders, women they didn't know began showing up. Within a few months, there were so many women asking to come that it was necessary to split into two groups.

The Idea Gained Momentum

Although early meetings were unstructured, the group steadily became more organized. They began with a series of four meetings and met every three weeks. Dr. Herbert Ratner, then health commissioner of Oak Park, Illinois, USA, and a good friend of Dr. Gregory White, led a meeting for fathers.

The name La Leche League was chosen in 1957. "La Leche" is a Spanish phrase (pronounced "la lay chay") that means "the milk."

THE WOMANLY ART OF BREASTFEEDING began as a course-by-mail in loose-leaf binder form, intended for use by mothers living too far away to attend LLL meetings. Vi Lennon remembers she couldn't see the need for a book at first, but letters from mothers all over the USA changed her mind. At first, every copy of the book went

In searching for a name for our new organization, we Founders were struck by the importance placed on breastfeeding by early Spanish settlers in America. In 1598, the settlers dedicated a shrine to "Nuestra Senora de la Leche y Buen Parto" [Our Lady of Happy Delivery and Plentiful Milk]. The words "happy delivery and plentiful milk" spoke profoundly of yearnings that are common to many mothers. Like women of old, we rejoiced in breastfeeding our babies and wanted to share our newfound knowledge with others. Even though our name came from a religious shrine, we unanimously chose to be a nonsectarian organization from the start. To us, "La Leche" [The Milk] became as much a symbol as a name. While it was chosen in part because the word "breastfeeding" was not acceptable at that time, in another sense our name's lofty origin reflected the importance we attached to the work we were undertaking.

The LLLI Founders, September 1997

out with a personal letter of encouragement. The first edition of THE WOMANLY ART OF BREASTFEEDING was revised and expanded into a blue-covered book in 1963. More than a million copies were sold in the eighteen years before it was revised in 1981. In 1983, this edition was licensed to New American Library (now Penguin USA), which now co-publishes the book and makes it widely available in bookstores. Subsequent editions were published in 1987, 1991, and 1997. THE WOMANLY ART OF BREASTFEEDING is available in eight languages—English, Spanish, German, French, Dutch, Italian, Japanese, and Polish.

In 1958, LLL NEWS began. Marian Tompson was its first editor, and compiling it was a family affair at her house. LLL NEWS continued as the LLLI member publication for twenty-six years until 1985, when its format was revised and expanded into NEW BEGINNINGS. LEAVEN, the LLLI journal for Leaders, began publication in 1965.

In 1963, for the first time, an employee was hired to help with the mail; LLL also rented its first one-room office. The organization drafted a constitution in 1963 and officially became La Leche League International in June 1964. The organization's international office is now located in Schaumburg, Illinois, USA. There, staff members process LLLI orders and memberships, handle inquiries, produce LLLI publications, keep up-to-date files of breastfeeding research, seek grants and funding, plan LLLI conferences, seminars, and workshops, manage LLLI Internet activities, and handle the administrative duties of the organization.

Many of the women who wrote to the Founders wanted to start LLL Groups in their own communities. They were encouraged to do so, and before long LLL News listed Groups in the USA, Canada, and Mexico. This rapid growth began to worry the Founders, since they wanted the organization to foster a particular philosophy of breastfeeding and mothering. They wanted mothers to find the same kind of information and encouragement wherever a La Leche League Group was formed. It became evident that a standard procedure was needed for those who were interested in starting Groups. Also needed were procedures to keep in touch with Leaders and Groups all over the world. These needs led to the establishment of the Leader and Leader Applicant (now Accreditation) Departments in 1964.

Also in 1964, LLL held its first convention at the Knickerbocker Hotel in downtown Chicago, Illinois, USA-quite an unusual undertaking for a group of mothers with babies. Since then, La Leche League International Conferences have been held in various US cities and in Toronto, Canada.

Thoughout the 1980s, LLLI and a number of LLL entities developed different working relationships and signed a formal document called the Agreement of International Principles of Cooperation. Signing the AIPC provided for these LLL entities to be affiliated with LLLI rather than part of the Division administrative structure. The six Affiliates are Canada, Ligue La Leche (Canada FranÁais), Deutschland, Great Britain, New Zealand, and Switzerland.

Each step in the growth and expansion of the organization was taken in an effort to continue meeting the needs of the mothers and babies who turned to LLL for breast-feeding help. The LLLOVE STORY (1978) and SEVEN VOICES, ONE DREAM (2001) provide a history of La Leche League's development.

The Organization Today

La Leche League International is a not-for-profit, nongovernmental organization incorporated in the state of Illinois, USA. Under the laws of Illinois (and in most other states of the USA and many other countries), not-for-profit organizations are required to have a Board of Directors to establish policies, hire an Executive Director (if needed), and ensure the legal and ethical integrity of the organization, including effective management of resources and continued focus on the mission of the organization. The details of the organization and functioning of the LLLI Board of Directors, including elections, officers and committees, can be found in the LLLI Bylaws and in the *LLLI Policies and Standing Rules Notebook* (PSR), which is available on the LLLI Web site or from your Area/Affiliate administrator.

Currently, according to the LLLI Bylaws, the LLLI Board is composed of members from the LLLI geographic zones and members at large. A minimum of two-thirds of the Board members must be Leaders. The seven zones are Europe, Eastern US, Western US, Canada, South Pacific and Asia, Africa and Middle East, and Latin America. Each Zone has at least one seat on the Board, with additional seats determined according to the Zone's percentage of the total LLLI active Leader population. Most Board members are nominated by the Zones and elected by the Board; the Board can also elect members at large, usually for particular knowledge and skills (for instance, accounting or law).

Today La Leche League is recognized internationally as the world's foremost authority on breastfeeding. LLLI maintains consultative status with the United Nations Children's Fund (UNICEF), maintains official working relations with the World Health Organization (WHO), acts as a registered Private Voluntary Organization (PVO) for the United States Agency for International Development (USAID), and is a founding member of the World Alliance for Breastfeeding Action (WABA). The Accreditation Council for Continuing Medical Education accredits LLLI to provide continuing medical education for physicians in North America.

In 2000, LLLI initiated a process of organization-wide evaluation and renewal. This process will help build LLL's capacity for learning and change, enabling LLL to be flexible in continuing to meet the need for breastfeeding information and support around the world.

As LLLI has grown into an international organization, the primary focus has remained on the personal one-to-one sharing of information and encouragement that provides a new mother with the confidence she needs to breastfeed her baby. As a Leader providing this personal support to mothers, you are vital to the fulfillment of the LLLI mission.

CHAPTER ONE

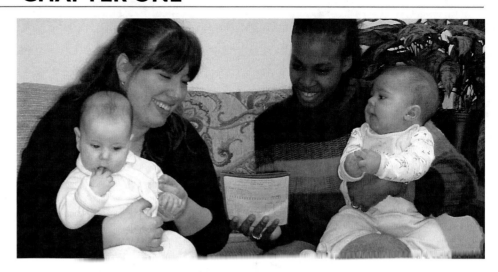

Mother-to-Mother Help

A Leader—an experienced breastfeeding mother—helps another mother with questions or concerns about breastfeeding, one mother to another. The one-to-one approach is the core of our work as La Leche League Leaders.

One of the most important things we do as Leaders is to help a mother build her self-confidence and trust in her own mothering instincts. In this way, the mother is empowered to solve many problems herself, by looking to her baby and responding to his needs.

Basic communications skills help us establish rapport with the mothers who turn to LLL for help. These skills also help us share information effectively in one-to-one situations and at Group meetings.

THE BASICS OF ONE-TO-ONE HELPING

Some of the key communications skills that Leaders find useful in one-to-one helping are discussed in this section.

Key Communication Skills
- Encouraging the mother to feel at ease
- Establishing a feeling of rapport with the mother
- Listening carefully to demonstrate genuine interest in helping
- Asking questions to clarify the mother's situation
- Helping the mother identify her feelings, where appropriate
- Offering information, making suggestions, and discussing options, so the mother can evaluate the advantages and disadvantages, and make up her own mind
- Recognizing the mother as the expert on her own baby

When LLL Leaders convey
warmth, sensitivity, and respect,
the mother who contacts LLL is
more likely to be receptive to
information and suggestions.

Encouraging the Mother to Feel at Ease

A warm, sincere manner and tone of voice will help put an anxious mother at ease.

When LLL Leaders convey warmth, sensitivity, and respect, the mother who contacts LLL is more likely to be receptive to information and suggestions. Some Leaders seem to have these qualities naturally. Most of us benefit from the opportunity to further develop these skills by being aware of the principles of good communication and practicing them.

Communicating Skillfully—Learning by Doing

Observing other Leaders

It is natural to learn from observing other Leaders—watching and listening to them at Series Meetings and noticing the tone and attitude they communicate, the way they address mothers' concerns, and how they present information and options.

Practicing with the Preview

"The Breastfeeding Resource Guide" and "A Preview of Mothers' Questions/Problems and Group Dynamics/Management" (also known as "the Preview"), which are parts of the preparation for leadership, provide ways to practice and gain confidence in communication skills.

Participating in Communication Skills Sessions

Opportunities to learn about and practice communication skills are often offered at local or Area workshops and LLL conferences by the Communication Skills or the Human Relations Enrichment (HRE) Department to Leaders, Leader Applicants, Group members, and other interested parties. (See **Communication Skills/Human Relations Enrichment Sessions,** pages 156 & 171.)

Establishing a Feeling of Rapport with the Mother

Pacing the conversation according to the mother's cues helps to build rapport. If a mother is crying, reassure her that it's all right to cry. Using her name frequently, and talking slowly and quietly may help calm her so that she can describe the specific problem. Trying to verbalize her feelings about what seems to be the problem may be appropriate. A sympathetic statement (for instance, "I can see it's been hard for you") can also help.

If a mother is crying, reassure
her that it's all right to cry.
Using her name frequently and
talking slowly and quietly may
help calm her so that she can
describe the specific problem.

Talking about personal experience

One of the strengths of La Leche League is that Leaders are or have been breastfeeding mothers. While it can be helpful for a mother to know that you have overcome a similar problem, it is best to be cautious in sharing personal experience.

Although we have valuable insight and may have relevant personal experience to share, the mother usually can't really listen to our information until she feels assured that her feelings and situation have been understood.

Even when the mother is ready to hear information, our personal experience may not be relevant to her situation. Just as we all react differently and make different choices, we can all feel very differently about similar situations.

When discussing feelings, it may occasionally be helpful for mothers to hear how you felt.

> *"I remember when I used to wonder if my baby would ever sleep longer than two hours at a time."*
>
> *"I was skeptical myself when I first heard you could let the baby show you when he was ready for solids."*

By keeping any sharing of your own personal experience brief, you will be able to refocus immediately on how the mother feels about her situation or the information and options you have shared.

Listening Carefully to Demonstrate Genuine Interest in Helping

Active listening can help clarify the mother's feelings, making it easier for you to understand the real question or problem and decide what information will be helpful to offer. It demonstrates to the mother that you are making an effort to understand her.

When you help a mother in a face-to-face situation, maintaining eye contact is an important part of active listening.

Whether you help in person or by telephone, rephrasing statements, naming feelings, and summarizing what the mother has said offers her the chance to confirm or to correct your understanding.

> *Rephrasing statements, naming feelings, and summarizing what the mother has said offers her the chance to confirm or to correct your understanding.*

> *"Let me see if I am following you. You said…"*
>
> *"Did you mean that….?"*
>
> *"You seem to be telling me that…"*
>
> *"I hear you saying that…"*

Naming the mother's feelings helps clarify

> *Mother: My baby cries all the time.*
>
> *Leader: That's really tough—you don't know what to do.*
>
> *Mother: Yes, it seems like I've tried everything to quiet her.*

Sometimes simply helping a mother clarify her feelings can help her solve her own problem.

For example:

> *Mother: Whenever I put my baby down, he cries. I considered using a baby sling to keep him close while I do housework, but my mother keeps telling me that I will spoil the baby if I don't put him down.*
>
> *Leader: You're saying that the idea of using a baby sling appeals to you but you're also worried that your mother may be right. She has a lot of experience with babies.*
>
> *Mother: You're right. I am so confused! What information do you have about spoiling babies?*

Phrases such as these help reflect feelings:

"*I sense you feel strongly (or worried or unsure or unhappy) about that.*"

"*You seem to be feeling . . .*"

"*You sound . . .*"

Responding without judging

When a mother feels your empathy and understanding, she is more likely to be able to accept suggestions.

Active listening is a useful tool, especially when a mother's choice or point-of-view is outside our personal experience.

For example, a mother boasts that her three-week-old baby takes two bowls of cereal a day but wonders why her milk supply seems to be decreasing. It might be tempting to tell her that it is too early to give solids. However true this may be, such an opening remark would probably make the mother feel criticized. This feeling might make her unable or unwilling to hear the information you have to offer.

When a mother feels your empathy and understanding, she is more likely to be able to accept suggestions. For example:

"*You're worried that your milk supply seems to be decreasing. We've found that the breasts need to be stimulated often by baby's sucking to maintain or increase milk production. Reducing the solids might encourage your baby to breastfeed more and bring your supply back up again.*"

If the mother is receptive, continuing with specific suggestions on what she can do to reestablish her milk supply will probably be helpful. Afterwards, she may be interested in discussing starting solids when the baby is older.

Every mother wants to do the best for her baby. The mother of the three-week-old baby who is already on solids is concerned about her baby's welfare. Since she has contacted LLL, she probably does want to continue nursing. Although you might think privately that it is a mistake to give cereal to such a young baby, expressing such thoughts interferes with the focus on the mother's concerns. The mother is more apt to be receptive to suggestions or alternative approaches when there is no hint of criticism.

Respecting differences

Mothers' backgrounds and experiences vary widely. A single mother's challenges are different from a married mother's challenges, and an adolescent mother's challenges are very different again. Different cultural backgrounds lead to different childbirth, breastfeeding, and child-rearing customs. Here are a few suggestions to keep in mind when talking to mothers whose experiences may be different from your own: (Additional suggestions may be found in the "Giving Effective Breastfeeding Help" chapter of THE BREASTFEEDING ANSWER BOOK.)

- Asking questions to find out more about the mother's support network avoids the assumption that a mother has a partner.
- Adolescent mothers have concerns that may not be obvious to an older mother—for example, feelings of fear and insecurity, or heightened concerns about appearance, weight gain, freedom, and peer opinions. When talking to an adolescent mother, it helps to try to look at the world through her eyes. It may be helpful to emphasize the benefits of breastfeeding to her as well as to her relationship with her baby.

- Customs regarding health, medicine, and sexuality may vary a great deal according to cultural background and religious belief. Suggesting a variety of alternatives in an objective way can help avoid suggestion of criticism.
- When recommending special breastfeeding equipment or any other purchases, it is important to remember possible economic differences and to give several options with different costs, such as renting instead of buying a pump, or using hand expression.
- Referring the mother to books that she might find helpful takes into account that parenting styles can be very different, even within the same cultural and economic group.

Asking Questions to Clarify the Mother's Situation

Many times the first question or situation a mother raises is not what is bothering her most. She may not identify other factors underlying her immediate problem. In some cases, a mother asks a testing question first to see what kind of reaction or information she receives, before she gains enough trust to share what is really bothering her.

For example:

> Mother: *My baby isn't getting enough milk!*
>
> Leader: *Why do you think he isn't getting enough?*
>
> Mother: *I'm nursing him all the time.*
>
> Leader: *That can be tiring! And you worry because he seems hungry all the time. Tell me more about your baby's nursing pattern.*

Open-ended questions can help both the mother and Leader better understand the situation

Questions that begin with "what" or "how" encourage more informative responses than questions that invite a "yes" or "no" answer. For instance, you might ask, "How is the baby getting along?" instead of, "Is the baby getting along well?"

Asking what the mother sees as the problem

Asking the mother about her perception of the problem helps you address her concerns more effectively:

> *"What do you see as the problem?"*
>
> *"How would you like to see this resolved?"*

Although you might identify an additional problem, it's important to address the mother's immediate concerns first. A mother may also bring up something that you consider a problem, but she does not. Keep in mind the old saying, "If it's not broken, don't fix it." If the mother is happy with the way things are, and the baby's health is not in jeopardy, it is not necessary to suggest that there might be a problem. (See **A Guide to Possible Clues**, page 19.)

MOTHER-TO-MOTHER HELP

Different cultural backgrounds lead to different childbirth, breastfeeding, and child-rearing customs.

Questions that begin with "what" or "how" encourage more informative responses than questions that invite a "yes" or "no" answer.

Helping the Mother Identify Her Feelings

Sometimes when a mother raises many different issues at once, it can be hard to know which to address first. If you rephrase the mother's feelings as you understand them, the mother will usually suggest where to go from there.

> *Mother: I guess I'm just going to give up on this breastfeeding. My doctor says John is gaining too slowly and that I shouldn't have to nurse him more often than every three hours. My two-year-old got hold of some aspirin while I was nursing John. I had been up all night rocking John so he'd sleep longer than two hours. I knew if I had to tell the doctor he was waking all night and nursing more often than every three hours, the doctor would want me to supplement and I'm just not going to do both. I'm just not!*

Rushing in with information and suggestions may be a tempting response. However, responding with empathy can help the mother identify her most pressing need.

> *Leader: You're bewildered. The baby doesn't seem to be doing as well as you had hoped. You are afraid that your doctor will tell you to supplement. Your other little one needs attention. That aspirin incident scared you! Now you really wonder what to do.*

This statement recognizes the mother's feelings. Notice the feeling words used: "bewildered," "afraid," and "scared." The Leader specifically mentions each area of concern; then the mother can indicate which needs attention first.

> *Mother: You're right. I feel like such a failure. I don't seem to be able to handle anything. The aspirin incident really shook me. I know what to do about that though. I'll just have to keep my two-year-old with me. I know that's what I'll have to do, but I'm so tired. Being responsible for anyone other than the baby is more than I can bear.*

> *Leader: When you're as exhausted as you are now, it seems hard to handle everything, but even as tired as you are, you've come up with a plan: keeping your two-year-old with you. You would like to be able to handle this, yet you're not sure whether you can keep yourself and your two-year-old together.*

> *Mother: That's it. I know the only thing to do is to keep him with me, but how will I manage with two children?*

Who would guess that the first thing on this mother's mind is suggestions for handling two children rather than how to increase her milk supply?

Notice how the Leader responds empathetically to the mother until she identifies her priorities. Even if the Leader labels the mother's feelings inaccurately ("bewildered," "afraid," "scared"), the mother will clarify these in her response. In this case, the Leader knows she's identified a major concern when the mother says, "You're right. I feel like such a failure."

The Leader continues with empathy until the mother says she needs help handling two children. The Leader can tell the mother is ready for suggestions because she specifically asks for information. It is important to wait for that moment before offering suggestions.

Rushing in with information and suggestions may be a tempting response. However, responding with empathy can help the mother identify her most pressing need.

Leader: Meeting the needs of two young children without getting overwhelmed is a big challenge for most new mothers. Some mothers find that using a baby sling to carry the baby around while tending the older child works well. By the way, it is easy to nurse the baby any time he likes when you carry him around. This may really help his weight gain, too—many newborns do need to breast-feed more often than every three hours to thrive.

MOTHER-TO-MOTHER HELP

Offering Information, Making Suggestions, and Discussing Options

Sharing information rather than giving advice

Giving advice often sends an unspoken message—a lack of confidence and trust. The assumption is that the listener needs to be told what to do. Advice usually begins with phrases such as:

> *"You should…"*
>
> *"You ought to…"*
>
> *"Why don't you…?"*
>
> *"You should have…"*
>
> *"Why didn't you…?"*
>
> *"You shouldn't have…"*

In giving information, making suggestions, and presenting options, we convey trust, which is the basis of any successful helping relationship.

Even if a mother asks for or is open to receiving advice, the result may not be helpful. Some possible outcomes are:

- The mother follows the advice and is successful.
  Possible result: The mother may not give herself credit for making the decision to use the information in the advice and for implementing it.
- The mother follows the advice and fails.
  Possible result: The mother may give all the responsibility to the Leader, and the Leader and LLL lose credibility.
- The mother rejects the advice and is successful.
  Possible result: The mother doesn't trust LLL's information, and the Leader and LLL lose credibility.
- The mother rejects the advice and fails.
  Possible result: The mother resents the Leader or becomes dependent on her and doesn't trust herself.

Giving information implies that the person receiving the information is qualified to make choices. In giving information, making suggestions, and presenting options, we convey trust, which is the basis of any successful helping relationship. Even when we may have more knowledge and experience about breastfeeding, it is the mother's responsibility to make her own decisions. (See also **The Art of Sharing Information without Giving Medical Advice,** page 11.)

Offering information

Mothers usually find it easier to accept information when you present it positively, highlighting benefits rather than stating negative consequences.

For example, "We have found that babies who have only human milk until about the middle of the first year after birth are far less at risk of developing allergies" is more positive than "If you give solids before the baby is six months old, he has a good chance of developing allergies."

Telling the mother the source of the information gives her the option of referring to it herself, if she wishes.

Deciding how much information to offer

When a mother has many difficulties or is struggling to handle her situation, it is often best to start with simple, specific suggestions that are easy to carry out. Even when it is clear that there are some deep, complicated causes for a mother's problems, small changes can be important and are usually more feasible.

For example, a mother who is overwhelmed by many pressures may be totally exhausted. The simple suggestion of napping with her baby may give her a way to get the rest she needs to renew her strength to face her other difficulties.

Even in less complicated situations, listening and then being selective in offering information is usually most effective. If the mother is worried about her baby or lacking confidence, her emotional state may not allow her to absorb very much new information.

Try singling out one or two suggestions that are most likely to help. Listen carefully to the mother, repeating those same one or two suggestions. Ask her to contact you later if these ideas don't help, or offer to contact her.

> Giving a little information at a time allows the mother to absorb it more fully, to react to it, and to ask questions.

Giving a little information at a time allows the mother to absorb it more fully, to react to it, and to ask questions. When she has time to talk and clarify her needs, you both learn more.

Making suggestions

Tactful ways of presenting suggestions leave room for individual preferences:

"Here's what other mothers have done in similar situations."

"How would you feel about…?"

"Many mothers have found…"

"Some babies seem to need…"

"You may find that…."

It may feel awkward at first to consciously word suggestions this way, but most Leaders find it becomes more comfortable with practice.

Another possibility:

"These ideas have worked with other babies. Try them if you think they might work for you. If you find success with something I haven't mentioned, please tell me so I can pass your idea on to other mothers."

This approach offers information, reminds the mother to use her own experience and intuition, and encourages her to share her ideas for the benefit of others.

Discussing options

When presenting options, you can encourage the mother to respond honestly by saying something like:

"Do you think any of these alternatives might work for you?"

"Could one of these options be modified to fit your family?"

Sometimes a mother may react negatively to a suggestion. It is important to respect the mother's feelings.

In this example the Leader and mother have already discussed the benefits of nursing her slow-gaining baby more often.

Mother: So you're suggesting not only to nurse more frequently—whenever the baby wants—but to use both breasts. I can manage that, at least during the day. But what will I do about nighttime? I really do need some sleep.

Leader: You're concerned about not getting enough sleep if you have to nurse frequently at night. Have you thought about taking the baby to bed with you?

Mother: You've got to be kidding! I don't think it's good to have a baby in bed with us. Surely you don't do that, do you?

Leader: You're surprised. I was, too, when I first heard that this does work for some families. Since you are not comfortable with it, let's consider other options. Have you thought of using an adult bed in the baby's room and going to him the first time he wakes? If you fall asleep while nursing, at least you would be getting some rest.

Mother: This sounds like it would work. And I certainly would welcome the sleep!

If the mother isn't interested in this suggestion, the Leader might offer another (a cradle or crib in the parents' room, for instance). She may also invite the mother to problem-solve: "Can you think of a way to adapt this idea so you can nurse during the night and still get rest?"

Recognizing the Mother as the Expert on Her Own Baby

At least once during a conversation try to say something like,

"It sounds to me as though you are really trying to understand your baby."

"Your baby is so lucky to have you for his mother."

"I can tell that you are aware of your baby's different cries and needs."

Positive feedback is an important reassurance and a confidence booster to the mother. The more specific you can be in giving positive feedback, the stronger the reassurance.

Breastfeeding difficulties often impact on the new mother's sense of self-esteem. Be aware of the mother's sensitivity to any suggestion of criticism.

Sometimes a mother may react negatively to a suggestion. It is important to respect the mother's feelings.

Encourage openness and honesty between the mother and her health care provider. Remind her that they are working as a team in safeguarding the health of the baby.

BREASTFEEDING QUESTIONS AND POSSIBLE MEDICAL IMPLICATIONS

When the Leader's Suggestions Differ from the Health Care Provider's Advice

Sometimes a Leader's suggestions differ from those of a mother's health care provider. Often there is no specific medical issue involved but rather a matter of breastfeeding management.

One example is the mother whose health care provider tells her that her slow-gaining baby shouldn't nurse more often than every three hours. The Leader can tell the mother that, "Many mothers have found that nursing more often improves weight gain," and reinforce this with references from LLL publications (backed by the LLLI Health Advisory Council). If the mother seems comfortable with the idea of nursing more often, the Leader could suggest she try it for a week or so, or until the baby's next check-up, and see if the baby's weight improves.

Encourage the mother to tell her health care provider what she is planning to do. If the more frequent nursing results in improved weight gain, the health care provider will learn more about breastfeeding from mother and baby in a positive way.

Encourage openness and honesty between the mother and her health care provider. Remind her that they are working as a team in safeguarding the health of the baby.

If the health care provider has suggested that there is a medical problem with the baby or if the mother seems reluctant to go against his or her advice, encourage the mother to call the health care provider and further discuss alternatives. Be sure the mother knows the background information that supports the recommendation of more frequent nursing. Perhaps she can offer to bring the baby in for weight checkups every week or two until the health care provider is satisfied with the baby's progress.

Encourage the mother to tell the health care provider how she feels: "I feel very uncomfortable about trying..." or "I will feel so sad if..." or "I would feel more comfortable trying..." Help the mother to decide for herself, speak for herself, and avoid saying "LLL says..." She can share the background material you have supplied with the doctor, or she can say, "I read... in..." or "A book I read suggests..."

Handling Medically Related Breastfeeding Questions

A mother who needs information about breastfeeding in a medically related situation may call you for two reasons. First, she recognizes that you, as a Leader, will be sympathetic and empathetic to her feelings. You listen and offer support. Second, she may seek to access the resources of LLL.

Leaders are not health care providers. The skills and insights you have gained as a mother and Leader give you a unique perspective that is helpful and reassuring to mothers who call. When asking a mother questions or offering information, it's important to keep your limitations as a lay counselor in mind and to know the difference between offering information and giving medical advice. Giving medical advice can result in discord with the medical community and possible legal problems for you and LLL.

It is your responsibility to be well informed and up-to-date on breastfeeding matters and to know where the relevant information can be found. If a mother asks about a medical situation that affects breastfeeding, such as newborn jaundice, mastitis, or medication use while breastfeeding, encourage her to check first with her health care provider.

In medically related breastfeeding situations, you can help mothers by:

- Offering information from LLL publications, and other appropriate resources
- Letting the mother know that there may be alternative ways of handling the situation, and
- Helping the mother work with her health care provider.

MOTHER-TO-MOTHER HELP

You can always feel free to say, "I don't know, but I'll check it out and call you back."

The Art of Sharing Information without Giving Medical Advice

Consider the situation of a mother who contacts a Leader by telephone; her baby is jaundiced. Her health care provider says she must wean because her milk is causing the jaundice. The mother does not want to stop breastfeeding and wants to know what she should do. How do you respond?

Listen and ask questions

Your immediate reaction may be to say, "You don't have to wean." Instead, find out as much as possible about the situation. How old is the baby? What has the health care provider said? Why does he or she think weaning is indicated? Is he or she referring to a temporary weaning? What is the health care provider's attitude toward breastfeeding? What does the mother think she should do? What does her partner think?

Sometimes a mother can provide her own answers if she only has someone who will listen. These questions may provide a good beginning:

"What did the doctor say?"

"Why do you think the doctor said that?"

"How do you feel about those suggestions?"

"What do you want to do?"

Avoid giving personal opinions

It may sound like a simple case of physiologic jaundice, and you may wonder why the health care provider insists on treating it like a medical problem. In many cases, even when bilirubin counts seem high, weaning is not necessary. Remember that as a Leader you are not qualified to diagnose the situation. You may not have all the facts. Maybe there is something that the mother is not telling you. Maybe the mother did not fully understand what the health care provider said. There may be more to the situation than is apparent.

Share information and resources

Quote accurately and objectively from THE WOMANLY ART OF BREASTFEEDING, THE BREASTFEEDING ANSWER BOOK, LLL pamphlets, and other sources. Let the mother know the source of the information so she can refer to it herself and perhaps share it with her health care provider, who may not be aware of the latest research and treatment options. Be sure to include the title page and full reference citations when providing partial references. Encourage her to refer to these resources by name rather than saying, "LLL says...."

When you tell the mother what others in similar situations have done, you might use phrases such as "The LLLI Health Advisory Council suggests..." or "Many mothers have found..."

Using the Leader's Log and Medical Questionnaire forms helps ensure that you have gathered enough information from the mother.

Contact a Professional Liaison (PL) Leader

If your local PL Leader doesn't have the information on hand, she will contact others, including her PL resource Leaders and the LLLI Center for Breastfeeding Information (CBI), and get back to you with additional information you can offer the mother. If you are in an online helping situation, you may also contact an Online Professional Liaison Resource Leader. (See **Support for the Leader Dealing with Medically or Legally Related Issues** and Chapter 6, **Keeping Up-to-Date.**)

Helping the Mother to Work with Her Health Care Provider

Most people, but especially pregnant women and new mothers, find it very stressful to be in conflict with a health care provider. The mother may need suggestions on how to achieve a frank dialogue with her health care provider. You can suggest to the mother many ways to help her encounter with the health care provider be a positive one.

- Think through her approach in advance—what is important to her, what concerns her,
- Practice her responses before she talks to the health care provider,
- Ask for a complete explanation of the treatment and how it is related to her baby, in particular—repeating the health care provider's statements in her own words can help the mother check her understanding,
- Make statements in a positive way,
- Try the "broken record" technique,
- Use tact, give respect and expect tact and respect in return, and
- Be confident!

Inform the mother that she has certain rights as a patient. In most situations a mother has a right as a patient to seek a health care provider who understands the benefits of breastfeeding. She can do this on her own or ask the health care provider to consult with a colleague who has had experience in this area. Inform her of this option, but leave the decision to her.

Questions about Medications while Breastfeeding

Leaders often receive calls from mothers who have questions about taking medications while breastfeeding. Perhaps they have been told a drug will be harmful to the baby; perhaps they have been told it will not be harmful and they want reassurance.

In some cases, a medication may be one that is commonly used or prescribed for breastfeeding mothers. In other cases, the medication is one that has been associated with some risk to the breastfeeding infant, or it is a new drug that has not yet been tested on lactating women.

The ultimate decision whether or not to take a medication and/or whether to continue or stop breastfeeding must remain with the mother in consultation with her health care provider.

Because of the wide variety of complex medical issues involved in treating any patient, neither LLLI nor any of its Leaders can give medical advice. However, you may be called upon to share medical information with a mother, particularly regarding questions about medications. For this reason, you may want to have a reference list of drugs on hand. THE BREASTFEEDING ANSWER BOOK includes "The Transfer of Drugs and Other Chemicals into Human Milk" published by the American Academy of Pediatrics Committee on Drugs. A Professional Liaison Leader will have additional resources on hand.

Since information on medications is updated periodically, be sure the reference you're using is current. Read the information verbatim without paraphrasing, interpreting, drawing conclusions, or giving medical advice. Tell the mother the name and date of the reference and any other sources listed.

Anyone who is concerned about drugs in human milk needs to consider three questions. If these are answered in open communication between physician and patient, most mothers' concerns can be resolved.

1. Will the drug harm the breastfeeding baby?
2. Will weaning harm the breastfeeding baby or the mother?
3. What are the options?

Too often only the first question is raised; the other two are equally important.

If a mother contacts you to ask about taking a specific drug, you can help her make a decision by asking:

- Has the medication been prescribed by a physician or other health care provider?
- Does the health care provider know the mother is breastfeeding?
- Has weaning been recommended?
- Has the mother asked about alternative drugs or treatments that would enable her to continue breastfeeding or about the possibility of postponing therapy?

If a mother has been advised to wean, but you have information that shows that other mothers have used this medication without harmful effects, you can provide this information along with the necessary background references so the mother can discuss the matter further with her physician.

If, after raising these issues with her physician, the mother is not satisfied, she may want to consider a second opinion, especially if the doctor insists that she wean her baby.

For legal and ethical reasons, a Leader should never:

- Make a statement about whether or not a particular drug is safe. Individual response to a medication may vary. You should only read to her verbatim what the medical references indicate about a medication's possible effects on lactating women and their babies.

MOTHER-TO-MOTHER HELP

The Leader needs to be aware of her limitations. Leaders are not doctors, psychiatrists, or marriage counselors.

- Tell a mother whether or not she should take a particular drug. This decision rests solely with the mother in consultation with her health care provider.
- Tell a mother whether or not she should wean her baby if she decides to take a particular medication. Again, this decision rests with the mother. You can provide background information to help the mother make an informed decision, taking care not to let your personal opinion enter the picture.
- Give a mother the name of another medication that she could take. This is a responsibility that is strictly the physician's and is not within the realm of a Leader's responsibility or expertise.

THE LEADER'S EXPERIENCE IN HELPING MOTHERS

When a Leader Doesn't Know the Answer

No matter how experienced you are as a Leader, situations or problems will arise for which you do not have an immediate answer. You can always feel free to say, "I don't know, but I'll check it out and call you back."

Fortunately, at times like these you can be confident of the resources available to help you find the information you need. La Leche League's many years of experience, its wealth of reference material, and its worldwide network of professional advisors provide Leaders with the information and expertise to respond to almost any breastfeeding question. (You can find more information on Leader resources in Chapter 6, **Keeping Up-to-Date.**)

When you encounter an unfamiliar breastfeeding problem, you may be tempted to immediately refer the mother to a more experienced Leader. An alternative is for you to call the more experienced Leader and find out what you need to know to help the mother. If you pass the call on to another Leader, you also pass up the opportunity to improve your helping skills and increase your own understanding of an unfamiliar situation. The Leader's Log and Medical Questionnaire forms help ensure that you have gathered enough information from the mother. (Sample **Leader's Log** and **Medical Questionnaire** forms are in Appendix 4.)

On the other hand, there are times when a mother would find it reassuring to talk to another mother who has been through a situation similar to hers. Mothers of twins, mothers facing specific illnesses, or mothers who have disability or whose babies have special needs often appreciate speaking to a Leader who has been in a similar situation. Your Area or Affiliate may keep a file of Leaders who have breastfed in specific circumstances. LLLI also keeps a Leader specialty file, which is available on the LLLI Web site.

A Leader may also want to discuss a mother's concern with a Professional Liaison Leader. The role of this resource Leader is covered in **Support for the Leader Dealing with Medically or Legally Related Issues,** pages 157-159.

When a Mother Asks for Help beyond LLL Expertise

Occasionally a mother may ask for help on a matter that does not pertain to breastfeeding or mothering. The Leader needs to be aware of her limitations. Leaders are not doctors, psychiatrists, or marriage counselors.

When a mother asks for non-breastfeeding help, tactfully tell her you don't know or aren't qualified to help in this instance. If possible, direct her to a more appropriate source of help.

Sometimes a Leader suspects that a person is abusing a child. Contact your support Leader or Professional Liaison Leader immediately, before taking action. In this way you benefit from another's objectivity and guidance before taking an action as serious as reporting the call to the authorities.

Personal Reaction to Helping Situations

Giving mother-to-mother help often brings personal satisfaction. When a mother and baby continue breastfeeding because you gave them the right information at the right time, it feels great to have played a part.

Sometimes, however, a mother may not continue to breastfeed. There may be times when a mother chooses not to accept any of the information and suggestions you have to offer, and decides to stop breastfeeding. Or a mother may not want to wean, but circumstances dictate that she must.

Many Leaders have found it helpful to have supportive responses ready for these times.

"That must have been a difficult decision."

"I'm so glad you're enjoying your baby."

"You sound happy, relieved, calm."

"If I can be of further help, or if you want more information, please call."

"I certainly wish that your nursing experience could have been more enjoyable."

Some general guidelines that you may find helpful:

- Affirm the value of any breastfeeding. "Even one nursing session benefits baby."
- Acknowledge any grief the mother is feeling.
- If it seems appropriate, assure her that she did not waste your time. "You wouldn't have felt you had done everything possible if you hadn't called."
- Let the mother know that mothering her baby is most important.
- Be tactful. Each mother's opinion of LLL is important. And when a mother feels positive about LLL, she may refer others to us.

Probably the best measure of how we, as Leaders, are doing our job is how the mother feels about La Leche League when her contact with the Leader is over. Did the Leader help her feel good about being a mother and meeting her baby's needs in the way that seemed most appropriate to her? This is especially true when a mother decides to stop breastfeeding.

You may be disappointed. Knowing firsthand the joy of breastfeeding, you can't help thinking about what the mother and baby are losing. You may wonder if there was something else you could have said or done that could have helped the mother continue the breastfeeding relationship.

MOTHER-TO-MOTHER HELP

Did the Leader help her feel good about being a mother and meeting her baby's needs in the way that seemed most appropriate to her?

These feelings are natural. It may help to talk about them with a support Leader. It may help to remind yourself that a Leader is not responsible for a mother's decisions. You help a mother work out problems by asking helpful questions and suggesting possible solutions; the mother makes up her own mind. The decision to breastfeed or not, or how long to breastfeed, is the responsibility of the mother and father, with input from their health care provider when medical issues are involved.

Discussing One-to-One Helping Situations with Another Leader

Many Leaders find it helpful (especially with their first few calls or for complicated questions) to consult with a co-Leader or other experienced Leader. Checking with another Leader gives an opportunity to review the approach used, the information provided, and how the mother responded. It also gives you a chance to benefit from another Leader's insights. The reinforcement you receive can help you feel more confident.

If a helping situation does not go as well as you would have liked, the perspective of another Leader can help pinpoint why you are dissatisfied and whether it might be better to try a different approach next time.

Confidentiality

Mothers come to LLL for breastfeeding information, just as they might approach a health care provider. It is important to respect a mother by keeping personal information private.

Keep identifying information confidential. This includes names, distinguishing family characteristics and any other information that does not pertain to the breastfeeding situation itself.

It's necessary to keep confidentiality in mind when:

- Consulting with another Leader about a helping situation,
- Discussing examples of questions mothers ask and ways Leaders respond with a Leader Applicant,
- Showing a Leader Applicant how to keep a telephone log,
- Describing a helping situation in a workshop, at a Chapter Meeting, or in an article for a Leader publication, and
- Talking about others' breastfeeding experiences at Series Meetings.

When mothers are reassured by a Leader's actions that helping calls and conversations are kept confidential, they can feel confident recommending LLL to others.

> When mothers are reassured by a Leader's actions that helping calls and conversations are kept confidential, they can feel confident recommending LLL to others.

HELPING BY TELEPHONE

One-to-one helping most often takes place in telephone conversations.

Advance Preparations Can Make Telephone Helping Easier

Materials to keep close at hand

- Leader's Log and pen,
- Medical Questionnaire forms,
- Reference materials such as THE WOMANLY ART OF BREASTFEEDING, THE BREASTFEEDING ANSWER BOOK, LLL pamphlets,
- Area Directory,
- Meeting information, and
- Stationery, envelopes and stamps.

If you have more than one telephone, it can be helpful to have pen and paper and a few Leader's Log sheets near each one.

Equipment

- A cordless telephone or extra long telephone cord and shoulder rest add comfort and flexibility.
- If older children tend to get noisy, phone jacks in a few places or a cordless phone may make it possible to find a quiet place for your conversation. Cordless phones are convenient but do not guarantee conversation privacy.
- Younger children might be kept busy and happy with a box of quiet toys or craft projects reserved for phone calls.

The Importance of the Written Log

- Taking notes during a telephone conversation helps you concentrate on what the caller is saying and keep track of important points. Careful note taking can help discover a pattern, identify conflicting information, or uncover a connection—the missing link to a perplexing question.
- A written log serves as a reminder should the mother call again and/or should you initiate a follow-up call.
- A written log offers legal protection to the Leader. Leaders who are recorded in the LLLI database are covered by liability insurance. Prompt response to the Leader dues notice ensures that your Leader status is recorded.
- A written record is important if a situation arises in which the information a Leader gave the mother is questioned.
- Notes may be more or less extensive, but for the above reasons should include at least: date; name and address and/or telephone number of the caller; the main suggestions you made; which documents you sent or gave as references. If the caller is not willing to identify herself, be sure to write the time of the call and any other identifying details that may come up in your conversation.
- For legal reasons, it is preferable to write with a pen rather than pencil.
- How long you should retain your Leader's Logs may vary depending on local law. Your Area or Affiliate may have a policy. If not, you might consult with your PL or support Leader.

Being Friendly and Accessible

A mother may feel awkward the first time she calls a Leader. She may find it difficult to talk to a stranger about a subject as personal as breastfeeding. If she is having difficulties, she may be feeling unsure of herself.

Some ways you can contribute to a positive beginning to the conversation:

- Smile (the smile will show in your voice),
- Respond in a friendly, interested tone of voice to convey that you are pleased the mother has called you,
- Express interest in the mother and her situation. For example (and when appropriate):
  "Congratulations on the birth of your baby."
  "What did you name your baby? What a beautiful name!"
  "Sounds like you're having trouble with breastfeeding. How can I be of help?"
- Be genuine; combine the helping techniques you've learned, your desire to help, and your own personality, and
- Use the mother's and baby's names during the conversation.

Throughout the conversation:

- Give your full attention. If a child needs your attention for something that won't take long you might ask the mother to wait while you take care of the situation. Otherwise, you might offer to call her back.
- Remove distractions where possible. Don't doodle, wash dishes, or shuffle papers.
- Be patient. Give the mother the time she needs to tell her story without interruptions.

Fussy Children and Telephone Calls

If your children are fussy while you are trying to talk to a mother, try to determine if there is an immediate need that can be satisfied, for example, by nursing or offering a drink of water.

Some Leaders keep ideas and materials handy for activities they can supervise while they talk with a mother. Others take a portable telephone to the play area and sit on the floor where the child plays.

These activities may hold a child's interest, especially when they are reserved for telephone-helping times:

- manipulative toys, such as beads and wind-up toys,
- magnets, such as refrigerator letters,
- children's video or audio tapes,
- play dough or modeling clay,
- a pan of water, sponge and unbreakable dishes, or
- collections (shells, buttons) for older children.

Sometimes children play happily until the telephone rings. Then they suddenly seem to need their mother's attention. Children often feel left out when we are on the telephone.

Many Leaders have found that verbally recognizing the child's feelings and talking about them as well as about the importance of helping other mothers helps their children accept telephone time.

A Guide to Possible Clues

The following list, compiled by Professional Liaison Leaders, may serve as a reminder of some of the details you might ask the mother to describe. In a difficult or unusual situation, this list could help uncover information that might suggest a solution to you and the mother.

Not all of these topics are applicable to every mother or situation. You will want to avoid the impression that you are bombarding the mother with questions. With practice, it becomes natural to interject relevant questions into the conversation.

- Mother's name and phone number or other contact information
- Baby's name and age
- Siblings and ages
- Birth weight and current weight
- Growth pattern: gaining weight, growing in length, head circumference?
- Frequency and length of breastfeeding sessions
- Is baby latched on well? Does mother hear swollowing? Are mother's nipples sore?
- Stool frequency, size, color, consistency
- How many wet diapers in 24 hours?
- Breastfeeding during the night?
- Using both breasts? switching too soon?
- How does baby act at the end of breastfeeding?
- Inverted nipples?
- Does mother feel the let-down?
- Engorgement?
- Is baby getting anything other than human milk? Water? Juice? Formula? Solids?
- Pacifier or thumb-sucking?
- Using nipple shield or bottle? what kind of nipple shield?
- Vitamins, iron, fluoride (mother or baby)?
- Medications—baby?
- Medications—mother: birth control pills; prescriptions (name and spelling of drug, dosage); over-the-counter drugs?
- Smoking (mother, other people in the house)?
- Baby's activity level: active; happy; contented; listless; fussy; sleepy?
- Baby's sleep pattern
- Recent immunizations?
- Family history of allergies?
- Schedule changes in the household: school; job?
- Stress-producing situations: death in family; relatives visiting; vacations?
- Family attitude toward breastfeeding
- Has baby been ill?
- Has mother been ill?
- How does mother feel: tired; frustrated; overwhelmed; anxious?
- Mother's diet; fluid intake; coffee, diet or regular cola; alcohol; cow's milk?
- Has baby seen a doctor? When? Doctor's name? What does doctor say?
- What does mother want to do?
- Has mother read THE WOMANLY ART OF BREASTFEEDING or LLL pamphlets?
- Does mother attend LLL meetings?

Handling Complicated Telephone Calls

Some helping calls are simple and straightforward. A mother calls and wants meeting information or asks a simple question. You express interest in the mother and her baby, provide information in response to the mother's query, and possibly offer additional information about publications and monthly meetings. The mother is satisfied and the call is over.

Other calls are more complicated. The mother is upset, the baby is not doing well, or the mother is confused by conflicting advice. Listening carefully and sensitively before offering information is critical. The communication skills described earlier in this chapter are especially useful when you encounter a complicated one-to-one helping situation.

Recapping the Discussion

Before ending a conversation with a mother, remember to recap. If the telephone conversation covered many subjects or if the mother was very upset when she phoned, it may be difficult for her to clearly remember what she has heard.

This is also a good time to tell the mother about THE WOMANLY ART OF BREAST-FEEDING or other LLL books and publications relevant to her situation. You can offer to send a copy of a pamphlet or tear-off sheet.

Be sure to invite the mother to the next Series Meeting. We want mothers to know that La Leche League can be a source of ongoing support, not just a telephone hotline where someone provides answers to breastfeeding questions.

A sincere, personal closing remark using the mother's name leaves her with a good feeling about LLL.

"It's been good talking with you, Jane. Do call me again and let me know how you are getting along."

Following Up with the Mother

Many Leaders find after a long conversation with a mother that there are one or two more things they wished they had asked or said. If you have recorded her telephone number, you can call her back. Another option is to enclose a note with the written material you send.

After giving telephone help, you may wonder how things worked out. Although Leaders usually ask mothers to call them back and let them know how they are doing, most mothers don't. Perhaps all went well and they saw no need to call. Perhaps they feel they'd be bothering the Leader. Another possibility is that the situation has not improved, and they are reluctant to telephone again.

At the end of the conversation, you could say:

"I'd really like to know how you are doing. Would you like me to telephone you on _____ (interval depending on the problem) to see how things are working out? What time would be most convenient?"

That way you have the mother's permission to return her telephone call at a later date. The mother could, of course, say that she would rather telephone you instead; she may be more likely to do so because you made it clear that you want to hear from her.

Some Leaders make a routine practice of placing a telephone call to mothers to make sure the mother received written material sent. It is important, however, to leave each mother the option of ending her contact with LLL if that is what she wishes. We can do that if we are sensitive to the mother's reactions when we offer to call her back.

> We want mothers to know that La Leche League can be a source of ongoing support, not just a telephone hotline where someone provides answers to breastfeeding questions.

If a Mother Phones at an Inconvenient Time

If a telephone-helping call from a mother comes when it's not a good time to talk, check if it's a true emergency. If it is, you can try to put the family on hold for a little while. If you don't do this too often and explain when you do, family members will usually understand. Even a young child can understand that another mother is upset.

If it's not an emergency, you can explain to the mother why you can't talk, take the mother's name and number and call her back, preferably at an appointed time—perhaps after some research about the mother's problem or question. Most mothers understand that Leaders have family needs, too.

It may not be a good idea to ask a hesitant new mother to call back or call another Leader. She may have made a big effort to make this telephone call and might not be able to get up the courage to telephone again.

An answering machine, when available, can be convenient when it is difficult to take telephone calls. However, since it can be frustrating for a mother to telephone a number of times and receive a recorded message, mentioning a time when calls would be most convenient or including another Leader's number on the recorded message may be helpful.

Be sure the message on your answering machine makes it clear to the mother that she has reached the Leader she is trying to contact by clearly stating your full name on the message.

Too Much Time on the Telephone?

Continual feelings of conflict between taking helping calls and meeting the needs of our children can indicate that we may be getting too many calls, spending too much time on each call, or both.

These suggestions can help.

- Let the mothers at the Series Meetings know your most and least convenient times to take calls.
- In the Group's welcome packets include LLL pamphlets and tear-off sheets on the subjects that generate the most calls.
- Use an answering machine to screen calls or ask your partner to answer the telephone and take messages when you are busy.
- Keep each call to a reasonable length. Except for a complicated situation, about ten to fifteen minutes is usually enough time. It's not necessary—or possible—to cover all aspects of breastfeeding in one call.
- If you find difficult to restrain call length, check whether it is you or the mother who engages a new topic during the conversation. Many Leaders mail pamphlets to reinforce basic information and offer extra detail.
- If a mother is calling about basics, encourage her to buy a copy of THE WOMANLY ART OF BREASTFEEDING.
- If she calls about trivial issues or those not related to breastfeeding or mothering, set limits on how often or how long you will talk.
- Be sure to send a meeting notice to every mother who calls. List the LLLI Web site on your meeting notice—some basic questions are covered there.

> Continual feelings of conflict between taking helping calls and meeting the needs of our children can indicate that we may be getting too many calls, spending too much time on each call, or both.

Handling Nuisance Calls

Nuisance calls can intrude on anyone's life, LLL Leader or not. Some calls are merely annoying, and some are downright scary. What should you do when you get a nuisance call?

- Trust your instincts. Does your gut feeling tell you that this call does not seem right?
- Are there no baby noises in the background, no indications that a mother really exists?
- End the call by saying you will call back at a later time or that you will have another, more experienced, Leader call the person back. Ask for the caller's number. Most nuisance callers will not give you a phone number or will give a fake one.
- Do not volunteer information about yourself, your family, or other Leaders. If someone wants meeting information and you are unsure of the motives, ask for the caller's phone number or address.
- Don't answer personal questions that make you feel uneasy. Asking questions back is a good method of tactfully avoiding this type of situation. Even basic questions to get more information can help confirm that a call is not legitimate or reassure you that it is genuine.
- If the caller asks for an uncomfortable level of details —for example asks you to describe exactly how to hold the breast for hand expression—you could ask for the person's address and offer to send an information sheet. You don't have to put a return address on what you mail. You could also suggest a book on the subject from the library or bookstore.
- Hang up. If the caller is verbally abusive, vulgar, or threatening, do not continue the conversation. Hang up immediately and contact your telephone company. Telephone companies may have a variety of ways to handle such calls, including referring you to the police and arranging for a method of call tracing. In many places it is against the law to threaten people, make obscene calls, or harass someone. Do not try to reason with the person or continue talking. By doing so, you are encouraging the behavior. Often this is what the person wants—attention and a reaction.
- Call your support Leader. It is important to report exactly what has happened. If the caller has contacted other Leaders, sharing information about the caller's methods may help to end the situation.
- Keep accurate information in your Leader's log. If the telephone company or police trace the call, they may need you to verify information. Without facts there is little authorities can do to help stop the calls. As soon as you get off the phone with a nuisance caller, write down the exact time and exactly what was said to you.
- Ask callers where they got your number. If it is from a source that seems to attract nuisance calls, look at other methods of publicity.
- If you are sure a call is a nuisance, do not call back. Don't think that you can convince nuisance callers to stop making such calls or reform them. You are just encouraging them to call again by giving them the attention they seek.
- If you are receiving repeated nuisance calls, you could let the answering machine screen all calls for a period of time, until the person tires of contacting you.

Keep in mind that the vast majority of calls are legitimate. As the police will tell you, most nuisance calls are harmless, even the obscene ones.

Just because a nuisance call is from a male caller does not mean that all male callers should be suspect. Many men call LLL for their partners; some call with their own questions. When a partner or friend calls on behalf of a mother, it can be helpful to give some basic information and encourage the person to ask the mother to call you back. The information the caller receives from a Leader can make a world of difference in how he supports the breastfeeding relationship. We don't want to create the mistaken impression that we give information to women only. If taking a telephone call from a man is uncomfortable for you, do as you would with any call that you do not want to handle: find another Leader in your Area who is willing to return the call.

HELPING ONLINE

Increasingly, one-to-one helping is taking place on the Internet.

MOTHER-TO-MOTHER HELP

There are many ways for a Leader to represent La Leche League on the Internet. Some Leaders work on Web sites for the Group, Area, Division, Affiliate, or LLLI; some Leaders answer questions via email through their Group Web pages or the online Help Form programs sponsored by LLLI and many Affiliates; others participate in LLL bulletin boards; and some Leaders host online meetings.

In many ways, helping by email is an extension of helping by telephone.

To find out more about these options, visit the La Leche League International Web site, at: **http://www.lalecheleague.org.**

Some files are password-protected, so that only Leaders can access them. Contact your local support Leader to obtain the passwords for Leader protected LLL Web pages.

Many mothers first encounter La Leche League through the World Wide Web. Email makes it possible for them to ask questions when a telephone call may be inconvenient or costly. In many ways, helping by email is an extension of helping by telephone. Note that it is optional for Leaders to put their email addresses on Group Web pages.

Skillful communication, using the Leader's Log, consulting as necessary with resource people, using published resources appropriately, offering information rather than giving advice, and considering the effect of our interaction are all important considerations whether we are helping in person, over the telephone, or by email. Leaders have an additional online resource in the LLLI Web site's collection of "Help Form FAQs," which provide sample answers to common email questions. This can be found in the password-protected pages of the LLLI Web site.

Most of the information in this chapter relates to helping by email as much as by telephone or in person. The following considerations may be especially relevant when helping by email:

Report email helping as you do telephone or other one-to-one helping.

- You will want to find ways to compensate for the differences between oral and written communication. It is important, for instance, to keep in mind that a written text lacks the warmth of the human voice;
- Email communication cannot be considered private;
- What you write can be altered and shared; print and attach the entire "conversation" to your Leader's log sheet; and also
- Copyright law applies.

Remember that you can consult with another Leader such as your support Leader or a Professional Liaison Leader (or Online Professional Liaison Resource Leader in Help Form situations) before responding to an email request for help. Report email helping as you do telephone or other one-to-one helping.

Representing La Leche League Online

Representing La Leche League as an accredited Leader is a wonderful way to further the mission of our organization, to:

> *Help mothers worldwide to breastfeed through mother-to-mother support, encouragement, information and education, and to promote a better understanding of breastfeeding as an important element in the healthy development of the baby and mother.*

It is also an awesome responsibility—one we as Leaders should never take lightly. For the first time, we as individual Leaders can represent LLL's philosophy to the entire world without leaving the comfort of home. It is important to remember this when we choose to reveal our Leader status online. Once the online audience learns someone is a Leader, everything she says from that point forward can be associated in their minds with La Leche League. For this reason, many Leaders choose not to disclose their Leader status online. Thus we avoid having to be "on duty" whenever we sit down to the keyboard. It is important to remember that we are the visible representatives of La Leche League; the manner in which we carry out our responsibilities—whether electronically or in person—reflects on the organization as whole.

Even if we do not explicitly advertise our Leader role, others will identify us as Leaders if we include "LLLL," "LLL Leader," "La Leche," or words containing triple Ls in an email address or signature. It is appropriate to have a separate email address and/or signature file for those times when we specifically choose to represent La Leche League. LLL position and job titles have no relevance outside the organization and we do not use them unless the title directly pertains to the reason for writing (e.g., an Area Conference Supervisor/Area Coordinator of Events announcing a conference speaker). Undistracted by titles, the audience can be comfortable contacting any Leader any time breastfeeding information is needed.

When Is It Appropriate to Identify Ourselves as Leaders?

There are many times when it is appropriate to identify ourselves as La Leche League Leaders, and the simplest test of this is to ask ourselves, "Am I representing La Leche League's purpose and philosophy and its reputation as the 'world's foremost authority on breastfeeding'?" Some situations where we can represent LLL in this manner online are:

- When answering LLL Help Forms,
- When answering personal email messages addressed to us as Leaders,
- When leading LLL-sponsored breastfeeding chats,
- When posting messages on Leader-only email lists, and
- When providing LLL information or resources on email lists for professional and/or lay lactation supporters.

When we help a mother through live chats, bulletin boards, or email we need to follow the same Leader guidelines we use in person or on the phone, providing information and suggestions to help that mother find the solution that will work best for her. Avoid furnishing the street addresses, phone numbers, or email addresses of others to any electronic forum. Send the information privately. It is appropriate and recommended to document messages posted as a Leader in our Leader logs.

Many Leaders subscribe to the LactNet email list. LactNet gives Leaders the opportunity to learn from others in the field of lactation and to help educate others about La Leche League and what we have to offer. It is also a wonderful way to help enhance LLL's image among health care professionals. Leaders who participate in LactNet or other non-LLL-affiliated breastfeeding forums must bear in mind that everything we post affects the image of LLLI. Therefore, it is vital to consult LLL resources (such as THE WOMANLY ART OF BREASTFEEDING, THE BREASTFEEDING ANSWER BOOK,

LEAVEN, and Professional Liaison Leaders) before posting any questions. Submitting questions to a non-LLL forum that are answered in LLL materials conveys the impression LLL does not provide its volunteers with adequate information to work with mothers. List members may infer that Leaders have not been trained adequately to check LLL resources before turning to a collection of busy professionals for help (LEAVEN, December 1998/January 1999, p. 120). When we post information as a Leader, it is important to provide full references. This not only gives the readers the information, but it also adds to the credibility of Leaders and the organization.

Is It Appropriate to Seek Breastfeeding Information Online to Help a Mother?

When someone chooses to contact us as LLL Leaders, it is because of our reputation for having a vast array of information to share. Our resources are excellent. We can handle the majority of situations we encounter when working with mothers and babies via the resources LLL provides us as Leaders. Now that so many Leaders around the world have access to computers, we answer questions even more quickly than ever before within our Leader support channels. The rare instance when outside online resources need to be accessed requires careful thought, so that we maintain the reputation as competent, knowledgeable volunteers whose expertise has been recognized for more than four decades. Just as in all aspects of our jobs as Leaders, it is our responsibility to make sure we have explored all of LLL's information before going outside the organization to help those who contact us.

Leader chain of resources (most recent edition available in Leader's language)

1. THE WOMANLY ART OF BREASTFEEDING,
2. THE BREASTFEEDING ANSWER BOOK,
3. LEAVEN, NEW BEGINNINGS (many articles available on the LLLI Web site), LLLI books, pamphlets, and information sheets or Affiliate Leader and member newsletters, pamphlets, and information sheets,
4. Area Leaders' Letters,
5. BREASTFEEDING ABSTRACTS or other LLL publications for health professionals (if accessible),
6. Professional breastfeeding resources available from LLLI by authors such as Hale, Riordan and Auerbach, Lawrence, etc.,
7. Professional Liaison Leaders,
8. LLL Online Professional Liaison Resource Leaders (OPLRs), and
9. Other breastfeeding resources, including online sources like LactNet in conjunction with PL Leader. (See **Using Non-LLL Resources,** page 165.)

We can contact PL Leaders whenever we are unsure of information, have questions, or if other resources are unavailable to us.

When Is It Not Appropriate to Identify Ourselves as Leaders?

- On non-breastfeeding email lists, bulletin boards, chats, or newsgroups,
- On breastfeeding email lists, in discussions that do not pertain to breastfeeding (e.g., circumcision, vaccinations, home-schooling),
- In discussions about appropriate medical/technical advice or information, and

- When expressing personal opinions or beliefs that are not representative of LLL, as readers may not be able to separate what reflects LLL's philosophy or policy from what does not.

What topics are not appropriate for discussion on public bulletin boards, email lists, newsgroups, and chat rooms?

- Leader or Group conflicts,
- Area Council business,
- Leader accreditation procedures or specific applications,
- Rumors, gossip, or speculation, and
- Denigrating or demeaning remarks about LLL, its facilities, services, or personnel. (Please note that respectful disagreement and honest discussions don't fall in this category.)

Electronic communication has allowed La Leche League to bring breastfeeding information to mothers who would otherwise not have access to it. It has increased the ease with which Leaders can communicate with each other. It has allowed those interested in lactation to benefit from worldwide networks of information and support. As we enjoy all that the new technologies have to offer, remember that common sense and LLL guidelines on how to help mothers are the best guides as we enter the world of LLL in cyberspace.

Nuisance Email

Leaders with email addresses listed on their Group Web pages sometimes get inappropriate email communications. Use the delete key to discard obvious "spam" messages.

Treat questionable messages carefully—you never know whether they might actually be sincere questions that are awkwardly worded. Many experienced online Leaders have found that simply replying with a very bland answer that refers the author of the email to a pertinent book or page on the LLLI Web site is an easy way to handle such questions. Other Leaders use a generic "address confirmation message" to confirm a sender's intent. You do not want to spend a lot of time on a question that is not genuine. In case the query turns out to be sincere, it is important to give at least a minimal answer and refer the questioner to resources for further information.

Some Leaders are unhappy to receive uninvited email as a result of being listed on a Web page—remember that these listings are optional. However, many Leaders find that the benefits of mothers finding the local Group, getting a question answered and then joining LLL, finding support when they need it, etc., outweigh the inconvenience of a few uninvited emails.

MAKING HOME VISITS

Although most mothers' questions can be answered over the telephone, some situations are more effectively handled in person. Sometimes a problem that takes several telephone conversations to figure out can be resolved immediately when you can see the mother and baby.

Some examples of situations that may be helped most efficiently by a home visit:

MOTHER-TO-MOTHER HELP

- The baby is refusing to breastfeed or having trouble latching on—it may be helpful to see the positioning, the mother's breasts, or the baby's latch-on.
- The baby is not gaining well and the usual management suggestions have not helped—positioning and latch-on techniques may need to be evaluated and/or demonstrated.
- A mother has persistent sore nipples and the usual over-the-telephone suggestions have not helped.
- A mother cannot attend a meeting or doesn't have access to a phone.
- Specialized techniques or breastfeeding-aid products are needed— it may be easier to demonstrate than explain over the telephone.

> Sometimes a problem that takes several telephone conversations to figure out can be resolved immediately when you can see the mother and baby.

Home Visits Are Optional

Whether or not to make home visits is a personal decision you make for yourself. Making a home visit is not part of the basic Leader responsibilities. However, home visits are covered by Leader liability insurance. You should be in good health, as should your children, if they will be accompanying you, or if the mother will visit you in your home. It is considerate to let the mother know in advance if you need to bring your children, and you will probably need to bring quiet toys to occupy them.

Other options for making sure the mother gets the help she needs:

- Consult with another Leader who can arrange to meet with the mother.
- If a Series Meeting is being held soon, and the mother can attend, you can give her personal attention either before or after the discussion. The timing of the meeting is an important factor, since some problems need immediate attention.
- It may be appropriate to refer the mother to a qualified lactation consultant or other health care provider. Your PL Leader can give you guidance about whether and how to make the referral. In this case you need to inform the mother that she may be charged a fee for services.

Whose Home?

If you choose to do a home visit, you might go to the mother's home or ask the mother to come to yours. Some Leaders may feel more self-confident in their own homes.

On the other hand, it may be difficult for a new mother to make arrangements to travel to your home with her baby. Furthermore, seeing the mother in her own home may provide you with some insight into factors that may be contributing to the mother's problems.

If you are making home visits for the first time, or feel unsure of yourself, you might ask the mother if another Leader may accompany you.

What to Take on a Home Visit
- THE WOMANLY ART OF BREASTFEEDING—bring the Group Library copy and/or a copy available for sale,
- THE BREASTFEEDING ANSWER BOOK,
- LLL pamphlets on relevant topics,
- Series Meeting information,

- Leader's log,
- Breastfeeding aid products you have on hand that may be useful with a particular mother's situation, and
- An LLLI or Affiliate Catalogue to refer the mother to books or products that may be helpful.

During a Home Visit

Begin by helping the mother feel at ease. Ask questions and empathize with the mother; check the information you already have and record further information about her concern. After you have gathered the information, discuss the concern or problem with the mother, and offer suggestions, carefully observing her responses.

Touching the mother or baby

If you need to touch the mother or baby, ask permission first, be gentle and respectful, and use appropriate hygiene by washing your hands thoroughly. Some Leaders prefer to bring sterile plastic gloves to wear, if they have access to them. Tell the mother exactly what you are planning to do and why.

In the rare instance that a mother asks you to nurse her baby, decline. This not only presents a health risk of cross-infection to the baby and to you, it also has the potential to undermine the mother's confidence in her ability to feed her baby herself at a time when she needs positive reinforcement.

When to proceed with caution

There are times when you will want to be extra cautious. If a particular situation makes you uncomfortable, consult with a Professional Liaison Leader or suggest that a health care provider see the baby immediately. Situations that warrant immediate intervention include, but are not limited to:

- a weak or listless baby,
- a tense, hypertonic baby (points his toes, arches, screams),
- a baby who is noticeably dehydrated (insufficient number of wet diapers, poor skin tone, dry mouth, dry eyes),
- a baby with very poor weight gain;
- a baby who is unable to suck, and
- anything out of the ordinary.

Following Up the Home Visit

Follow-up is important after a home visit. You can ask the mother to call in two or three days. If the mother forgets to call, you can call her. Usually things are going better for the mother by that time. If more help is needed, you can often give it over the telephone.

> If you need to touch the mother or baby, ask permission first, be gentle and respectful, and use appropriate hygiene by washing your hands thoroughly.

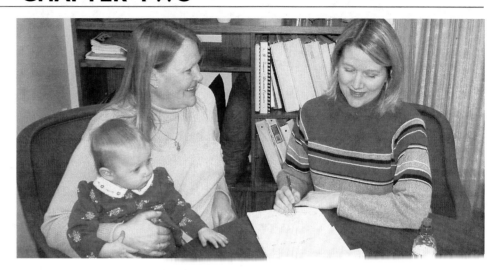

CHAPTER TWO

Preparing to Lead a Meeting

CHOOSING A FORMAT

From the beginning, Leaders have found that Series Meetings are most successful when the mothers attending the meeting do most of the talking. The goal is to have experienced mothers sharing rather than experts teaching.

A study in 1983 confirmed the wisdom of this approach when it concluded that lecture is not the most effective teaching method for adult learners. This survey reported that adults retain:

- 10% of what they read
- 20% of what they hear
- 30% of what they see
- 50% of what they see and hear
- 80% of what they say
- 90% of what they say and do

A Series Meeting works best as a flexible, guided discussion:

- Flexible, to meet the interests and needs of those attending the meeting;
- Guided, so the Leader can fulfill her responsibility to offer breastfeeding information; and
- A discussion, because we believe that people benefit from active participation.

Two discussion formats, the conversation-style and the round robin (each person speaking in turn), are most commonly used to lead Series Meetings. Sometimes a visual or discussion aid is included.

Conversation-Style Discussion

A Series Meeting works best as a flexible, guided discussion.

In a conversation-style format, the discussion is opened with a prepared question. Participants respond from their experiences, offer ideas in response to what someone else has said, or ask other questions. You might respond with a nod or give a brief affirmation. You might fill in with more information. If something a participant says is misleading or contrary to LLL's views, tactfully provide appropriate information; you might also ask for additional points of view from others.

This format is called *conversation style*, because it is like a conversation between you and the participants. The conversation flows naturally and spontaneously with you as moderator, guiding the discussion to cover the intended points. Your response to contributions helps participants see LLL's ideas through a variety of experiences and points of view.

If the Group is enthusiastic and talkative, one well-phrased question at the beginning of the discussion may stimulate enough conversation to cover the topic well. If the discussion stalls, you can continue by using one or more of several follow-up questions prepared in advance. You can also invite Group members who would be comfortable talking about their experiences to describe what they did in a particular situation.

Advantages

- Communication flows naturally between meeting participants in a conversational way.
- No one feels pressured to speak; no one feels the need to wait her turn.
- You have flexibility in directing the discussion. You can use more structure or less structure, depending on how talkative the participants are.

Points to consider

- You need to be well prepared, to have follow-up questions ready, and to know which Group members you can call on to contribute to specific areas of discussion.
- You need to be observant and ready to guide the discussion, so that talkative participants do not dominate it and quieter people who have something to say have adequate opportunities to speak.

Round-Robin Format

A conversation-style meeting is a free-flowing conversation between you and the participants.

In a round-robin format, you open the discussion with a question that is then answered by each participant in turn. In a variation of this format, you pass out written questions; participants read them in turn for the whole group to discuss.

As in the conversation-style format, you respond as appropriate, adding LLL's point of view as needed.

Advantages

- If the meeting is small to medium size (fewer than fifteen attendees), everyone has a chance to participate.

- Since each participant talks, everyone has an opportunity to get to know something about the others.
- More reserved mothers have a chance to contribute to the discussion.
- This format offers built-in predictability and the momentum of the discussion is certain, as each person speaks in turn.

Points to consider

- Participation may be less spontaneous. Some people may not speak until their turn, even if they have pertinent comments at other times. Others may feel pressured because they would rather just listen to the discussion.
- Participants may anticipate their turn, and not pay close attention to what others say.
- If the meeting is large (more than fifteen), those at the end of the circle may not get their turn. Or, the meeting may continue so long that attention begins to wane and some people find it inconvenient to stay.
- Responses may become repetitious.

Using Visual or Discussion Aids

Some Leaders like to use a visual aid to open a discussion topic or emphasize a point. Babies are the best eye-catching visuals of all. Usually there is no lack of babies at a meeting.

You might also want to bring specific items. For example, a fresh banana could be compared with a jar of banana baby food. A visual aid can also be used as the basis for the entire discussion, for example, a poster listing key words and phrases or showing pictures of the main points.

A discussion aid, on the other hand, uses words or an activity rather than images. For example, participants could name an advantage of breastfeeding beginning with the sequential letters in the word *breastfeeding*. Or they could imagine what their babies might name as their favorite advantage of breastfeeding.

Both visual and discussion aids can be used with round-robin and conversation-style meeting formats.

Advantages

- Visual or discussion aids help keep the discussion focused on the topic.
- A concrete symbol or an activity can make it easier for a mother to follow the discussion if she needs to turn her attention to her baby at times.
- Aids increase interest and can add a change of pace to meetings.

Points to consider

- The aid, rather than participants' questions and concerns, can sometimes become the focus of attention.
- Visual aids require careful preparation.
- Activities that require writing may be difficult for a mother who is holding a baby, or whose first language is different from the language of the meeting, or who is not comfortable reading and writing.
- The approach may become overly cute or gimmicky, making communication less spontaneous.

(See **Signs and Posters** page 58.)

PLANNING MEETINGS

In a round-robin format, a question is answered by each participant in turn.

Visual aids and discussion aids can be used as the basis for the entire discussion.

One Topic or More?

Some Leaders prepare more than one approach to the meeting topic and then make the decision as mothers arrive.

It may be impractical to try to cover in depth more than one general topic, such as "Avoiding Common Breastfeeding Difficulties" in Meeting 3 or "Starting Solids" in Meeting 4. Instead you might plan to focus on one or two areas of a chosen broad topic. As you plan, keep in mind how many participants usually attend and their anticipated needs. For instance, "Planning and Getting Breastfeeding Off to a Good Start" and "Avoiding Plugged Ducts and Breast Infections" for Meeting 3 may be too much for a short meeting with lots of children present, but it may work well at a quieter meeting.

One way to cover two topics is to divide the meeting into two separate parts. Some Leaders choose an informational focus for the first part, such as "Getting Breastfeeding Off to a Good Start" or "Starting Solids: When, What, How," and add a more personal focus for the second part, such as "Learning to Trust Our Instincts" or "Coping with Parenthood as a Couple." Others might use the first part of the meeting for a general topic, such as "Advantages of Breastfeeding," and the second for a focus suggested by participants, for instance, "Breastfeeding and Health."

By preparing two parts, you may find that you are able to meet the needs of both the newcomers and the regulars. The newcomers may want information, while the regulars may be more interested in the emotional side of breastfeeding. With this method, newcomers will find that LLL offers both information and support.

A Change of Plan

Occasionally, you may carefully plan a meeting only to discover at the meeting that your plan won't work with the women who have come. Perhaps the discussion topic turns out to be inappropriate. For example, the pregnant women for whom you planned the discussion on birth plans were unable to attend. Perhaps many more mothers came than expected. Perhaps time for the second part of the discussion ran out because participants had so much to contribute during the first part.

Flexibility is the key. Meeting the needs of the mothers, particularly newcomers, is the top priority. You may need to change topics just before, or even in the middle of a meeting, so the discussion can meet the needs of those present. Some Leaders prepare more than one approach to the meeting topic or more than one focus and then make a choice as mothers arrive. Your skills and confidence for doing this will increase with practice.

Deciding on a Focus

The focus guides your choice of information to include in the discussion.

The Series Meeting Guides (See **Series Meeting Guides** in Chapter 3) list many points you can cover for each meeting topic. The first step in planning a meeting is to narrow the possibilities by deciding on a focus. The focus guides your choice of information to include in the discussion.

One way to decide on a focus is to think about who will likely attend and plan according to what their questions or concerns might be. Be prepared to respond to different interests, especially those of the newcomers.

If, for example, in planning for Meeting 2, you know that pregnant newcomers will be attending, a good choice for a topic might be "How Childbirth Choices Can Affect Breastfeeding." If the newcomers have small babies, "The Basics of Breastfeeding" might be more appropriate. If you expect new mothers with small babies to attend

Meeting 4, "Nutrition for the Nursing Mother" or "Starting Solids" might be a good focus. If there will be mostly mothers of toddlers and no newcomers, "Weaning" or "Toddlers and Nutrition" might be a more appropriate focus.

If you don't know who will attend the meeting, planning two alternatives might be helpful.

PLANNING MEETINGS

When Planning a Meeting, Consider:

- Who will be there?
- Will the women at the meeting be regular attendees or newcomers?
- Are they pregnant with a first or subsequent child?
- Have they nursed before?
- Are they employed?
- How can you achieve a balance between breastfeeding information and mothering philosophy?
- Will some people attend the meeting essentially for basic breastfeeding facts and techniques?
- Will others attend primarily for mothering support and reassurance?

(See **Balancing Information and Emotions,** page 40.)

Choosing the Points to Cover

After deciding on a focus, the next step might be to make a list of the points to cover during the discussion. This makes it easier to formulate questions that will draw responses from participants.

Planning and practice can help you develop the skill of asking effective questions.

For example, if you decide the focus of a particular Meeting 2 will be "Getting Breastfeeding Off to a Good Start," you might choose the following points to cover:

- How soon—advantages of nursing right after birth,
- How often—advantages of unrestricted nursing,
- Avoiding supplements,
- Avoiding sore nipples, and
- How to know baby is getting enough.

Next to certain points in your notes you may find it helpful to write the names of participants who would be willing to be called on when needed. For example, you may know of someone who overcame sore nipples by adjusting her baby's position at the breast.

Wording Questions

After you decide on the points to cover, you can prepare a question to open the discussion. Supporting questions can also be prepared and used as needed to keep the discussion moving and draw out points not yet mentioned.

Planning and practice can help you develop the skill of asking effective questions. The basic principles below can help you develop questions that stimulate discussions and bring out responses that support LLL information.

Ask open-ended questions

Questions that begin with **what** and **how**, and to some extent **who, when, where,** and **why,** elicit descriptive responses rather than one-word answers. Other helpful words include **describe, outline,** and **summarize**.

> *"Describe some ways you have found to meet baby's nighttime needs while meeting the needs of the rest of the family."*

> *"How have you handled comments about your desire to keep your baby close by?"*

Avoid questions that appear to have one right or best answer.

> *"What is the best way to get breastfeeding off to a good start?"*

While this question may be intended to draw out a variety of important points, the mothers may interpret it as a question that is asking for a single, best answer. Some people will be reluctant to respond, not wanting to be wrong. A better question might be:

> *"What are some ways you found (or are planning) to help get breastfeeding off to a good start?"*

Make Questions Applicable to the Whole Group

Keep the needs of a variety of participants in mind so that everyone will feel included in the discussion: women pregnant with their first child, first-time mothers, experienced breastfeeding mothers, mothers with other little ones at home, single mothers, employed mothers, etc.

A woman who is pregnant with her first baby may feel left out by a question that does not apply to her, for example:

> *"What are some ways that have helped you to get breastfeeding off to a good start?"*

By slightly changing the question, you can make it apply to all:

> *"What helpful hints about breastfeeding a new baby have you read about, heard about, or tried?"*

Help first-time pregnant women feel included and encourage them to join the discussion by specifically inviting them to bring up their questions and concerns.

Choose Questions That Draw on Experiences

Discussion questions can ask for opinions, information, or experiences.

- Asking for **opinions** can make it more difficult to bring out accurate information.
- Asking for **information** directly can make the meeting sound more like a class.

- Asking for **experiences** encourages women to talk about what they have gained from their personal experiences, at previous meetings, and from reading.

PLANNING MEETINGS

Because it is important to present specific breastfeeding information at meetings, it is tempting to use questions that ask for this information directly.

"What is natural weaning?"

"How can you tell when your baby is ready for solids?"

Wording questions this way may leave the impression that you are testing the participants to see how much they know, rather than leading a discussion.

Most test-type questions can easily be reworded. For example, you might start with a general question such as:

"What do you think of when you hear the term 'natural weaning'?"

"If you've started your baby on solids, what let you know she was ready? If you're wondering when to start solids, how do you think your baby will let you know it's time?"

If you want to bring out specific points during the ensuing discussion, you can direct a specific question to a mother who will be comfortable sharing her experience.

When Necessary, State Information Directly

Sometimes the discussion does not bring out important information. You might try a direct information question. Or you might go ahead and state the information, which others might not have.

For example, after a number of mothers talk about their experiences, you may take the opportunity to draw general conclusions. Or you can use one mother's response as a springboard to give more detailed information.

> You can use one mother's response as a springboard to give more detailed information.

"We've been talking about how to avoid sore nipples by positioning. THE WOMANLY ART OF BREASTFEEDING and our pamphlet on positioning explain a few more points in detail. Here are a few that haven't been covered yet..."

"You mentioned, Olga, that one of the reasons you decided to breastfeed was that human milk is the most natural food for babies. Would you like to say more about some of the nutritional qualities that are important to you?"

When you are aware of how the wording of questions and statements can affect responses, it is fairly easy, with a little practice, to guide meetings. Participants can leave feeling they have been part of a group discussion where they learned practical information about breastfeeding backed up by others' personal experiences.

Opening the Meeting
Introduction and announcements

Start the meeting promptly. Promptness tells participants that they are important and what LLL has to offer is important. Because the opening of the meeting leaves partic-

> The introductory remarks focus attention on the meeting topic and help participants prepare for the discussion.

ipants with an impression of LLL, carefully plan what you will say. The beginning of the meeting needs to project warmth and your confidence, respect for others, and preparation.

It is also an opportunity for the other participants to get ready for the discussion. Experienced mothers, new mothers, and mothers-to-be, each with their own personal thoughts and concerns, may be at the meeting. The introductory remarks focus attention on the meeting topic and help participants prepare for the discussion.

The meeting opening could include the following:

- Introduce the Group Leader(s) so participants can identify who officially represents LLL.
- Briefly describe LLLI's history and purpose.
- Mention something about the local Group.
- Introduce the Group workers: Librarian, Treasurer, Hostess, etc. Allow a moment for each to say something about her job and how she can be of help.
- Explain LLL membership.
- Provide information about the meeting facility: which rooms may be used, the location of the toilet, etc.
- Explain that meeting babies' needs is a priority we all understand. Mothers can feel free to move around the room during the discussion. Invite mothers of older babies to stay close to their little ones to keep them happy and attend to their needs.
- Invite participation in the discussion and caution against side conversations.

> *"We are all here to share our breastfeeding and mothering experiences. Because what each person has to say is important, please share your comments with the whole group and refrain from side conversations."*

Encourage participants to ask questions. Because the discussion covers specific topics, you may need to reassure them that no one needs to wait for a specific meeting to ask her question. You could mention that mothers can raise questions during the discussion or, if a mother prefers, she can talk to a Leader individually during refreshment time. Some Leaders leave the last few minutes of the meeting for questions on any breastfeeding topic.

Don't rush the opening of the meeting. Participants are getting settled. Qualifying statements and other important information can be made directly after introductions when the attendees are focused on the meeting. To avoid giving the appearance that these details are an inconvenience, refrain from statements such as, "Now that we have all that out of the way..." or questions such as, "Did I leave anything out?" An efficient, confident opening can set a positive tone for the rest of the meeting.

Qualifying Statements

> Membership and the qualifying statement are an integral part of the spoken introduction.

A qualifying statement at the beginning of each meeting:

- Informs participants that Leaders, as official representatives of LLL, speak for La Leche League;
- Invites participants to accept or reject, agree or disagree with what they hear at the meeting; and

• Makes it clear that there is no one right way to practice mothering through breastfeeding, that there is no "La Leche League way;"

"At this meeting we'll discuss a variety of ideas. Please keep in mind that each person here speaks from her own perspective. As a Leader, I represent LLL and offer LLL information."

"La Leche League is interested in supporting and encouraging you in your breastfeeding and mothering experience. Some of the ideas may be new to you. Feel free to take what seems right for you and leave the rest."

"LLL believes that mothers know their own babies best. We offer suggestions from our experience and that of many other mothers. If there's something you don't agree with, please do come back and continue to participate. We all have different ideas and opinions, and we welcome yours at our meeting."

PLANNING MEETINGS

Announcement Sheet

One option that can save valuable meeting time is to provide some of the information normally included in the opening in written form. The announcement sheet could include information about:

• Group Leaders' names and telephone numbers,
• LLL history and purpose,
• Membership,
• Area and other conferences,
• Group Library books,
• Group and/or other LLL fundraisers,
• Group activities and other meetings, such as Enrichment, Toddler, Couples Meetings, and
• Qualifying statements.

Because of their importance to LLL everywhere, membership and the qualifying statements are an integral part of the spoken introduction, even when participants also receive this information in written form.

Check with your support Leader about review procedures for announcement sheets and handouts. She can also offer suggestions for content or appearance. (See also **Group Newsletters,** page 100; **Copyrighted Materials,** page 101; and **Appendix 1: LLLI Policies and Guidelines.**)

Personal Introductions

A good time for participants to introduce themselves can be right before the discussion. Not only does this give them the opportunity to get to know a little about each other, it also helps them warm up to participating in the discussion.

Set the tone by starting the introductions, giving your name, your children's names and ages, and/or your due date, if relevant. Then each participant in turn can introduce herself.

Many Leaders like to include a short-answer question in the personal introductions.

Many Leaders like to include a short-answer question in the personal introductions. The question may be of a general nature, or it may pertain to the meeting topic. When introducing yourself first, you can answer the question briefly so the mothers realize that short responses are expected. This will allow plenty of time for the topic that will follow. Sometimes mothers bring up issues that merit discussion later in the meeting. Take note of these issues and ask the participants later to go into detail.

"How did you first hear about La Leche League?"

"What's your favorite way to relax?"

Word questions so that it is not necessary for mothers to say how many months or years each baby breastfed. This will avoid an atmosphere of competition over who nursed the longest. Some participants might not have thought about breastfeeding beyond the first few months. Affirm that each breastfeeding experience is unique and that our goal is to help each mother have what she would deem a successful breastfeeding relationship.

Opening the Discussion

To transition into the discussion, consider announcing the topic both before and after the introductions. State the broad topic, for example, "Welcome to the meeting. Our topic today is the Advantages of Breastfeeding." Next, define the topic by explaining the focus and whether the meeting will be divided into parts.

You can open the discussion by asking a question or asking participants to describe an experience. Stating LLL philosophy before asking can be helpful to the Group.

La Leche League believes that for the healthy, full-term baby, breast milk is the only food necessary until the baby shows signs of needing solids, about the middle of the first year after birth.

Clarifying LLL's philosophy in advance allows newcomers to choose whether to talk about personal experiences or opinions that differ from LLL. For example, you can avoid putting a mother in the position of mentioning that she started solids at six weeks and then finding out that LLL doesn't recommend this. The mother may be comfortable sharing this information and asking questions later in the discussion, but she should have the right to decide if, when, and how she does this. This doesn't mean that we discourage mothers from mentioning or discussing any aspects of their personal experiences that differ from LLL recommendations.

Ending the Meeting

Every meeting should end on a positive note. You can prepare a closing in advance, perhaps modifying it in light of the actual course of the meeting. Some Leaders like to end with a short quote from THE WOMANLY ART OF BREASTFEEDING, a bit of LLL philosophy, or a touching moment shared by a mother.

Consider the following:

- Invite participants who have questions to speak with you during refreshments.
- Focus closing remarks on what was accomplished rather than what was not.
- Refer mothers to THE WOMANLY ART OF BREASTFEEDING, and Group Library books for more information.

- Briefly summarize the key points of the discussion and mention the focus topic.
- Make announcements and reminders, including time, place, and topic of the next meeting.
- Thank everyone for coming, as well as the hostess and those who brought refreshments.
- Make sure everyone knows that a Leader is available between meetings and how to contact you, a co-Leader, or LLLI.
- Add a short reminder about membership dues.

Lasting Impressions

Keep in mind that the atmosphere of respect, the heart of mother-to-mother support, is as important as the information imparted at meetings. One of our goals is to provide an environment where mothers can learn about breastfeeding from one another. Our primary message is the importance of each mother to her baby and how breastfeeding enhances this relationship. We hope that each mother leaves with a strong belief, trust, and confidence in her own instincts.

> We hope that each mother leaves with a strong belief, trust, and confidence in her own instincts.

LEADING AN EFFECTIVE DISCUSSION

Opening Questions

One of the greatest fears a Leader may have is that her carefully prepared questions will meet with long, uncomfortable silences. She may interpret this as meaning that she failed in some way to get the discussion moving. This is usually not true. Silence and hesitation can be normal in the early stages of discussion.

Before or after you ask a question, prepare for this natural pause by suggesting that participants take a moment to think of a response. Several studies have shown that this wait-time usually averages only a few seconds. Deliberately increasing wait-time can increase length of responses, number of volunteers, and confidence reflected in the answers. By allowing a reasonable silence, you let people know that it is all right to take the time to think before speaking.

If the silence continues, you can ask the Group why nobody seems to want to speak. This allows participants to express their confusion about the question, their reluctance to appear irrelevant or foolish, or their need for background information. You can also mention what you think the hesitation might be. "It may seem risky to be the first to respond." This may free a participant to take the risk. You can also simply give an answer for the question yourself, invite others to add to it, and then continue with the meeting.

Encouraging Participation

You can use several techniques to acknowledge the importance of each participant's contribution and encourage participation.

> Acknowledge the importance of each participant's contribution and encourage participation.

- Check the seating arrangements before the meeting to make sure the circle can include everyone.
- Explain words some people may not be familiar with. A newcomer may feel left out if she doesn't understand terms such as *let-down*, *areola*, *colostrum*, *oxytocin*, and *rooting reflex*.

- Maintain eye contact with speakers; show attentiveness with other nonverbal signals such as smiling and nodding.
- In almost all situations, let the speaker finish without interruption; wait to make a comment or ask for clarification.
- If a participant speaks too softly for others to hear, repeat the question or the comment to the Group.
- Give positive reinforcement and feedback. A nod of the head or a word of support can encourage continued participation.
- Watch for nonverbal signals or body language that may indicate someone wants to respond or ask a question.
- Encourage Group members to socialize with newcomers. This can foster a sense of friendship and belonging and can help sell memberships.

Balancing Information and Emotions

Be sensitive to a mother's need to discuss breastfeeding's broader effects on life, as well as breastfeeding's emotional side.

Most mothers come to their first LLL Series Meeting primarily to learn about breastfeeding. Some attend meetings during pregnancy to find out how to get breastfeeding off to a good start. Others begin attending after their babies are born to find out how to overcome a breastfeeding difficulty or to sort out conflicting advice.

These are important needs. Be sensitive to mothers' needs to discuss breastfeeding's broader effects on life and its emotional side. Perhaps breastfeeding is going well for a mother, but her family or friends are critical. Maybe she is suffering from a lack of self-confidence despite all objective indications that her baby is thriving. Knowledge of the basics of breastfeeding and a positive attitude are both important.

Covering two general topics at each meeting gives you the opportunity to provide balance between information and feelings. If you cover only one topic, or you choose two factual topics, you may have to make more of an effort to include both information and the emotional side of breastfeeding.

One way to do this is to prepare at least one question to draw more feeling-related responses. For example, in a discussion about breastfeeding's advantages, you could purposely prepare a question to highlight the emotional advantages or plan to bring them up yourself. One part of the discussion could integrate "Learning to Trust Our Instincts" with a more informational topic.

In some Groups the discussions often center on the emotional aspects of breastfeeding. In this case, you may want to plan ways to balance the emotions with research. You may rely on THE WOMANLY ART OF BREASTFEEDING, fact sheets such as LLLI's annual *Facts about Breastfeeding,* or other LLL published pamphlets to interject factual information.

Accepting and Respecting Each Mother

Establishing and maintaining an atmosphere of respect is crucial to effective learning and open communication, and it can be a real challenge. It is not always easy to show respect for a person's opinion when we disagree with it. Sometimes it helps to focus on the feelings behind the decision or opinions.

For example, a Leader can empathize with a mother who feels pressured to feed her baby solids at six weeks on her doctor's advice, but she does not have to agree with her reasons for following the advice.

"Sounds like you are feeling pressured by advice from your doctor and everyone around you. Are you torn between what they say and what you hear at these meetings?"

Your empathy shows your respect for the mother.

Another example might be a mother who spends long hours away from her baby and believes hers is an ideal situation. Most Leaders have strong feelings about a baby's need for his mother's presence. This can make it difficult for some Leaders to keep their own feelings in the background when helping a mother who leaves her baby for extended periods of time. It may help to remember that you are not responsible for changing a mother's mind.

Consider the following situation. A mother in the circle is a newcomer with a young baby. She expresses her delight over their breastfeeding relationship, which involves the mother being away at work for long hours and the baby receiving pumped milk.

You could respond with appreciation for the woman coming to the meeting and for her devotion to using human milk:

"Wow, what an undertaking! I'm so glad you came tonight and brought your baby. She looks like she's doing beautifully. I'm sure there are other employed mothers who'll be glad to hear how you manage pumping and working."

Others may pick up on your respectful attitude and follow suit with their responses to the mother.

Use the same open, accepting body language no matter how different or unusual a mother's choices may seem to be. Sometimes personalities can be irritating, making it difficult to be accepting. Remember how easy it is for a mother to pick up on what you might think is a subtle signal to a co-Leader.

The mother attending her first LLL Series Meeting is usually full of hope that she's doing the right things for her baby. She may be vulnerable to what you say. To help her feel good about what she's doing for her baby and keep an open mind about what she hears at the meeting, use your voice and manner to convey respect.

You convey respect when you:

- Listen,
- Ask questions,
- Talk with the other person and learn from her experience.

Conveying respect in these ways can also help you gain a deeper understanding of the situation. In a sensitive situation, you might want to wait to offer suggestions when they could seem less threatening.

If the women attending the meeting truly feel respected and supported, they will be receptive to the information LLL has to offer, and the Group will thrive. An effective Group is one in which participants are comfortable exchanging ideas.

Encourage all mothers to attend Group meetings, whether or not they agree with LLL philosophy. Our primary goal is to provide each mother with sound knowledge; she will proceed according to her own beliefs, values, and personality. Leaders can offer ideas and suggest possibilities, but we cannot and should not presume that all mothers will find LLL philosophy attractive or that all families will incorporate the philosophy into their lives in the same ways.

PLANNING MEETINGS

Handling Strong Feelings, Doubts, and Disagreements

To the mother, you are La Leche League. Being sensitive to others' feelings and respecting each mother is important, no matter how different her ideas may be. Offer your knowledge and experience without appearing to tell her what she should do. Each breastfeeding and mothering choice is rightfully the mother's to make.

> Offer your knowledge and experience without appearing to tell anyone what she should do.

Be sure that mothers understand that you are offering possibilities and suggestions, not dictating a certain way of breastfeeding or mothering. Emphasize throughout the discussion that each breastfeeding couple, each family, is different. Avoid blanket statements and words such as never, must, should, always, everyone, and all babies. It is possible to make a point and still allow room for exceptions by saying:

> *"Many mothers have found…"*

> *"Some babies…"*

> *"THE WOMANLY ART OF BREASTFEEDING suggests…"*

> *"The LLLI Health Advisory Council says…"*

THE WOMANLY ART OF BREASTFEEDING is filled with examples of these kinds of statements.

As the discussion progresses, watch individual reactions in the Group. Look for agreement, curiosity, disagreement, disapproval, skepticism, impatience, or hostility. Take cues from body and facial reactions. If you note disagreement, encourage mothers to verbalize their doubts. It is much easier to help someone who expresses doubts than to help someone who is silent.

Before responding to strong statements try to focus on the speaker's feelings:

> *"It sounds to me like you're feeling anxious about your new role as a mother. Many of us felt that way when we were expecting our first babies."*

> *"You seem to feel rejected by your older child."*

> *"You're really feeling torn between your baby's needs and your own."*

Express the value of each person's contribution to the discussion and follow through with more information by asking the Group for support, clarification, or different experiences.

> *"Thanks, Eva, I'm glad you mentioned that. Has anyone else had a similar experience?"*

> *"Yes, it really is hard to delay solids when your pediatrician isn't supportive. You had this experience, too, Mary, didn't you? How did you work it out with your doctor?"*

Try to observe the meeting from a new participant's point of view. What does she see and hear? Happy, talkative mothers casually breastfeeding their contented, happy babies? Or strange ideas that seem foreign to her? What is she feeling? Can you guide the discussion to the new mother's questions without making her feel unduly self-conscious? Can you, in some way, give her the message that you were once new to LLL Series Meetings and that you, too, had doubts about breastfeeding?

> *"It must be puzzling to you, Joyce, to hear all these people talk about how much they enjoy motherhood and yet hear them talk about the difficulties they've had with breastfeeding. When I first came to meetings, I didn't know how I felt about these different ideas."*

You may feel threatened when a mother expresses negative feelings, but when a mother speaks openly, opportunities to help her increase. Sometimes people need to know that it is all right to have these feelings before they can go on to try some of the suggestions that the Group presents.

"You seem discouraged now because you wonder if you will ever again get enough sleep."

"You feel frustrated, Ellen, when you hear your baby crying just after you have put him down. You can't think of what more you can do to help him."

Controversy can be a challenge; it also has positive aspects. It can be a sign of open, honest discussion. Questioning can help attendees become more aware of LLL's philosophy and the reasons behind our suggestions. This can also increase your awareness of how the women in the Group perceive La Leche League. Disagreements also challenge you to use the skills you have learned.

In the midst of a controversy:

- Keep in mind that there is no need to apologize for LLL philosophy.
- Take a moment to pause and think positively. Listen to and respect each person's opinion and feelings.
- Don't allow the mother who raised the controversy to be attacked by others. Be tactful and positive.
- You may want to remind the Group about the goal of the meeting and the need to stay within the meeting time frame.
- You can offer to discuss the matter on a one-to-one basis outside of the meeting.

Responding to Contrary Information

When a participant's comments include information different from LLL views, you can make a statement that emphasizes the importance of respecting another's decision whether we agree or not.

"We each have different opinions and different family situations. What works for one family might not work well in another."

"I'm glad that worked for you."

Then offer appropriate LLL information in a tactful, non-threatening way:

"Many mothers find that…"

"The LLLI Health Advisory Council recommends that…"

"La Leche League recommends… because…"

You can also ask how others have handled similar situations.

These tips can help:
- Respond to the participants in a positive manner.
- Ignore comments that indicate minor differences with LLL information.
- If the topic seems to be of interest to one participant in particular, suggest that you can continue the discussion with her after the meeting or over the telephone.
- If the participant persists with the discussion beyond the point where others are comfortable, say that it's time to go on to another topic and shift body and eye contact to someone else.

PLANNING MEETINGS

Controversy can be a challenge; it also has positive aspects.

When comments include information that differs from LLL views, you can emphasize the importance of respecting another's decision.

• If appropriate, very carefully interject humor. It is never appropriate to direct humor at a participant, present or not.

Group Dynamics

Encouraging shy or quiet participants

Using eye contact and a friendly manner may encourage a shy, quiet mother to participate. Remember, too, that a newcomer may only appear shy; her lack of knowledge may make her hesitant to ask questions at first.

Some women are not comfortable speaking in a group and will never be very vocal at LLL meetings. They come to listen. They may be more comfortable speaking on an individual basis during refreshments or between meetings.

Helping everyone get a chance to speak

At LLL Series Meetings, we encourage all to participate in the discussion and need to make sure that everyone who has a comment to offer gets a chance to speak.

At meetings, we need to make sure that everyone who has a comment to offer gets a chance to speak.

When a talkative participant takes over, it is not easy to regain control of the discussion. Occasionally you may actually have to interrupt her, cutting in when she takes a breath. However, you can also use both body language and words to direct the Group's attention elsewhere. As you turn away from the mother, pick up on what she has said and use it as a beginning for the next topic. Ask a direct question of another mother who looks as if she has something to say. If nothing else works, you may have to say:

> *"I know you're really excited about your experience. I want to talk with you more about it, perhaps during refreshments."*

Or sum up her comments, thank her for her important contribution to the discussion, and shift to a new topic:

> *"Thank you, Mary. Your large family has certainly given you a variety of nursing experiences. And now we need to talk about getting the baby off to a good start in the hospital."*

If there's any indication that the mother feels offended or left out, seek her out at refreshment time and talk with her.

Sometimes it is possible to prevent a talkative participant from dominating before she gets started on a particular subject. For example, if someone tends to dominate meetings with her own experiences and you know she has a horror story about her early breastfeeding experience, at the beginning of Meeting 2 you could say something like:

> *"Tonight we're going to discuss childbirth choices and the early days of breastfeeding. We've all had different experiences—some more positive than others. During the discussion let's focus on how our childbirth experiences helped get breastfeeding off to a good start."*

Some people continually bring up events that seem to be of little consequence. Sometimes just avoiding eye contact with a person who is doing this will cut down on what others consider irrelevant comments. If you casually turn your body away and look toward someone else, it can tend to slow her down without being offensive. Often, talking with someone over refreshments helps to fulfill her need to relate experiences that are significant to her.

When side conversations persist

To keep side conversations to a minimum, you might say something like this at the beginning of the meeting:

> *"We are here to exchange ideas. Typical of people who are enthusiastic about a subject, we love to talk! Because we are in a group, let's try to make it possible for all to hear and contribute, by taking turns."*

PLANNING MEETINGS

Use other more direct and forceful techniques carefully and sparingly, because they can hurt feelings.

> *"You and Jane seem to have an idea…"*

> *"Would you like to add something to what Mary has said, Judy?"*

> *"Did you have something to share, Nan?"*

You might also be able to stop side conversations by pausing and asking:

> *"Can everyone hear what Sara is saying?"*

Try using eye contact and frowning for side comments of a disrespectful nature, giggling, or open hostility.

After a meeting in which side conversations were a problem, think about the root cause. Perhaps the weather or recent world or local events disturbed the usual atmosphere. Perhaps the Group is getting too large and the meeting needs to be split. Maybe the way the chairs were arranged contributed to the problem. Or perhaps there were too many toddlers present to keep the discussion on track. Discovering the cause can help you make adjustments for the next meeting.

Preventing arguments

Sometimes you can prevent an argument from occurring if you notice someone seems emotionally charged. You can ask the mother making a challenge to answer her own question.

> Mother: *Do you really believe that a baby benefits in any way from nursing past six months?*

> Leader: *Barbara, what are your feelings on this?*

It may then be necessary to use one of the techniques described in the sections **Handling Strong Feelings, Doubts, and Disagreements,** page 42, and **Responding to Contrary Information,** page 43.

If an argument does arise, you can use a hand gesture to ward off further comments: you can hold your hand up in stop position or wave your hands as if aiding someone in distress. You might need to signal verbally as well. A humorous remark about the Group's disorder may help direct attention away from the argument itself. You can then attempt to guide the discussion in a positive direction.

> *"We're not going to agree about everything. Let's try to get back to the real message in what Mimi is saying: that there are times when she really doesn't think breastfeeding is worth it. Can anyone else add something to her comment?"*

> Sometimes you can prevent an argument from occurring if you notice that someone seems emotionally charged.

Sometimes you may need to cut in and summarize:

> "It's obvious that this is important to you both and worth taking time to work through. Perhaps after the meeting would be a good time. Right now, let me see if I can summarize what you are saying…"

You can summarize in a sentence and go on to connect the summary to the meeting topic, LLL information, or to the idea that what works for one family might not for another. You could then return to the meeting topic, perhaps with a new question.

When LLL expertise is overshadowed

> If a health care provider implies an expertise superseding that of LLL, the Group may turn to her instead of you.

A female health care provider or student is always welcome to attend meetings as an interested woman. Sometimes a participant who is a nurse, doctor, lactation consultant, or other health care provider uses medical or technical terms as she tells about her experiences. If she implies an expertise that supersedes that of LLL, the Group may turn to her instead of you.

One way to counter this situation is by mentioning that Leaders are experienced breastfeeding mothers who have received LLL training so they can provide technical knowledge as well as mother-to-mother support. Leaders help families to have satisfying breastfeeding experiences.

Our first responsibility at Series Meetings is to mothers and babies. Helping mothers to feel comfortable in an atmosphere that is conducive to open discussion is most important. Keep the discussion directed toward the mothers' needs.

When health care providers who are also mothers are favorably impressed with LLL meetings, their visits can have far-reaching benefits for LLL's relationship with the medical community. They may also acquire valuable information they can share with breastfeeding patients. Then, through these health care providers, breastfeeding mothers and babies will receive more support!

However, when a doctor, male or female, asks to attend a Series Meeting in a professional capacity, arrange a separate meeting instead. Series Meetings are not an educational tool for medical professionals. At a special meeting a doctor could meet with Leaders, ask them questions, and discuss the services LLL offers breastfeeding mothers.

Keeping LLL's purpose clear

> Our goal is to offer information and support to women who want to breastfeed their babies.

All women in LLL are interested in breastfeeding, and many are involved in other causes as well. A mother may feel moved to bring a cause especially close to her heart to the attention of her friends in her LLL Group.

When a participant brings up a topic that has nothing to do with LLL objectives, have a ready-made statement that LLL has a primary purpose: breastfeeding information and support.

> "As an organization, LLLI is neither for nor against any other cause. Our goal is solely to offer information and support to women who want to breastfeed their babies."

Empathize with the mother's feelings and proceed with the regular discussion.

"Lina, I can understand your deep concern on this matter. However, LLL takes no stand on this issue. At this meeting, our focus is breastfeeding and mothering through breastfeeding. Outside the Series Meeting would be a better time to talk about that."

This might be a good time to mention another benefit of meetings—an opportunity to develop friendships. If the Group holds Enrichment Meetings, you might bring these up as a way to encourage further involvement in the Group and to transition out of a discussion that has strayed from the subject of breastfeeding. If a person is attending seemingly with the purpose of promoting a business, talk to her privately about LLL meetings not being a forum for that.

Deciding when to talk about your own experience

LLL meetings should be a place where everyone can communicate information and experiences. Focusing too much on one person's experience can present a limited picture of LLL information and philosophy and of how these might fit into others' lives.

Talk about your own experience sparingly to avoid inadvertently setting yourself up as a model others believe they are expected to imitate. However, sometimes a description of your experience can be valuable. Perhaps a mother is feeling alone in a situation that only she and you have in common or needs the long-term mothering perspective only the mother of an older child can give.

You can appropriately bring up your own experience after others have talked about theirs, as an affirmation of whatever point was raised. Take care to do so in a way that does not presume that another mother would necessarily respond in the same way. (See also **Talking about Personal Experience,** pages 2–3.)

> **PLANNING MEETINGS**

> You can appropriately bring up your own experience after others have talked about theirs, as an affirmation of whatever point was raised.

Knowing When to End the Meeting

An hour to an hour and a half is usually about the right length of time for the meeting. Remember that participants may feel they have to stay until the meeting breaks.

Being sensitive to these factors can help you end the meeting at the proper time:

- **Clock time.** If many toddlers are present, it is best to keep the meeting on the short side. Leave participants involved rather than frustrated by a chaotic meeting.
- **Topic completion.**
- **Side conversations and body language.** Chatting among participants, moving around, and avoidance of eye contact during discussion may be clues that it's time to wrap things up.
- **High noise level.** Unchecked noise is very irritating. If it's bothering you, it's probably bothering others, too. Remind mothers to take care of their children's needs. Bad weather, a small room, or one with poor acoustics can intensify a noise problem. Try a short break, or keep the discussions brief and use lots of summarizing.
- **Participants' fatigue.** Watch for signs of physical discomfort and take a break so pregnant women aren't sitting too long. End the meeting with an invitation to talk more over refreshments and to look for more information in the pamphlets and Group Library books.

Special Considerations for Large and Small Meetings

The small meeting

Seating arrangements can help both the small or large meeting be more accommodating to the participants.

A small meeting, one with fewer than six participants, can sometimes be more of a challenge than a large meeting. Participants may feel more on the spot. These ideas can add a spark to a small meeting:

- Sit around the kitchen table. If more mothers arrive, change to the regular meeting set-up.
- Use an informal meeting structure. Think of it as a get-together rather than a meeting, and keep the introductory remarks conversational.
- Focus on the people who attend, not on how many didn't. Emphasize the positive aspects of a small meeting: "We can really get to know each other." "We have time for lots of questions." "We can go into our topic in more depth."
- Encourage LLL membership to help people develop a sense of belonging and commitment.
- Encourage Group Library use by frequent reference to LLL books. If a mother takes home a book, she'll be more likely to return to a meeting.

The large meeting

Gratifying as it may be to have more than 20 people arrive for a meeting, sheer numbers can make it difficult to allow time for everyone to participate in the discussion. Speaking personally to everyone may be impossible. These suggestions may help make this situation more manageable:

- Plan ahead. A carpeted meeting room has better acoustics. Eliminate noisy toys. Plan to keep the meeting on the short side, no longer than an hour.
- Watch or ask a co-Leader to watch for signs of unanswered questions and talk with those mothers after the meeting.
- Ask for help from Group members. If you haven't had the opportunity to ask for help in advance, approach them just before the meeting.
- Consider suggesting seating arrangements: mothers with small babies closer to the Leader, and mothers of active toddlers in the back or to the side, where they can get refreshments and supervise their children.
- Divide into two discussion circles if more than one Leader is present and a separate room is available. If there is a consistently large turnout of fifteen or more and there are enough Leaders, the Group should consider splitting into two Groups. (See **Splitting a Group,** pages 130-131.)
- Use "buzz groups." After introductions, small groups can discuss different aspects of the topic. Each group reports back to the whole Group. With this arrangement, everyone can participate; during reporting time you can comment on ideas. This method works best if there is a Leader available for each buzz group. If there are not enough Leaders to have a Leader in each group, the Leader can circulate from group to group. This method is helpful if the meeting is being held in a language that is not the first language for many of the attendees. Do not be surprised if the groups stray from the discussion topic. Although they may be off topic, they are developing friendships with other breastfeeding mothers, which can increase their brastfeeding success.

OLDER BABIES AT MEETINGS

Reactions to Breastfeeding Toddlers

La Leche League encourages mothers to bring their breastfeeding babies to Series Meetings and also toddlers who would be unhappy away from their mothers. A Series Meeting may be a new mother's first encounter with toddler breastfeeding. This could be an eye-opening experience for her. If you notice a strong reaction from a newcomer, talking openly about it can help.

> *"It is unusual in our society to see children breastfeeding past babyhood, but worldwide, it is quite common. We encourage each mother to make this decision according to what feels right for her and her family."*

When it is your toddler who is breastfeeding, you might want to use the approach LLL co-Founder Edwina Froehlich found successful:

> *"If I happened to be sitting next to a mother whose eyes bulged as she watched my toddler nurse, I would cheerfully remark that her baby probably wouldn't nurse as long as mine and she shouldn't worry. If a mother commented she hoped her baby would wean before he reached that age, I would reassure her that he probably would. I figured I couldn't be too far off saying this, because I knew by then that when a mother truly wants her little one to wean, she usually can accomplish it. But I'd tell her that since Peter and I enjoyed his nursing, I saw no reason to say no to him.*
>
> *"The idea behind this approach is the same one in THE WOMANLY ART, which was written not for the experienced mother but for the first-time mother. Our goal was to offer her as much information as she would need to get her off to a good start, rather than overwhelming her with all the ups and downs a parent can encounter. There is no sense in spending time at a meeting trying to convince a first-time mother of a young infant of the importance of not making arbitrary decisions about weaning. Her own feelings for her baby, if she gets off to a good start, will do more to convince her than anything else will of the child's need to continue at the breast as long as he seems to want to."*

Pointing out books and other LLL resources to a participant who seems shocked by extended breastfeeding can allow her to look into the idea without targeting her. You may want to talk about these reactions with experienced mothers in the Group outside of the meeting. Together, you might decide on approaches that are sensitive to the reactions of new mothers. Approaches might include more discreet nursing and reiterating the positive aspect of extended breastfeeding. Also discuss the possibility of older toddlers being happier if left with someone else while mother attends the meeting. Some may insist on nursing because they are bored.

Advance Planning for Toddlers

With a little planning, a Leader can help all participants, including the mothers of toddlers and the toddlers themselves, enjoy the meeting.

A safe environment

Safety is critical when little explorers are present. If the meeting is in a home, a reminder telephone call to the hostess and a last-minute check before the meeting starts can avoid a wide range of problems. If the hostess does not have toddlers of her own, you can help her with childproofing tips.

PLANNING MEETINGS

A Series meeting may be a new mother's first encounter with toddler breastfeeding.

Find out beforehand whether the hostess has any room restrictions. If she does, remember to inform mothers where the play area is located. Easy accessibility of children to their mothers is important. It is also wise to remind mothers that each is responsible for her own child. Stress that meetings are informal and that it's all right to walk around or give a hungry little one a drink or snack, where appropriate, so that a mother with a restless toddler will feel comfortable to meet her child's needs.

If the meeting is held in a public facility, you, and perhaps some Group workers, will want to arrive early to check the room for safety.

Refreshments with toddlers

Keeping in mind that toddlers enjoy eating and tend to make messes, carefully consider what refreshments to offer. It is your responsibility to find out where the hostess or facility allows food and to tell the participants. Leave the meeting space clean when you are finished. Promote clean-up time with the mothers as an extended opportunity to socialize.

Minimizing Toddler Problems

Occasionally, toddlers may seem to outnumber mothers at a Series Meeting. In this case you need to keep the meeting short for everyone's sake. Even a short meeting is too long for some toddlers. Be prepared for some toddler-related escapades and be ready to show an extra dose of patience to the toddlers and their mothers.

> Be prepared for some toddler-related escapades and be ready to show an extra dose of patience to the toddlers and their mothers.

A short announcement at the beginning of a meeting can help ward off potential problems. Set the tone by alerting participants to potential disturbances. A first-time mother may be unaware that in a roomful of little ones her toddler might suddenly become possessive of his toys. Remind participants that young children do not always understand about sharing and ask each mother to keep an eye on her child with that in mind.

Sometimes a toddler who comes to meetings is noisy, pushes other children, or bites. In these cases, consider what to suggest to help the child, how to help the mother, and how to protect the other little ones in the group.

Encourage the mother to vigilantly monitor her toddler. Each mother watching her own child can keep the problem to a minimum. Befriending the mother and dialoguing with her about solutions may help both her and the Group. Reassure her that you know she is trying her best. By commenting in an understanding way to a mother that it must be frustrating when she sees her child pushing another child, you give that mother the chance to express her fears and feelings and talk about ways to help the child learn more appropriate behavior.

LLL meetings may be the only place where a mother with a disruptive toddler feels welcome. Make a point of mentioning the toddler's positive qualities to the Group. Encourage mothers to openly love their children in spite of their sometimes unlovable behavior.

When toddler noise threatens to overrun the meeting, some Leaders find it helpful to use a nearby separate room where a co-Leader or Group member can focus attention on the children. By attending to the children rather than the meeting, these adults help keep the noise level down. They can lead quiet play activities and help resolve problems before they escalate. They may intervene to prevent little ones from getting hurt, but if a toddler needs his mother or some loving guidance, the mother should handle this. As always, mothers are responsible for their own children.

In some daytime Groups that usually have large numbers of children, each mother pays a small amount to help cover the fee for a mother's helper. The helper is not a babysitter; she knows that the children are welcome to toddle back and forth to their mothers.

When you comment on the mothers' abilities to meet the needs of their children and be involved in the meeting, you encourage mothers' comfort in responding to their children's needs in public situations.

When You Bring Your Own Toddler

When you bring a toddler along, you show mothers that everyone is responsible for meeting the needs of her own children, including you.

Delegating meeting set-up to Group workers can allow you to settle your child before the meeting starts. For example, the Greeter passes out nametags and welcome packets, the Librarian sets up the Library, the Treasurer makes sure sale items are in place. Keeping drinks, snacks, toys, and books nearby helps reduce the number of times it is necessary to get up.

If leading an entire meeting and giving your little one needed attention is difficult, a co-Leader could take over partway through, perhaps when a topic focus changes or as needed. This is easier when you and your co-Leader plan the meeting together and know what points are going to be discussed.

A lone Leader with a needy toddler might try to schedule meetings at a time when her toddler will be happy staying with someone else. Sometimes a child who would be miserable left at home is delighted if his father takes him out instead, especially if they leave home before mother leaves for the meeting. You could try hosting a series in your home, so that the father could care for your child in another part of the house and bring him to you if necessary. If the meeting is in the evening, this might allow enough time for you to lead the meeting until your toddler is ready for bed, then you could invite the mothers to have refreshments while you settle him in.

Sometimes a lone Leader cannot leave her toddler and he is unhappy at meetings. Changing the meeting time might help. The toddler may do better during an earlier or later part of the day. Another idea is to take along an older child as a mother's helper. A Group member might pour a drink or help with a toy while you lead the meeting. If the situation becomes stressful, contact your support Leader for suggestions.

> When you bring a toddler along, you show that everyone is responsible for meeting the needs of her own children.

Too Many Children?

While breastfeeding babies and toddlers who need to be with their mothers are always welcome at meetings, mothers sometimes continue to bring older toddlers and preschool-age children after they have reached the age and maturity when they would be happier at home.

Sometimes a mother continues to bring her child out of habit. Sometimes she is comfortable leaving her child at home on other occasions but brings the child to LLL meetings because she thinks it is expected. Sometimes she brings her child along because the child asks to see the babies or wants to play with toys at a new house.

The primary concern of the Group is to meet the needs of the newcomers. Newcomers, especially women expecting their first babies, may feel overwhelmed by

> Newcomers may feel overwhelmed by the noise and confusion of large numbers of children.

the noise and confusion of large numbers of children. The children themselves may be happier at home with their fathers or another caregiver. When their mothers are more interested in what's being said during the discussion than in paying attention to them, older toddlers and preschoolers may become bored with the meeting and misbehave.

Restricting toys at meetings to those that interest only babies or toddlers may result in fewer preschoolers asking to come. If mothers bring their older children to meetings for the purpose of socializing, suggest that they set up informal playgroups instead.

If large numbers of children disrupt meetings and the advance planning suggestions do not help, dialogue with the mothers to find solutions for how to make a meeting more enjoyable for everyone. This open dialogue may prompt the mothers to discover new ways that they can attend to their children or may even prompt them to find ways to leave them at home. In these situations it is important that you set an example by leaving your own older children at home. Recognizing when a child is ready to stay at home while mother is away could be a topic for discussion at an Evaluation or Enrichment Meeting. One Leader used this guideline for her own children: the preschooler who needs to be with mother is a preschooler who is willing to stay close and play quietly. She told her child that if he comes along, he must be willing to sit in her lap.

SETTING THE SCENE: WHO, WHEN, WHERE, WHAT, AND HOW

Who

Women and children first

All women are welcome at La Leche League Series Meetings. Any woman interested in breastfeeding, whether she is pregnant, breastfeeding, or just hoping to learn more, may attend. This includes grandmothers! Breastfeeding babies and toddlers who would be unhappy away from their mothers are also welcome.

Fathers

> With input from Group members and your support Leader, you can decide how and when to invite fathers.

Traditionally, Series Meetings have been open only to women. In some situations, women might be uncomfortable breastfeeding their babies or reluctant to ask certain questions in a mixed group. A single mother or a mother whose spouse is not interested in attending might feel out of place if others at the meeting were all couples.

Some Groups hold two series: one for couples and one for women only. Other Groups include fathers at Series Meetings. With input from Group members and awareness of the population served by the Group, and in consultation with your support Leader, you can decide what is best for the Group.

Fathers can be included in meetings in several ways:

• Invite fathers to participate in all meetings.
• Invite fathers to certain meetings in each series, for example, Meeting 2.
• Offer a fifth meeting for fathers at the end of each series.
• Offer optional meetings, such as Couples Meetings or fathers' nights.

One Group, which held both morning and evening meetings, decided to invite fathers to their evening meetings. This worked especially well, because several mothers lived out of town and were driven to the meeting by their husbands, who previously had been left to wait for them outside the meeting area. When fathers began attending, the Leaders did not change their meeting format. They simply added two more considerations to their plans:

- They arranged for an additional room where a mother could breastfeed her baby in private and still hear the meeting.
- They tried to find a hostess whose husband would be home during the meeting, so that if just one other man came he wouldn't feel out of place.

Reporters

To preserve the privacy of participants, we do not invite reporters to regular Series Meetings. We don't want to close the door on good publicity, however. If a reporter wants to know more about LLL and/or interview Group members, there are alternatives. You could invite the reporter to a Chapter Meeting or hold a mock meeting with experienced mothers and Leaders. Checking in with your support Leader before the meeting is a good idea. Your support Leader may have suggestions that can help you develop beneficial contact with the media.

When
Selecting a meeting day

New breastfeeding mothers need to be able to count on getting information and encouragement on a regular basis. Holding Series Meetings at a regular time, for example, the third Wednesday of each month, enables new mothers to get the help they need. Make every effort not to cancel a meeting.

If there are several Groups in the locality, each Group can choose a different time to meet, thereby meeting the needs of a variety of families. Likewise, if a Group has several Leaders, Leaders can branch off to offer other meetings at other times. Whatever time works best for you and the mothers in the Group is appropriate.

Evening or Daytime Meetings?

Mothers may prefer daytime meetings because:

- They do not interrupt evening family time.
- Traveling to the meeting and finding the site can be easier during the day.
- Babies, toddlers, and mothers are often at their freshest in the daytime. Mothers may be better prepared to meet their child's needs and participate in the meeting.

Evening meetings may be preferable because:

- More mothers who work outside the home can usually attend.
- Older toddlers and preschoolers may be happier staying at home in the evening with a father or caregiver. Fewer children at meetings can mean less noise and confusion, making it easier to hear the discussion.

PLANNING MEETINGS

If a reporter wants to know more about LLL there are alternatives to regular Series Meeting.

When selecting a meeting date and time, whatever works best for you and the mothers in the Group is appropriate.

Relocating or postponing meetings

If a change in location is necessary, contact as many mothers as possible to notify them of the change.

What if the hostess calls on the day of the meeting to tell you someone in her family is ill? What if the Leaders all get sick on the day of the Series Meeting? Perhaps the weather is bad, and travel conditions are hazardous. What should you do?

If the hostess is unable to host the meeting, do your best to relocate. Contact as many mothers as possible to notify them of the change. A note posted on the door of the original home can redirect people and save the hostess from having to answer the door. Perhaps a Group member can wait at the original meeting location to redirect mothers and drive them to the new location if needed.

If you are unable to attend, a co-Leader, a Leader from a neighboring Group, or a Leader on reserve may be available to help out in an emergency. If there are no other Leaders nearby, you may need to postpone the meeting. Expected participants will need to be contacted about the change. A note on the door of the meeting location will inform attendees who could not be contacted. In some areas, local radio stations are willing to announce meeting changes.

What if something happens at the last minute, after people are already en route to the meeting, for example, if there is an accident? In a situation like this a Group member would explain that in the absence of the Leader there is no official LLL Series Meeting, although people may want to stay and talk. If questions come up during the discussion, the Group member can suggest people contact you or she can offer to relay their questions to you so you can contact them.

Some Groups have an understanding that if the temperature dips below a certain level or it snows heavily, the meeting is automatically postponed to the following week on the same day. Some Groups follow school closing schedules: if there is no school because of bad weather, the meeting is automatically postponed or cancelled. If this change comes up often, announcing it on meeting notices will warn participants beforehand.

Perhaps the meeting date can be changed to accommodate a lone or isolated Leader's holiday plans. Even if attendance is temporarily low during the vacation season, getting together regularly can be very valuable for those who do come.

Where

A home or a public place?

Whenever possible use the same location for a complete series to eliminate misunderstandings and extra telephone calls.

Many LLL Groups meet in private homes, with the meeting place changing each series. Other Groups hold their meetings in a public place in the same location series after series. The Leader and the Group workers can decide which works best for them. Whenever possible use the same location for a complete series to eliminate misunderstandings and extra telephone calls.

Advantages of a home

- A warm, personal atmosphere can be conducive to conversation.
- The physical setting is usually appropriate, with carpets and comfortable chairs.
- Good acoustics and a small meeting area usually make it easy for participants to hear.
- Mothers have the opportunity to give the Group some short-term help by hosting meetings.

- Seeing you or Group members in their home settings can help dispel the super-mother myth some new mothers may believe.

Points to consider when deciding on a private home for Series Meetings:

- Is the home easy to find and close to town?
- Will parking be a problem?
- If a participant or child is injured is there a liability issue?
- Will there be another willing hostess for the next series? Is the home baby- and child-proofed?
- Will there be interruptions from people not participating in the meeting?
- Is there a backup plan in case the home is not available for the meeting?

PLANNING MEETINGS

Hostess Letter

You could use a hostess letter to begin discussion with a mother who has agreed to hold meetings in her home. The letter could serve as a pre-meeting checklist as well.

Dear _____,

Thank you for generously offering your home for our next series of meetings.

For our meeting we will need seating for about ___ mothers, a table for the Group Library, and a table or counter for refreshments. Traditionally, our hostess provides the beverage, cups, and napkins for each meeting and stores the Group Library books and bulletin board during the series. Other mothers are asked to provide snacks. Does this arrangement suit you?

Here are some practical things to consider as you prepare your home for a meeting:

Cleaning—Crawling babies and toddlers are safer on a clean, uncluttered floor.

Toys—Keep in mind that children of various ages may attend the meetings. If possible, have a few safe and quiet toys available; most mothers will bring a few. Please put away: riding toys; toys that play music, ring, bang, etc.; toys with long handles, like bats, brooms, swords; toys with tiny parts; toys your child may find difficult to share.

Pets—For the health and well-being of both your pet and the little ones present, please close the animal out of the meeting area.

Safety—You may have already baby-proofed your house. Please double-check for open stairs, dangling electrical cords, breakables, etc. Feel free to close doors to other rooms in your home. A Leader will remind mothers that they are responsible for their own children, but little ones can be quick.

As hostess for this series, you are invited to attend our Group Evaluation Meetings, held on _____ at _____.

Thank you again for welcoming us into your home. Any questions—just call.

Sincerely,

_____(Leader's signature, name and phone number)

Advantages of a public place

- You don't need to find a new place for the Group to meet each series.
- Publicity is easier, since meeting notices can state the location rather than instructing mothers to call.
- You can choose a central location that is easily available to more people.
- Newcomers may feel more comfortable coming to a public place than to the home of someone they do not know.
- Meeting surroundings are usually safe and clean.
- There is never a need to cancel or relocate due to illness or emergencies in the hostess's family.
- Public places usually offer good outside lighting, consistent snow removal in winter months, reliable heating and air conditioning.
- Meeting in a public place may be considered a sign of credibility. If meetings are held in a reputable place, people may assume that groups that meet there are reputable, too.
- If storage is available on site, the Group workers may be able to leave their supplies there between meetings, taking them home only when it is convenient or necessary.
- In some venues, there may be more meeting space for large meetings.

Points to consider when deciding on a public place for Series Meetings:

- Is there a fee for the meeting room?
- Are comfortable chairs available? Folding chairs or those with attached desktops can be uncomfortable for pregnant or nursing women.
- Can the meeting room be childproofed? Can breakables or hazardous objects be moved out of the meeting area and replaced afterward? Are windows, doors, railings, stairs, and heaters safe for little ones?
- Are toys available; if not, can they be stored or brought there for meetings?
- Is storage available for the Group Library?
- Are the toilets clean and convenient to the meeting room?
- Does the facility allow food and drink in the meeting room?
- Is the parking lot well lit and ample? Is public transportation available?
- Do acoustics allow participants to easily hear the discussion?
- Is the meeting room carpeted? Bare floors can be cold. They also can be slippery and dangerous for small babies and toddlers.
- Does the facility require proof of liability insurance? The facility owner or manager can let you know if proof of insurance is required to hold meetings in the facility. Note: A Group can obtain this proof of insurance by contacting LLLI.

What to Bring?

Identifying the meeting place

A welcome sign on the door is a signal to those looking for the meeting.

Consider one of the following suggestions to make sure the meeting place is easy to identify:

- LLL sign, windsock, banner, or flag near the door.
- LLLI logo silhouette in a lighted window.

- Welcome sign on the door. Although it may not be readable from afar, it can be a signal to people who are looking for a meeting place. If it says, "Welcome to LLL—Walk in," it also relieves the hostess of door duty, silences the doorbell, and eliminates waiting outside in cold or rainy weather.

PLANNING MEETINGS

Nametags

Nametags can help participants get to know one another and identify the Leader(s) and Group workers.

Nametag ideas:

- Strips of wide masking tape with names in permanent marking pen.
- Nametag stickers.
- File cards threaded with yarn or string to hang around a participants' necks.

Any baby-proof style nametag works well. Check for small or sharp fasteners, and use nontoxic marking pens. Make sure names are easy to read; for this reason, some Groups use only first names in broad tip marking pen.

Information packets

Information packets for newcomers can include a welcome letter, membership information, member publication sample, and one or two LLL information sheets. Some Groups compile two different packets, one for pregnant newcomers and one for the newcomers whose babies have already been born. Consult your support Leader about review procedures for materials created by the Group. She can offer suggestions for content or appearance. Using only LLL materials in these packets will avoid confusion about what LLL believes or recommends. (See also **Introductory Packets of Information,** pages 123-124.)

Resources at hand

In addition to the Group Library, you may want to bring to meetings your personal, marked copies of resources such as THE WOMANLY ART OF BREASTFEEDING, THE BREAST-FEEDING ANSWER BOOK, and THE LEADER'S HANDBOOK. You might also want to bring information sheets and pamphlets to give to mothers with specific concerns.

Refreshment time

Refreshments are optional and can be served before, during, or after the meeting. Refreshments offer an opportunity for attendees to mingle which can strengthen the Group.

Some Groups find that serving refreshments for about fifteen minutes before the meeting helps to break the ice. By mingling, you may hear stories or concerns from the participants that will help in facilitating the discussion. Offering refreshments at the beginning also provides a chance for people who arrive early to look over the Group Library and return books while others get settled. Some Groups encourage refreshment refills at any time; others prefer to minimize interruptions. In any case, water or a nutritious beverage should be available at all times for thirsty breastfeeding mothers.

If you choose to have refreshments and one-to-one chats at the beginning, make it clear that you will also be available to talk to participants after the meeting.

A refreshment period during the meeting can provide a needed break if babies or toddlers get restless or fussy. It can also allow time for easing any tensions that might come up during the discussion.

Serving refreshments after the meeting allows people to talk further about the meeting topic or ask questions mother-to-mother. You can meet with mothers individually or mingle with those new to the Group. (See also **Refreshment Coordinator,** page 92.)

Signs and posters

Notices on bulletin boards and posters can help illustrate LLL ideas and information. They save time by reinforcing points made in a meeting as well as making announcements and reminders. They can be used to:

- Welcome new mothers and their babies by name,
- Announce births or display snapshots of mothers and babies,
- Illustrate how membership dues are used,
- Display new LLL pamphlets,
- List titles and prices of books available for sale,
- List the titles of books, pamphlets, and information sheets especially relevant to the meeting topic,
- State breastfeeding facts or advantages,
- Show family photos that include breastfeeding,
- List breastfeeding tips,
- Illustrate nutritious snacks for expectant or nursing mothers and toddlers, and
- State LLL concepts relevant to the meeting.

(See **Using Visuals and Discussion Aids,** page 31.)

You can purchase a display board or make one by covering wood or heavy cardboard with fabric. Hinged display boards will stand alone. Card pockets can hold brochures.

Posters can be made in all sizes and shapes. Lettering needs to be large and heavy enough to be visible across the room. Laminating with clear plastic adhesive helps preserve posters. If using professionally produced photos, be sure to recognize the photographer by including his or her name.

Our goal to help women breastfeed is sufficient for all our attention at LLL functions. In regard to notices and posters created for the meeting, it is important not to distract participants with visuals representing other causes, no matter how worthwhile.

Sales at meetings

You can acquaint mothers with LLL-published information by displaying LLLI books and other printed materials at meetings. For many Groups, books sales, memberships fees, and the annual World Walk for Breastfeeding fundraiser provide enough money to pay Group expenses. Each mother who attends the Group deserves the opportunity to buy a membership and a copy of THE WOMANLY ART OF BREASTFEEDING. Other books published by LLLI can also be important sources of information; do not hesitate to recommend them. Items sold at Series Meetings should fulfill the goal of helping a mother have a satisfying breastfeeding experience.

If the Group sells breastfeeding-aid products, you can mention this at meetings, especially if a mother wants to discuss a situation in which one of these products would be useful. However, sales of these products should be handled on an individual basis, in order to avoid giving the impression that all breastfeeding mothers need them. Consult with your support Leader about any non-LLL products, such as baby carriers or slings, that the Group would like to sell at meetings. She can help you consider and evaluate any disadvantages. Displaying them separately from LLL books and products can

Notices on bulletin boards and posters can help illustrate LLL ideas and information.

Items sold at Series Meetings should fulfill the goal of helping a mother have a satisfying breastfeeding experience.

reinforce that our primary purpose is to provide information and support. To protect LLLI, baby carriers purchased for resale must carry product liability insurance.

You may want to announce fundraising activities at Series Meetings. To keep the time and focus on helping mothers, however, schedule and plan these activities outside of the meeting or after the formal part of the Series Meeting. (See also **Fundraising Coordinator**, page 92, and **Fundraising Activities**, page 108.)

PLANNING MEETINGS

How
Arranging the seating

Seating in a circle or semicircle helps to promote free-flowing discussion. Double-check the view from all seats before the meeting. A participant may have a more difficult time relating to the meeting if her seat is in a place that causes her to feel excluded. Also, when participants can see each other, it is easier to keep everyone's attention during the discussion.

Pick a seat where you can make eye contact with all participants. Many Leaders find that it is easier to lead a meeting from a hard chair that offers good support, rather than from a soft chair or sofa. Co-Leaders can be most effective interspersed among the other participants. Suggest to Group members that they sit interspersed with newcomers, rather than all together.

When participants can see each other, it is easier to keep everyone's attention during the discussion.

Meeting countdown

Although you are responsible for meetings, Group workers or members can help with many of these tasks.

Although you are responsible for meetings, Group workers or members can help with many of these tasks.

A week before the meeting

- Notify people—individually and with public notices—of the meeting.
- Remind those with overdue Library books to return them.
- Confirm who will bring refreshments.
- Plan the room layout with the hostess.

Day of the meeting

- Prepare the home or meeting place for guests. Are extra chairs needed? Is the floor clean and free of clutter? Is the meeting area baby-proofed?
- Make sure the meeting place can be easily located, especially if the meeting is held after dark.
- Check supply of nametags and welcome packets.

A half-hour before the meeting

- Check the seating arrangements. Plan for an arrangement that promotes free-flowing discussion.
- Set up the Group Library and books and items for sale. Prepare the area for refreshments.
- Put an "LLL" sign on or near the door.

Some Leaders follow a checklist as they prepare for each meeting; others delegate certain tasks to Group workers, who might create their own checklists.

Sample Countdown Checklist

- Chairs arranged in a circle or semicircle
- Group Library set up
- Sale items displayed
- Membership information available
- Refreshments ready
- Handouts available
- Attendance sheet ready with pen
- LLL sign, banner, flag, or windsock posted
- Area designated for coats, baby wraps
- Nametags ready
- Welcome packets ready
- Signs showing the way to the toilet and "No Smoking" sign posted
- Quiet toys available

Following Up the Meeting

- Many Leaders complete the meeting report at an Evaluation Meeting and send it to their support Leader immediately thereafter. Some Leaders prefer to do it right after the meeting.
- Process memberships immediately so that new members will receive the member publication as soon as possible.
- Some Leaders send a congratulations card to new parents as soon as they learn of the birth of a baby. This can be followed up with a telephone call a few days later.
- Some Leaders write personal notes to each new attendee, explaining the function of the Group and welcoming her to it.
- Some Groups send a follow-up letter to all newcomers.

Dear [insert the mother's name],

We're glad you attended our recent La Leche League Series Meeting! All interested women are invited to our meetings. Feel free to bring a friend or relative with you. Remember that we also welcome your breastfeeding baby or toddler at meetings.

Refreshments are available during the meeting. We appreciate donations of simple, nutritious snacks; let us know if you would like to help us in this way.

La Leche League provides mother-to-mother support. We appreciate your participation during the discussion; it is vital to the meeting. The Leader is a trained volunteer and experienced breastfeeding mother. She is prepared to offer practical breastfeeding information during meetings and between meetings as well. Just call [Leader's name and contact information].

THE WOMANLY ART OF BREASTFEEDING is available for loan or purchase at meetings. It is a valuable resource for breastfeeding mothers, with a wealth of breastfeeding and mothering information. Our meetings are based on its content.

We hope La Leche League has been and will continue to be of help to you. You help La Leche League by attending meetings. Without you, there would be no Group. You also help by paying dues to become a La Leche League member. Membership holds many benefits for you as well as La Leche League. A membership form is included with this letter.

We hope to see you at our next meeting. It will be on _____ at _____.

Sincerely,

_____ (Leader's name, signature, phone number)

CHAPTER THREE

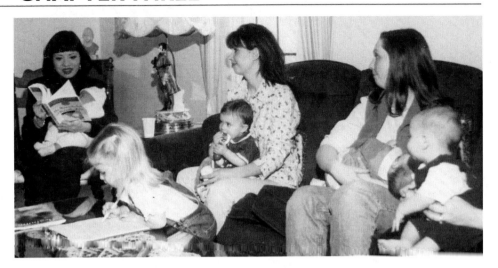

Series Meeting Guides

MEETING PLANS

The Series Meeting Guides offer a basic approach to meetings that promotes open, interactive discussions. THE WOMANLY ART OF BREASTFEEDING includes LLL's common core of knowledge from which Leaders support, inform, and encourage breastfeeding families at meetings. The Meeting Guides provide a sense of uniformity while inviting personalization and variety, just as with meeting ideas passed from Leader to Leader.

The standard series of four meetings progresses chronologically:
- The decision to breastfeed—Meeting 1: Advantages of Breastfeeding
- Birth and the first few weeks of baby's life—Meeting 2: The Family and the Breastfed Baby
- The normal course of breastfeeding—Meeting 3: The Art of Breastfeeding and Avoiding Difficulties
- Introducing solids and the weaning process—Meeting 4: Nutrition and Weaning

The Series Meeting titles repeat, series after series, yet each meeting is unique due to the ever-changing mix of participants, growth of the children, and families' ever-changing needs. Although the general topic is predetermined, you can choose a more specific focus based on the anticipated participants and their needs.

APPROACHES

Some Leaders plan meetings on a monthly basis, allowing for the most flexibility if changes in the schedule arise. Planning monthly gives you the opportunity to continue addressing the interests and needs of the mothers from one meeting into the next, or to try something new.

Another way to plan meetings is a theme approach. A theme gives a series continuity from meeting to meeting. Within the context of the theme, each meeting can be adapted to meet the needs of the participants.

For example, if "Expectations" is the theme, meetings might have the following titles and discussion questions:

Meeting 1—Great Expectations: Breastfeeding Benefits Everyone

What benefits are you expecting from breastfeeding? If you are an experienced breastfeeding mother, what benefits have you noticed that you didn't expect? How does breastfeeding help you fulfill the expectations you have for yourself or that others have of you?

Meeting 2—Realistic Expectations: A New Baby in Your Family

What does your family expect of the new baby? …of you? What do you expect from your partner when your baby arrives? …from your other children? …from yourself? What can make these expectations realistic?

Meeting 3—What to Expect: Knowing What's Normal and Avoiding Problems

What avenues did you/are you using to learn about breastfeeding? Are there people in your life who are teaching you about breastfeeding? What difficulties did you anticipate you might have with breastfeeding? (What difficulties do you anticipate you might have with breastfeeding?) If you have breastfed a baby, what did you do to avoid difficulties?

Meeting 4—Guess Who's Coming to Dinner? Beginning Solid Foods

What emotional and physical needs does a meal provide to you? What do you do to help accomplish that? During pregnancy, how long do/did you expect to breastfeed? If you have breastfed or are breastfeeding a baby, compare your original expectations with your expectations now. How have they changed?

Some Leaders plan meetings a year at a time to reflect meeting variety and promote LLL as a continuing source of new information. The twelve meeting titles each offer a different focus based on the meeting number in the series. By advertising a yearly plan, you no longer have to explain that every meeting is different. Some Groups find this has a financial advantage, since the meeting notice can be developed and bulk mailed once a year.

Both the theme approach and yearly plan can limit flexibility in choosing topics based on the needs of the people attending a particular meeting. The more specific the meeting title, the less flexibility you will have, since the focus needs to reflect

> The Series Meeting titles repeat, series after series, yet each meeting is unique due to the participants' everchanging needs.

the title. A flexible meeting plan allows for spontaneity and offers the freedom to meet the needs of the participants.

Even though the meeting title suggests a focus or topics for that meeting, no mother should have to wait for a specific meeting to answer her question. Perhaps her question can fit into the meeting topic. If not, you can alter the focus or suggest talking together at refreshment time. Some Groups set aside the first few minutes of each meeting to respond to specific questions, especially if they are not directly related to the meeting topic. You might say something like this during introductory remarks:

> *"Please don't go away with your question unanswered, even if it doesn't pertain to the subject of this meeting."*

A flexible meeting plan allows for spontaneity and offers the freedom to meet the needs of the participants.

SERIES MEETING GUIDES

Using the Meeting Guides

Each Meeting Guide includes two sample prepared meetings and several possible focuses for less structured meetings. Each offers discussion plans and possible questions to carry the discussion along. The Meeting Guides are ready to use and can be adapted as the meeting progresses. Feel free to use the prepared meetings as they are, adapt them, or compose your own ideas from other Leader resources. By frequently enriching your Meeting Guides and staying up-to-date on the latest information and meeting format ideas, you can add spark to meetings. This benefits the participants and helps keep your own enthusiasm high.

Add spark to your meetings by frequently enriching your Meeting Guides and staying up-to-date on the latest information and meeting ideas.

(Also see **Planning and Leading Optional Meetings,** pages 172–190.)

References and Resources

THE WOMANLY ART OF BREASTFEEDING is a Leader's primary source for breastfeeding information and LLL philosophy. Within each of the Meeting Guides, specific chapters of THE WOMANLY ART OF BREASTFEEDING (WAB) are referenced. These chapters offer detailed information that will support and enrich the meetings.

In addition to THE WOMANLY ART, many other resources will help you in planning a meeting. An article in a member publication may be used as the basis for a meeting. Leader publications often offer meeting ideas. LLL-published books and pamphlets can spark meeting ideas and provide supporting information. LLLI's Web site, **www.lalecheleague.org,** is also a wealth of expanding information and support for families and Leaders, and includes a collection of meeting ideas.

Within each meeting guide is a section called, "Additional Resources," which lists LLLI-published books and pamphlets that offer information pertaining to that focus. Titles in uppercase letters signify books that are published by LLLI. Titles in italics signify pamphlets or tear-off sheets that are published by LLLI. A few books not published by LLLI are listed as suggested resources for specific meeting focuses. The titles of these books are in italics and the authors are named.

The resources that are listed can be made available during the meeting. These resources need to be updated as new information is published by LLLI or becomes available in your language. You might also want to display relevant titles from the Group Library as a way of further engaging the participants in the Group.

MEETING 1: ADVANTAGES OF BREAST-FEEDING

References from
THE WOMANLY ART
Chapter 1—Why Choose Breastfeeding?
Chapter 18—The Superior Infant Food
Chapter 19—How Breastfeeding Affects a Mother

Additional resources:
Breastfeeding Makes a Difference, 1196–17
Breastfeeding Makes a Difference, 568–27
Breastfeeding: Baby's First Immunization, 565–27
Facts About Breastfeeding (Annual)

Prepared meeting

Alternate Titles: The Benefits of Human Milk, Why Breastfeed Your Baby?

Introductory questions

- What's one advantage of breastfeeding that attracts you?
- What particular advantage influenced your decision to breastfeed?
- If a friend or relative told you she was pregnant, what would you tell her about breast-feeding?
- What is one advantage that has been particularly helpful with this/that child?
- Was there an advantage of breastfeeding that surprised you?

Discussion

Ask discussion participants to expand on the physical and emotional advantages for baby and the physical and emotional advantages for mothers. You might list advantages on a big pad of paper as the mothers talk. You might pass out photographs from magazines or household items that would inspire participants to think of advantages. You could also highlight passages in THE WOMANLY ART OF BREASTFEEDING, mark the pages with tabs, and pass the book around for participants to read from. Below are advantages that can serve as examples if the participants get stuck.

Best for baby

Physical—Colostrum: immunities; defense against infection; laxative effect to pass meconium, stimulating hunger and milk supply; decreases absorption of bilirubin; high in protein. Mature milk: only food needed for the first six months; supplies all necessary nutrients in proper proportion; digests easily. Promotes good health and optimal development: antibodies from mother; protects against infections; hydrates baby during illness and speeds recovery; reduces risk of allergies; reduces risk of obesity later in life; reduces incidence of Sudden Infant Death Syndrome; higher IQs; develops hand-eye coordination; promotes proper jaw, tooth, and speech development.

Emotional—Satisfies hunger immediately. Mother and baby togetherness: builds strong ties of love; ensures lots of close physical contact; suckling at the breast is comforting to baby when fussy, overtired, ill, or hurt.

Best for mother

Physical—Continues natural reproductive cycle of conception, pregnancy and childbirth. Hormones stimulated by suckling contract the uterus, reducing the risk of hemorrhaging. Aids in natural weight loss. Night feedings are easier, less disruptive. Prolactin relaxes, making mothering easier. Reduces risks of breast and uterine cancers. Saves time and money. Trips away from home are easier, no worry about baby's food. Delays return of fertility.

Emotional—Mother feels physically relieved of milk; hormones make her calmer and more relaxed, adding to mother's enjoyment of baby; being able to physically satisfy and comfort baby increases mother's self-confidence; greater closeness increases mother's perception of her baby's needs.

Follow-up questions

- How does breastfeeding help you put people before things?
- How does breastfeeding help meet the challenge of caring for a new baby?
- What would a mother miss if she decided not to breastfeed her baby?
- What are some advantages of breastfeeding to siblings?
- What advantages of breastfeeding are important to you today that perhaps would have been less important a generation ago?

Prepared meeting–Alternative Plan

Alternate Titles: The ABCs of Breastfeeding, Advantages of Breastfeeding from A to Z

Introductory questions

- When was the first time you saw someone breastfeeding?
- Can you name an advantage that begins with the first letter of your child's name?
- How is breastfeeding helping you love and enjoy your baby?
- How has the experience of breastfeeding changed you?
- What were/are your expectations about breastfeeding?

Introduction

Ask each participant to write on a piece of paper an advantage that is important to her. Collect these pieces of paper and save them for later in the meeting.

Discussion

Create a list of breastfeeding advantages by using the letters in the alphabet. You will need a flip chart, poster, or large piece of paper to write on so that everyone can keep track of the advantages. While going through the alphabet, add the written advantages offered by the participants. To make the game a little more challenging, ask the mothers to come up with an additional advantage for each letter. Here are some examples:

A—Always available, avoiding allergies
B—Bonding
C—Colostrum, comfort
D—Delicious!
E—Ear infections reduced, eye-hand coordination
F—Frugal, fresh, fewer health problems
G—Growth
H—Healthy, happy baby
I—Immunities, intelligence, illnesses fewer, immediate
J—Jaundice risk lower
K—"Kangaroo care" for premature babies
L—Laxative, less constipation
M—Money saved
N—Nighttime parenting easier
O—"Outage" of power but baby can still have a warm meal
P—Periods delayed, peace of mind
Q—Quick
R—Rest
S—Simple, safe, sterile
T—Travels well, temperature always right
U—Use of breastfeeding reduces risk of some cancers
V—Viruses result in "custom made" milk
W—Warm fuzzies
X—"Xactly" what the baby needs, when he needs it
Y—Yummy smell of breastfed infants
Z—Zero chance of forgetting baby food

Follow-up questions

- How does breastfeeding affect the way you parent?
- Why did you decide to breastfeed, and what helps you to continue?
- How do LLL meetings support you in your breastfeeding relationship?
- Can you describe a situation when you were especially glad to be breastfeeding?
- What would your baby say is the most important advantage?

MEETING I: ADVANTAGES OF BREAST-FEEDING

SERIES MEETING GUIDES

References from
THE WOMANLY ART
Chapter 1—Why Choose Breastfeeding?
Chapter 18—The Superior Infant Food
Chapter 19—How Breastfeeding
Affects a Mother

Additional resources:
Breastfeeding Makes a Difference, 1196–17
Breastfeeding Makes a Difference, 568–27
Breastfeeding: Baby's
First Immunization, 565–27
Facts about Breastfeeding (Annual)

MEETING 1: ADVANTAGES OF BREAST-FEEDING

Additional resources:
MOTHERWISE: 101 TIPS FOR A NEW MOTHER, 148-12
THE FUSSY BABY, 1169-12

When Babies Cry, 310-17

Possible Title/Focus
How Breastfeeding Affects Mothering
Questions
- How has breastfeeding enhanced the way you parent?
- How do you feel when you breastfeed?
- When did breastfeeding become natural for you?
- What doubts or worries did/do you have about breastfeeding?
- What do you hope to gain from breastfeeding?

Discussion: In this meeting, you might discuss the benefits of prolactin, bonding, tuning into baby's needs, and building confidence in mothering.

Possible Title/Focus
Coping with Others' Attitudes about Breastfeeding
Questions
- Whose attitude about breastfeeding affects you the most?
- What was the best advice about breastfeeding you received from a friend or relative?
- How does breastfeeding help you meet your baby's nighttime needs?
- How have you dealt with something that our society sees as a disadvantage of breast-feeding?
- Give an example of positive or negative coverage of breastfeeding in the media.

Discussion: In this meeting, you might discuss society's misconceptions about breastfeeding, how a mother can breastfeed discreetly, and how the attitudes of family, friends, and health care providers can have an effect on the breastfeeding relationship. It is important to accentuate the positive and find opportunities to build the mother's self-confidence.

Possible Title/Focus
Breastfeeding Facts
Questions
- Why do you think it's important to be aware of the advantages of breastfeeding?
- Were physical or emotional advantages a greater factor in your decision to breastfeed?
- What advantage of breastfeeding did you find that was unexpected?
- Has breastfeeding altered the way you look at the world?
- How does breastfeeding help you to understand your baby's needs?

Discussion: Ask each participant to select a *Facts about Breastfeeding* sheet from assorted years. Ask each participant to share one or two items on the fact sheet. While each participant talks, you can record a phrase summarizing that advantage on a poster board. A different approach is to make small posters using photos that highlight an advantage. On the back, you could paste facts from *Facts about Breastfeeding* sheets that pertain to that advantage. Pass the posters around and ask participants to read the facts.

Prepared meeting

Alternate Title: Preparing for Birth and Breastfeeding

Introductory questions

- What have you done/did you do during pregnancy to make the early weeks after birth easier?
- What have you done/did you do during pregnancy to prepare for breastfeeding?
- What does a mother need to think about before the baby comes?
- What was the best suggestion someone gave you for the early weeks?
- What have you done/would you do differently in subsequent pregnancies in planning for your birth and breastfeeding?

Discussion

For the following three areas of preparation for a new baby, pass out cards, each with a point on it for participants to read and discuss. Or write the three main points on a board and ask mothers to fill in the list and discuss.

- Research: information about breastfeeding, birth plan, finding a support network, figuring out how to...
- Equipment: clothing, furniture, and accessories; is a pump necessary?
- Technique: latch-on and positioning, normal newborn behavior, care of mother and baby, avoiding and overcoming problems.

Follow-up Questions

- Describe your favorite clothing for ease of breastfeeding.
- What do you consider essential for your favorite breastfeeding spot?
- Who gave you support when you were breastfeeding for the very first time? What did they say or do to help you feel good about breastfeeding?
- What special needs do you/did you and your baby have at first?
- How is life different after the baby is born?

SERIES MEETING GUIDES

MEETING 2:
THE BABY ARRIVES: THE FAMILY AND THE BREASTFED BABY

**References from
THE WOMANLY ART:**
Chapter 2—Plans Are Underway
Chapter 4—Your Baby Arrives
Chapter 5—At Home with Your Baby
Chapter 6—A Time to Learn
Chapter 10—The Manly Art of Fathering
Chapter 11—Meeting Family Needs

Additional resources:
BREASTFEEDING PURE AND SIMPLE, 803–12
GROWING TOGETHER: A PARENT'S
GUIDE TO BABY'S FIRST YEAR, 158–12

Preparing to Breastfeed, 563–27

MEETING 2: THE BABY ARRIVES: THE FAMILY AND THE BREASTFED BABY

References from
THE WOMANLY ART:
Chapter 2—Plans Are Underway
Chapter 4—Your Baby Arrives
Chapter 5—At Home with Your Baby
Chapter 6—A Time to Learn
Chapter 10—The Manly Art of Fathering
Chapter 11—Meeting Family Needs

Additional resources:
BREASTFEEDING PURE AND SIMPLE, 803–12
GROWING TOGETHER: A PARENT'S GUIDE
TO BABY'S FIRST YEAR, 158–12
MOTHERWISE: 101 TIPS FOR A
NEW MOTHER, 148–12

Preparing to Breastfeed, 563–27
When You Breastfeed Your Baby, 306–17
When Babies Cry, 310–17

Prepared meeting

Alternate Title: There's a New Baby in Your Life

Introductory questions

- Who were the people in your life who provided the emotional support you needed in the first months?
- What advance plans have you made to make life easier at home once your baby is born?
- Tell about one change having a baby has made in your life.
- People often talk about a "good" baby. How would you describe a good baby?
- What item(s) have you gotten/did you get while pregnant that will help with breast-feeding?

Discussion

"There's a new baby in your life, how do you…" This discussion can generate many tips that are useful for pregnant mothers who are wondering what life is like with a new baby and for mothers with young children who need fresh ideas. On the front of small cards write: "How do you…" and on the other side of each card write one of the following activities. Pass the cards out and ask the mothers to share their answers.

- take a shower?
- cook dinner?
- go grocery shopping?
- eat?
- drive?
- go shopping for clothes?
- use a public restroom?
- sleep?
- take care of older children?
- clean your house?
- get your hair done?
- have time alone with your partner?
- get exercise?
- breastfeed in public?
- relax?

Follow-up questions

- What other activities were challenges for you with a new baby? What did you do?
- What special needs did you and your baby have at first?
- How can we handle the feeling of being overwhelmed by baby's needs?
- What special interests or hobbies did you have before the baby arrived? What did you do about these (hobbies/interests) in the first few months after your baby arrived?
- How can we keep ourselves focused on those things we really value?

Possible Title/Focus
Getting Breastfeeding Off to a Good Start

Discussion
Often this discussion brings up local hospital policies and how they affect the early days of breastfeeding. You can let mothers know that they have the right to ask for optimal conditions. However, it is equally important that they understand that an ideal situation is not a prerequisite to breastfeeding. You can encourage mothers to communicate with the hospital staff about policies. You can also call on mothers whom you know have had a wide range of birth experiences and ask how they have worked to have successful breastfeeding relationships.

Questions
- What have you done or are you doing to help breastfeeding get off to a good start?
- What early breastfeeding experience did you have that you did not expect?
- What made/makes you anxious about breastfeeding in the early days? What do you know now that would have made those days easier?
- What have you and those around you done to make the early days of breastfeeding go more smoothly?

Possible Title/Focus
Adjustment of Older Children

Discussion
The birth of a baby affects all family members. Discuss preparations and attitudes before and after a baby's birth that can help make the adjustment easier for siblings. Acknowledge that jealousy and regression are normal and that children need to find acceptable outlets for the expression of their feelings.

Questions
- What have you done/can you do before the birth to prepare a sibling for the baby's arrival?
- How can you help the older child to still feel loved and needed?
- Who in your family had a difficult time adjusting to the baby's arrival? How did you help?
- What are some ways to handle bringing home a new baby to siblings?
- How can you help every child within the family to feel special and yet understand that the baby's needs come first?

SERIES MEETING GUIDES

MEETING 2: THE BABY ARRIVES: THE FAMILY AND THE BREASTFED BABY

References from
THE WOMANLY ART:
Chapter 2—Plans Are Underway
Chapter 4—Your Baby Arrives
Chapter 5—At Home with Your Baby
Chapter 6—A Time to Learn
Chapter 10—The Manly Art of Fathering
Chapter 11—Meeting Family Needs

Additional resources:
BREASTFEEDING PURE AND SIMPLE, 803–12
GROWING TOGETHER: A PARENT'S GUIDE
TO BABY'S FIRST YEAR, 158–12

Preparing to Breastfeed, 563–27
When You Breastfeed Your Baby, 306–17
Is Baby Getting Enough? 566–27
Establishing Your Milk Supply, 527–27
Breastfeeding Tips, 1168–27

MEETING 2: THE BABY ARRIVES: THE FAMILY AND THE BREASTFED BABY

References from
THE WOMANLY ART:
Chapter 8—Breastfeeding and Working
Chapter 9—Making a Choice

Additional resources:
Nursing Mother, Working Mother
by Gale Pryor, 4–7

A Mother's Guide to Pumping Milk, 991–17
Balancing Act, 1164–17
Working and Breastfeeding, 1220–27
Storing Human Milk, 555–27
Breastfeeding Tips, 1168–27
(See also **Employed Breastfeeding Mothers Meeting,** pages 184–188.)

Possible Title/Focus
Working and Breastfeeding

Discussion
Women who plan to return to work outside the home after their babies are born are often concerned about what they can do before birth and in the early weeks to make working and breastfeeding go more smoothly. Some meetings will have primarily stay-at-home mothers. Other meetings will have primarily working mothers. Other meetings will have a mix. With all, it is helpful to focus on what all mothers—those who do and don't work outside the home—have in common. Almost all mothers have scheduling challenges, and many mothers have used pumps occasionally or for special circumstances. If the experienced breastfeeding mothers in the Group have not faced the challenges of breastfeeding and working outside the home, stories from member publications can be helpful in adding to the discussion.

Questions
- What adjustments have you made at work to help with breastfeeding and pumping?
- What would your ideal work situation look like?
- What pumps or other products have been helpful to you?
- If a mother has read a book about working from the Group Library, would she be willing to comment on or give a review of the book?
- What changes have you experienced in your working and breastfeeding career?

References from
THE WOMANLY ART:
Chapter 2—Plans are Underway
Chapter 4—Your Baby Arrives

Additional Resources:
Breastfeeding after a Cesarean Birth, 327–17
The Birth Book by William and Martha Sears, 46-7

Possible Title/Focus
How Childbirth Options Can Affect Breastfeeding

Discussion
Because a home birth allows a mother to bypass the schedules and restrictions of hospitals, many mothers are enthusiastic about this option. Check with your support Leader or a Professional Liaison Leader about legal restrictions and provisions regarding home birth in your community, state, province, country, or region.

A new mother can experience a range of emotions, from elation at having a new baby to discouragement that the birth experience wasn't what she expected. Encourage diversity of reasons for choosing various birth options. Invite mothers in attendance who have had multiple birth experiences to speak about their positive experiences.

Questions
- What are some decisions you have made about your birth that you think will have a positive effect on the early days of breastfeeding?
- What are some things about your baby's birth and breastfeeding that you have talked over with your health care provider?
- What childbirth options have you found that allow for minimum separation between you and your baby?
- Which childbirth choices would you make differently next time?
- How can you/did you include your family in the birth experience?

Prepared meeting

Alternate Titles: Avoiding Common Difficulties: Using LLL Information

Introductory questions

- Is breastfeeding easier or harder than you expected?
- What is a question about breastfeeding to which you have never received a satisfactory answer?
- What is one remark you remember hearing that helped keep you breastfeeding when you were still learning and unsure? (Record these answers and reread them at the end of the meeting for a positive conclusion!)
- Tell us one of the ways you are learning to breastfeed.
- Where do you get your determination to breastfeed?

Discussion

Gather several LLL-published information sheets that address common difficulties and put them in a basket from which participants can take one. Tear-off sheets might be folded in thirds with the title showing. Invite participants to choose a sheet and take a moment to read (or "skim") it. Ask them to give mini-reports, pointing out what LLL suggests about handling or avoiding that difficulty. Then encourage the participants to share their personal experience. At a meeting with all repeat mothers, ask them to pick books they have read from the Group Library that address common difficulties and discuss them.

Common difficulties or concerns could include:

- Sore nipples
- How to know if baby is latched on well
- How to know if baby is getting enough milk
- How to know if baby is getting too much milk
- Plugged ducts/breast infections (mastitis)
- Jaundice
- Fussy baby
- Baby biting
- Nursing strike (not natural weaning)
- Mother or baby ill
- Worries about what is normal

Follow-up questions

- Why continue to breastfeed if you experience difficulties?
- Did you have any preconceived ideas that caused you to have problems with breastfeeding? What did you do to change?
- What was a problem you expected while you were pregnant that was not a problem when you were breastfeeding?
- What support do you need most during breastfeeding? If you are pregnant, what support do you need most in making your decision and preparations to breastfeed?
- What resources do you find the most practical to turn to when you have questions about breastfeeding?

SERIES MEETING GUIDES

MEETING 3:

THE ART OF BREASTFEEDING AND AVOIDING DIFFICULTIES

References from
THE WOMANLY ART:
Chapter 3—Your Network of Support
Chapter 4—Your Baby Arrives
Chapter 5—At Home with Your Baby
Chapter 6—A Time to Learn
Chapter 7—Common Concerns
Chapter 20—About La Leche League

Additional resources:
LLL pamphlets and tear-off sheets cover a variety of topics that relate to this meeting.

MEETING 3: THE ART OF BREASTFEEDING AND AVOIDING DIFFICULTIES

References from
THE WOMANLY ART:
Chapter 3—Your Network of Support
Chapter 4—Your Baby Arrives
Chapter 5—At Home with Your Baby
Chapter 6—A Time to Learn
Chapter 7—Common Concerns
Chapter 20—About La Leche League

Additional resources:
GROWING TOGETHER: A PARENT'S GUIDE TO BABY'S FIRST YEAR, 158–12
THE FUSSY BABY, 1169-12

Breastfeeding Tips, 1168–27
When You Breastfeed Your Baby, 306–17

Prepared meeting

Alternate Titles: The Normal Course of Breastfeeding, Questions Mothers Ask, Is It Normal or Does It Need Attention?

Introductory questions
- What was your question or concern when you first contacted LLL? If this is your first contact with LLL, what brought you here today?
- What is something you've heard about breastfeeding that you are not sure about?
- What cues does your baby (or your body) give you when it's time to breastfeed?
- What suggestion would you give a friend who was planning to breastfeed?
- Tell us one thing your baby does that he was not doing last month. How has this affected breastfeeding or your relationship?

Discussion

Offer the following statements to participants, asking if each seems normal or needs attention. The statements can be printed on individual cards or written on a board so everyone can see. Some situations may be normal at one stage of breastfeeding but need attention when they arise at another stage. Remind participants that situations that need attention are not necessarily abnormal. Encourage mothers to trust their instincts based on knowledge of their babies, to ask questions, and to seek out answers that will work for their families. Remind mothers that they may also want to contact their health care providers if they have concerns or worries about their baby's health.

Discuss some of the statements below in depth. Choose situations that will be relevant for the mothers at your meeting.

- My baby is eight months old and still shows no interest in eating solids.
- My breasts are uncomfortably swollen. They feel heavy, hard, warm, and sensitive, as if they are ready to burst!
- My baby breaks out in a rash every time I eat peanuts.
- My baby is two weeks old and exclusively breastfed. He had two wet diapers today, and he hasn't had a bowel movement in three days.
- My baby cries uncontrollably for hours every night.
- I never feel the let-down sensation, and my breasts don't leak.
- My baby keeps biting when we nurse.
- I have no interest in being intimate with my partner. Whenever we are intimate, it's really uncomfortable for me.
- My newborn sleeps all the time. He won't wake up to nurse.
- My baby makes noise when he breastfeeds.
- My baby won't take a bottle.
- Yesterday my breasts were big and full. Today they are soft.
- My baby is six months old, and I still haven't had my period.
- My toddler is breastfeeding like a newborn!
- Breastfeeding was going along just fine, but in the past few days my breasts are extremely sore when my child nurses. (pregnancy, menses, yeast)
- I think I have the flu. My breast is sore and red and I ache all over.
- My six-week-old baby is nursing all the time. It seems like as soon as one feeding is over, it's time for another one. He nurses for 30 minutes at a time!

Add to or revise these concerns to meet the Group's needs.

MEETING 3:
THE ART OF
BREASTFEEDING
AND AVOIDING
DIFFICULTIES

SERIES MEETING GUIDES

The Normal Course of Breastfeeding

Issues that are part of the normal course of breastfeeding can include (though not necessarily in this order):

- Engorgement
- Establishing supply
- Adjusting to the nursing relationship (establishing ease and pattern)
- Growth spurts
- Teething
- Starting solids
- Mother's menses return
- Common problems, e.g., mastitis, sore nipples, nipple confusion, thrush
- Next pregnancy
- Extended breastfeeding
- Weaning

Follow-up Questions

- What did you think life would be like with your baby, and what is it really like?
- How can you learn to trust your instincts and discover that you know your child best, when breastfeeding seems like such a scientific process?
- Why is it important to listen to your instincts when it comes to breastfeeding?
- What has your child taught you about breastfeeding? Have subsequent babies taught different lessons or created different answers?
- How can the range of "normal" be different for mothers?

MEETING 3:
THE ART OF BREASTFEEDING AND AVOIDING DIFFICULTIES

Additional resources:
Common Breastfeeding Myths, 226-17

Possible Title/Focus

Breastfeeding Myths and Facts

Introductory questions:

- Where have you heard breastfeeding myths?
- What other myths about breastfeeding have you heard?
- What conflicting advice have you received about caring for your baby?
- What is a funny piece of advice about babies that you got from a family member?
- How do you handle comments that show disapproval for your way of caring for your baby?

Discussion

On one side of small cards print one myth of breastfeeding. On the other side of each card, write its corresponding fact. Myths and corresponding facts can also be printed on separate cards to be played as a matching game. Some Leaders prefer to let the mothers verbalize the truths. Pass these out to the participants to read and discuss. Some examples could be:

Myth—"Never wake a sleeping baby."

Fact—"A hungry baby may be too weak to indicate his need for food."

Myth—"If the baby isn't gaining well, you may have low quality milk."

Fact—"Studies have shown that even malnourished women are able to produce milk of sufficient quality and quantity to support a growing infant."

Additional resources:
LEARNING A LOVING WAY OF LIFE, 159-12
GROWING TOGETHER, 158-12
MOTHERWISE, 148-12
FATHERWISE, 933-12

Possible Title/Focus

Becoming a Mother: Adjusting to Parenthood

Questions

- How is motherhood different from what you thought it would be?
- What is the biggest adjustment you needed to make before the baby arrived? How about after the baby arrived?
- How has becoming a parent affected your attitude and lifestyle? What changes do you anticipate?
- Name one positive way you or your lifestyle has changed since you've had your baby.
- How can breastfeeding make the adjustments easier? Or, how has breastfeeding affected your parenting?

Discussion

Many new parents find that their day-to-day pattern of living is altered. They often restructure their priorities to accommodate the baby, for instance by simplifying housekeeping and meals, and modifying usual activities. Changes can be hard to make and harder yet to accept. One of your challenges is to guide a discussion that looks at these changes positively and yet acknowledges common feelings. At a La Leche League Series Meeting participants can see happy mothers and babies bringing joy to each other and talking about the positive side of mothering, childcare, and family life.

MEETING 3:
THE ART OF BREASTFEEDING AND AVOIDING DIFFICULTIES

SERIES MEETING GUIDES

Additional resources:
NIGHTTIME PARENTING, 160-12
THE CUDDLERS, 155-12

Possible Title/Focus
Nighttime Parenting

Discussion

Discuss attitudes and expectations as well as ways to satisfy baby's nighttime needs that are least disruptive of sleep. Respect each family's individuality and acknowledge that each family must find nighttime solutions that are most comfortable for them. What works well in one family may not be appropriate for another.

A mother who is waking up frequently with her baby is very vulnerable. She is tired and frustrated, maybe even frantic. She may need an opportunity to talk things out after the meeting, one-to-one with a Leader.

Questions

- How do you make night breastfeeding easier?
- Other than getting enough sleep, what worries do you have about meeting your child's nighttime needs?
- How have you found ways to meet your need for sleep, your baby's need to be close to you, and your baby's physical needs?
- What has worked and what hasn't for your family? How has that changed with time?
- What are some reasons your baby wakes at night?

Possible Title/Focus
THE WOMANLY ART OF BREASTFEEDING

Discussion

Display copies of THE WOMANLY ART OF BREASTFEEDING from the Group Library and book sales area for this meeting, to promote LLL as a resource. This meeting can enlighten participants about LLL information and philosophy, sell memberships and THE WOMANLY ART OF BREASTFEEDING, and promote volunteerism and an interest in leadership.

Questions:

- How is breastfeeding your baby an "art"?
- If you have been to other LLL Series Meetings, what are they like?
- Why go to LLL meetings if you don't have a question? Or, what continues to draw you to meetings?
- Tell us about something you've heard or seen at Series Meetings or read in THE WOMANLY ART OF BREASTFEEDING that was a surprise to you.
- What would you say to a friend or relative about LLL?

MEETING 4: NUTRITION AND WEANING

References from THE WOMANLY ART:

Chapter 12—Nutritional Know-How
Chapter 13—Ready for Solids
Chapter 14—Weaning Gradually, with Love
Chapter 15—Discipline Is Loving Guidance

Additional resources:

WHOLE FOODS FOR THE WHOLE FAMILY, 151–12
WHOLE FOODS FROM THE WHOLE WORLD, 152–12
WHOLE FOODS FOR BABIES AND TODDLERS, 1002–12

Nutrition and Breastfeeding, 309–17

Prepared meeting

Alternate Titles: Improving Family Nutrition

Introductory questions:

- Is there something in your diet that you feel especially good about that you would like to share?
- In your family, what problems have you had to overcome in your efforts to improve everyone's diet?
- What are some ways you have cut food costs without sacrificing quality?
- How does your diet compare to the way you ate when you were a child?
- Did you improve your eating habits during pregnancy? How?

Discussion: Bring to the meeting two paper grocery sacks marked "Not So Great" and "Getting Better." Before the meeting, fill the bags with items from your kitchen. At the meeting, pull out items from each bag as visual aids for carrying the discussion.

Learning about nutrition can be both challenging and fun. The goal is to offer a stimulating discussion on good nutrition, while leaving each mother free to choose whether or not she wants or needs to change her family's pattern of eating.

While taking out items from the "Not So Great" bag, discuss these points with the participants:

- An LLL Leader is not a nutritionist, nor is she on the perfect diet. When you show that these items came from your home, you show that you are also trying to improve and maintain healthy eating habits.
- Remind mothers to think of their eating habits over a long time, such as months and weeks, rather than focusing on what they ate that day.
- Avoid being extreme in your choices and telling scare stories about food choices. Referring to foods as garbage or junk might offend mothers who include them in their regular diets.

While pulling from the bag marked "Getting Better," discuss these points:

- Make it clear that "Not So Great" and "Getting Better" are not a comparison of good and bad; neither category is an extreme.
- Point out that LLLI does not have an official position on vegetarianism, boycotting artificial substances in food, eating organic food, or other special diets.
- Avoid reading labels or discussing technical terms and complex food charts.
- Prompt mothers to share tips on healthier eating during the various stages of pregnancy and breastfeeding. This might include the nauseated weeks of pregnancy, quick meals, feeding toddlers, eating on a budget, challenges to healthy eating while traveling, and introducing whole foods into your family's diet.

Focus the discussion on nutritious foods that can be found at the local grocery store. Mothers are often concerned about high food costs. Explain that processed foods generally cost more and are less nutritious. Fresh and whole foods are often the healthiest and most economical choice. You might also have available copies of the WHOLE FOODS FOR THE WHOLE FAMILY cookbook and ask mothers who use the book to tell the group about a favorite recipe.

Follow-up questions:

- What resources do we have locally to find foods that are as close to their natural state as possible?
- Tell us about a meal that is healthy and economical that your family enjoys.
- What are some ways that you introduce healthier foods to your family?
- What have you done to make food preparation (buying, cooking, cleanup) easier for yourself?
- How has having a child changed your attitude about nutrition?

Prepared meeting

Alternate Titles: Weaning: Four Chambers of the Heart

Introductory questions

- What concerns you the most about weaning or not weaning your child?
- How long did you originally think you would breastfeed your baby? How have your views changed?
- If your baby could decide, how do you think he would want weaning to happen?
- Other than nutrition, how does breastfeeding meet the needs of your child?
- With whom have you discussed weaning? How did it come up, and what was said?

Discussion

On a large poster board draw a large heart. Divide the heart into four sections. Label each quarter with one of the following descriptions:

- Child's reasons to continue
- Child's reasons to wean
- Mother's reasons to continue
- Mother's reasons to wean

Ask the mothers to find reasons to fill up the heart. For example:

- Child's reasons to continue: tastes good, feels good, time with mother
- Child's reasons to wean: too busy, likes variety of other foods
- Mother's reasons to continue: easy, good nutrition, cancer prevention
- Mother's reasons to wean: needs space, return to work, next child

When each chamber is full, mothers can see that the decision of when to wean is filled with emotions. With each perspective the mother can weigh the pros and cons. Having equal space for each chamber respects different decisions and thoughts about weaning and continuing to breastfeed.

Avoid a contest in which mothers compare length of breastfeeding. Too often this backfires by creating the impression that the longer a mother has breastfed, the better mother she is or the more welcome she is at LLL Series Meetings. Be ready to offer specifics about weaning with an emphasis on continuing to meet the baby's emotional as well as nutritional needs.

Follow-up questions

- What do you like best about breastfeeding your child at this age? How have your ideas changed since he was an infant?
- As your child loses interest in breastfeeding, how has his father's role changed?
- How do you cope with family and friends saying, "Is that baby still nursing?"
- As your child outgrows the need to breastfeed, how can you meet his needs in other ways?
- How did you feel the first time you saw an older child breastfeed?

MEETING 4: NUTRITION AND WEANING

SERIES MEETING GUIDES

References from THE WOMANLY ART:
Chapter 12—Nutritional Know-How
Chapter 13—Ready for Solids
Chapter 14—Weaning Gradually, with Love
Chapter 15—Discipline Is Loving Guidance

Additional resources:
HOW WEANING HAPPENS, 142–12
MOTHERING YOUR NURSING TODDLER,157–2
MAGGIE'S WEANING, 721–12

Approaches to Weaning, 307–17
Does Breastfeeding Take Too Much Time? 291–17

MEETING 4:
NUTRITION AND WEANING

**References from
THE WOMANLY ART:**

Chapter 12—Nutritional Know-How
Chapter 13—Ready for Solids
Chapter 14—Weaning Gradually, with Love
Chapter 15—Discipline Is Loving Guidance

Additional Resources:
WHOLE FOODS FOR BABIES AND
TODDLERS, 1002–12

Baby's First Solid Food, 303–17

Additional resources:
LEARNING A LOVING WAY OF LIFE
The Discipline Book by William Sears, 2–7

Possible Title/Focus
Starting Solids

Discussion

This discussion topic includes the wisdom of waiting until around the middle of the first year to introduce solids and awareness of and respect for each baby's individuality. There are many variations in readiness, appetite, and temperament. Visual aids representing readiness signals may help the discussion; these could include baby's interest in solids, emergence of teeth, hand-eye-mouth coordination, and sitting up unsupported.

Focusing the meeting on individual readiness may help mothers who have already introduced solids feel respected for their choices. When a mother asks for specifics about which foods should be started at what time, you might refer her to THE WOMANLY ART OF BREAST-FEEDING, and WHOLE FOOD FOR BABIES AND TODDLERS or other LLL-published resources.

Questions

- As your baby has grown older, what are the signs you've looked for to know he needs more than mother's milk?
- Once you have gotten your baby off to the best start by breastfeeding, how do you plan to continue as your baby graduates to solid food?
- What myths have you heard about babies and solids?
- When it was time to start solids, how did you feel about it, and how did it work out?
- Why would you continue to breastfeed once your baby starts solids?

Possible Title/Focus
Discipline Is Loving Guidance

Discussion

Your member publication may help to facilitate this discussion. Print the concept regarding loving guidance on a board for the Group to see. Ask the participants to discuss what this means to them. You might also want to ask participants to discuss parenting books they've read from the Group Library and the tips they've received from those sources.

When the meeting focuses on positive discipline, mothers feel respected and proud of their choices. We can present the principles that underlie loving guidance as a way of life for ourselves as well as how we interact with our children. Our goal is to affirm each mother's sensitivity to her baby's needs, encouraging her confidence in her ability to know what's best for her child.

Questions

- What helps you to remember that loving guidance is worth it?
- How does breastfeeding promote a loving way of life?
- One of the toughest comments to deal with is being told you are spoiling your child. How does that make you feel, and how can you deal with it?
- What suggestions do you have for keeping your priorities in order?
- How are you developing a parenting style that feels right?

Possible Title/Focus

Extended Breastfeeding

Discussion

An important point to keep in mind with this meeting is to not encourage competition about breastfeeding duration. To some mothers, breastfeeding beyond three months is extended breastfeeding. A discussion that promotes LLL resources and shows respect for mothers' knowing their babies best can be enlightening and inviting to both pregnant women and mothers with young babies. Discussing society and family expectations can help bring out concerns. Focusing on baby's needs can help mothers feel confident in their choices.

Questions

- When you were pregnant, how long did you think you would breastfeed?
- How does breastfeeding your toddler continue to meet his needs?
- What is your toddler or preschooler's word for breastfeeding when you are in public?
- What would your child's favorite benefit of breastfeeding be?
- How have your attitudes about breastfeeding and parenting changed as your child has grown?

Additional Resources:
HOW WEANING HAPPENS, 142-12
MOTHERING YOUR
NURSING TODDLER, 157–12;
MICHELE, THE NURSING TODDLER, 147–12
(See also **Toddler Meetings,**
pages 174–80.)
MAGGIE'S WEANING, 721–12

SERIES MEETING GUIDES

CHAPTER FOUR

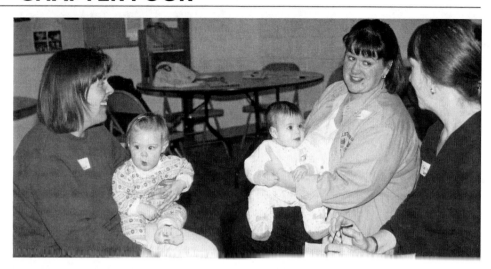

Managing the LLL Group

EVALUATION MEETINGS

Regular Evaluation Meetings contribute to smooth running and effective Groups, making working together easier and more fun for both Leaders and mothers. Taking care of Group business, getting to know each other, and discussing topics of mutual interest are important parts of the agenda.

While Series Meetings are geared to the newcomer, Evaluation Meetings provide opportunities for mothers to be involved in the management of the Group and opportunities for the Group to focus on the breastfeeding and mothering interests of mothers who regularly attend meetings. They can enhance the network of information, encouragement, and support for regular Series Meeting participants as their babies grow. For many Group members, Evaluation Meetings are the highlight of the month.

Benefits of Regular Evaluation Meetings

Evaluation Meetings provide opportunities for Leaders to:

- Get to know mothers and to encourage mothers to get to know one another better;
- Promote and support members' enthusiasm for LLL and interest in the LLL Group and LLL philosophy;
- Gather information to fill out the monthly Group report;
- Evaluate the effectiveness of the Series Meeting;
- Develop plans for future meetings and show how members can contribute to the meetings;
- Share and/or delegate Group management jobs and involve Group workers in Group management;
- Stimulate interest in leadership;

- Help Leader Applicants learn about Group management; and
- Discuss parenting topics of mutual interest.

Who, When, and Where?
Who attends Evaluation Meetings?

Some Groups limit Evaluation Meeting attendance to Leaders, Leader Applicants, and Group workers. Other Groups include the hostess of the series or those involved with a special event or activity such as the World Walk for Breastfeeding. Some Groups invite all LLL members (attendance is a benefit of membership). Other Groups invite all mothers who have attended at least a series of four meetings. Occasionally Leaders who want to stimulate enthusiasm and find volunteers for Group jobs issue an open invitation to all mothers.

When you invite a mother to attend Evaluation Meetings, let her know the purpose of these meetings and why you would like her involvement.

Babies and toddlers are part of Evaluation Meetings. Allow for toys, snacks, and space to play, and encourage mothers to attend to their children as needed.

When to hold Evaluation Meetings

Planning a set day and time each month for Evaluation Meetings can increase participation. It saves the effort of choosing a time and day to meet each month, because the meeting becomes part of everyone's schedule. Some Groups schedule the Evaluation Meeting within a week of the Series Meeting, while memories are fresh. Evaluation Meetings don't have to be at the same time of day as the Series Meetings. Participant availability is key.

For some Groups, a morning meeting is ideal. The children are rested and the afternoon is free for other activities. In other Groups, especially if older children attend afternoon preschool or kindergarten, the afternoon is better. If there are many older toddlers and preschoolers to consider, or if some of the women have jobs during the day, it may be more convenient to hold evening Evaluation Meetings.

It is a good idea to start on time and set an approximate ending time for Evaluation Meetings. Usually an hour and a half to two hours is long enough to finish Group business and the enrichment program.

Where to hold Evaluation Meetings

Many Groups will need to take toddlers' and preschoolers' needs into consideration. A home with toys and a safe play area makes a good choice. Some Groups meet in a park during warmer months of the year.

Some Groups choose a permanent location for their Evaluation Meetings, for example, the community meeting room where the Series Meetings are held. Other Groups schedule an Evaluation Meeting hostess for each series. Perhaps a mother cannot accommodate Series Meetings in her home but can host a smaller group.

Setting the agenda

The agenda for the Evaluation Meeting includes evaluating the Series Meeting, planning for the next one, and discussing Group business. Within that frame-

> Evaluation Meetings promote and support enthusiasm for LLL.

work, let the conversation flow! An Evaluation meeting is where participants can ask questions, air concerns, and gain support beyond the Series Meetings.

Evaluating the Series Meeting

It's a good idea to take a few minutes at the beginning to discuss why Evaluation Meetings are important to the effectiveness of the Group. This is helpful to a mother attending for the first time and reminds everyone of the shared responsibility for the Group. Together they can consider the meeting discussion and the Group's atmosphere and work out ideas for maintaining or improving the quality of Series Meetings.

There is always room for improvement, and there are always things to learn from each meeting. If participants were enthusiastic, felt free to talk, ask questions, and offer suggestions, and they received LLL information and support, the Series Meeting has met its goals.

The Evaluation Meeting is an opportunity for Leaders and mothers who feel responsible for the effectiveness of the Group to offer observations about what is going well and what can be improved. Encourage problem solving, keeping in mind the Group's goal of helping mothers breastfeed.

Some Leaders develop an outline that they use as a guide during the Evaluation Meeting and then as a checklist when they write to their support Leader.

MANAGING GROUP

Sample Evaluation Meeting Outline

This is a sample outline to help you complete your records and monthly Group report and to guide discussion during the evaluation meeting: adapt it to suit the Group, District, or Area.

Series Meeting date and time:

Leader(s) who led the Series Meeting:

Attendance Statistics

> Leaders:
>
> Leader Applicants:
>
> Group workers: (list names)
>
> New attendees (list names)
>
> New members this meeting: (list names)
>
> Returning Members (list names)
>
> Returning Non-members (list names)
>
> Visitors: (list all, including fathers)
>
> **Total Adults:**
>
> Babies (to one year):
>
> Toddlers (1 to 3 years):
>
> Children (3+):
>
> **Total Children:**

Meeting

> Assess:
>
> Discussion questions used

Perception of and response to needs of new mothers

Flow of discussion

Use of Group Library books and pamphlets in discussion

Consider:

What went well (continue)

Concerns or problems (plan for follow-up)

Group finances

Membership

One-year membership

New

Renewals

Six-month membership (if offered)

New

Renewals

Sales

WOMANLY ART OF BREASTFEEDING

OTHER LLL BOOKS

Fundraisers or other income

Other Sales

Group debts (if any)

Bank Balance(s), including savings

Group management

Reports from Group workers

Hostess or facility

Books on hand for sale

Library inventory

Materials to order

Optional activities (with consultation as needed)

Special meetings: Toddlers, Couples, etc. (attendance)

Fundraising/World Walk for Breastfeeding

Speaking engagements (attendance)

Enrichment topic (optional)

(See **Enrichment Meetings** in Chapter 7, page 173.)

Regularly Reviewing Group Jobs

Some Groups ask each Group worker to give a status report on her area of responsibility at every Evaluation Meeting. In other Groups, workers ask or answer questions as they arise.

Regular review of Group jobs is a way to recognize the Group worker's sense of responsibility and allows the Leader and Group workers to talk about whether changes are in order. For example, the Refreshment Coordinator might comment on the number of mothers volunteering to bring snacks, whether food choices reflect the

> Regular review of Group jobs recognizes the contribution of Group workers.

nutritional message of LLL, the need to simplify her job or suggestions to expand it. The Librarian might want to report on or invite discussion about book circulation, ways to encourage greater library use, problems with overdue books, book transport or storage.

Coordinating Group orders

Since shipping and handling costs are charged for each order sent, most Groups place orders at regularly planned intervals rather than each time a Leader or Group worker needs books, pamphlets, or Group supplies. Ordering in bulk quantities can save money, too. Neighboring Groups may wish to place orders together, to take advantage of discounts.

Leaders and Group workers can bring their lists for the Group order to the Evaluation Meeting. The Treasurer can complete the order, a Leader can sign it, and one of the Leaders can take responsibility for placing the order. (See Appendix 2: **Ordering Information.**)

MANAGING GROUP

Planning special functions

Evaluation Meetings provide the perfect opportunity to discuss, plan, and then assess other Group functions, such as optional special meetings (Toddler Meetings, Couples Meetings, Employed Breastfeeding Mothers Meetings, Teen Mothers Meetings), family picnics, World Breastfeeding Week/World Walk for Breastfeeding, or other fundraising events.

Enrichment Topics at Evaluation Meetings

An enrichment topic at Evaluation Meetings can add extra enthusiasm to the Group. An important benefit of these meetings is the close contact among Group members and the support LLL provides them.

Enrichment can complement Series Meetings by covering topics of interest to mothers of older babies and toddlers. (See **Enrichment Meetings** in Chapter 7, page 173 for topic suggestions.)

Some Groups hold Enrichment Meetings separately from Evaluation Meetings. Evaluation Meetings are scheduled regularly, while Enrichment Meetings may be planned to meet Group needs and interests.

Reporting is part of a Leader's basic responsibility and provides an important barometer of LLL's overall health.

Reporting

Reporting is part of a Leader's responsibility.

In the same way that an experienced mother's insight helps other breastfeeding mothers, a Leader's report can help other Leaders. Your knowledge can reach beyond your neighborhood, your city or town, your Area and even to other parts of the world. Ideas from your reports are shared with other Groups through the support network of LLL.

Over the course of several months, reports also provide an assessment of the vitality of the Group and trends. For example, a series of reports might indicate that the Group Treasury balance is steadily falling; you, your support Leader, and/or Group workers might identify reasons and generate solutions together. Regular reports might show that the Group is drawing more and more newcomers. You, your support Leader, and/or

Group members might look at some of the reasons; then you could pass on the ideas that increased attendance to other Groups.

Information from regular reports also provides an important barometer of La Leche League's overall health. It is important to know the number of mothers La Leche League Leaders are reaching through meetings, telephone helping, online helping, and other contacts. Figures from your report become part of local, national, and international reports. These statistics are used to publicize the extent of work done by LLL volunteers. They are also used in writing grant proposals to secure funding for LLL projects that help us reach more mothers. In addition, they help LLL allocate resources to meet current and future needs. For example, an Area or Affiliate might use the statistics on Leaders' one-to-one helping contacts to decide if it needs to recruit and train more Professional Liaison Leaders.

The report can take different forms. Because a brief summary of the Series Meeting gives your support Leader an opportunity to add a different perspective to the questions and problems the Group is considering, you might write a letter about the Series Meeting and the work of the Group. Many Leaders use the notes taken during the Evaluation Meeting as the basis for a report.

Whatever format(s) you use, include:

- Statistics on:
  attendance at Series Meetings and Evaluation Meetings,
  membership, and
  mothers helped by telephone, email, and in person
- Group Treasury figures (including sales)
- Information about:
  the Series Meeting,
  enrichment/discussion topic at the Evaluation Meeting,
  Leader and Group activities,
  participation in Leader continuing education, and
  problems, questions, and/or concerns.

(See the sample **Evaluation Meeting Outline** on previous pages.)

Who completes the report?

Although you, as the Group Leader, have final responsibility for making sure reports are completed and submitted, a Leader Applicant or Group worker may help fill them out. A sample **Monthly Activity Report Form** is included in Appendix 4. Your support Leader can tell you if there is a standard monthly report form that Leaders are expected to use in your Area or Affiliate.

SHARED LEADERSHIP

When there is more than one Leader in the Group, you can divide responsibilities and share the workload. Co-leading is a partnership; there is no junior or senior Leader.

Clear communication is vital for effective sharing of Group responsibilities.

Shared leadership mainly concerns two aspects of Leader work: leading Series Meetings and managing the Group. Working together in the Group includes open discussion, goal setting and planning, decision making, problem solving, and evaluation on an ongoing basis.

Co-Leaders at Series Meetings

Two or more Leaders can share leading a Series Meetings in several different ways:

1. One Leader plans and leads the business portion of the meeting—introduction, the history and purpose of La Leche League, LLL membership, information about the facility, reminders about meeting babies' needs, the importance of participation, personal introductions by the mothers, etc. Another Leader plans and leads the Series Meeting topic.
2. One Leader leads both parts of the meeting; the other assists. The assisting Leader helps keep the discussion on track by adding additional points of information and discouraging side conversations or by taking over the discussion if the other Leader's attention is needed elsewhere. Co-Leaders need to be familiar with the meeting plan.
3. Each Leader leads a different aspect of the business and or topic part of the meeting. For example, one Leader can focus on the emotional aspects and the other on the practical information of a topic.

Advantages of Co-Leaders at Series Meetings:

- Mothers have the opportunity to enjoy different leading styles.
- Mothers get to know more than one Leader.
- The meetings benefit from the creativity and enthusiasm of more than one Leader.
- Leaders can focus on topics and areas of topics that interest them.
- Leaders may feel more relaxed, knowing they can rely on each other.

Series Meeting responsibilities can be divided in many ways, depending on the number of Leaders in the Group and the availability of each Leader. Some Leaders decide on a plan by the series, others plan by the year. Some co-Leaders plan informally—over the telephone or by email; others find that decisions can be more easily worked out at periodic Leaders' Meetings separate from monthly Evaluation Meetings. (See **Leaders' Meetings** in the following pages.)

Co-Leaders and Group Management Responsibilities

Each Leader has unique interests, talents, energy levels, and family situations. Leaders, mothers, and the Group benefit when co-Leaders appreciate these differences and work together to accommodate one other.

Effective sharing of Group responsibilities hinges on several factors:

- All Leaders know who is responsible for each job. Clear communication is essential.
- All Leaders follow through on their appointed jobs. It may help to check with each other regularly—at Leaders' Meetings if you have them—to allow for changes that could mean a Leader would have more time to offer, may need help, or wants a change in job assignment.
- Jobs rotate in an agreed manner among Leaders. You may need to plan short- and long-term goals together and identify where your interests and skills would be most effective.

MANAGING GROUP

At different times, your personal lives allow more or less time for LLL work. You may find yourself able to do lots of work or barely be able to keep up with the basics. When you work together as a team, you provide and receive the kind of support that enables you to keep your interest and participation in the Group, and your cooperation strengthens the Group.

Deciding on a Listed Leader

The Listed Leader is the official contact person for the Group. All correspondence and Group account invoices are mailed to her; her address is the Group's mailing address. She is responsible for sharing all correspondence from LLLI or your LLL Office and the Area with the other Group Leaders.

Since written and computer records need to be changed each time the Listed Leader changes, it is best to not rotate this job unless necessary. When a change of Listed Leader is necessary, complete and send in the appropriate Leader Change of Address/Status Form to your Area and your LLL Office. If you do not know the correct form to use, your support Leader will be able to help you.

(A sample **Leader Change of Address/Status Form** is included in Appendix 4.)

Overseeing Group Jobs

Communication with Group workers may be simpler when each works with a specific Leader. Your work in overseeing a Group job includes explaining the responsibilities of the position to the Group worker, answering questions, and helping her as necessary and appropriate.

Delegating jobs is important. It provides opportunities for women in the Group to use their skills for the benefit of the Group. It helps mothers learn more about LLL and LLL leadership. At the same time, you get to know the mothers more closely. Delegating work can also make it easier for you to balance your LLL commitments with family needs. By sharing the Group's workload, you can have more time for the jobs only Leaders can do.

Leaders' Meetings

Getting together periodically for Leaders-only meetings can be a useful aid to clear communication. Leaders' Meetings provide an opportunity for you as co-Leaders to talk among yourselves about important issues such as:

- How much time each of you can commit to the Group
- Group goals
- Series Meeting leading schedule
- Group management issues
- Whether you all want to engage in or suggest the Group engage in optional activities such as special meetings, fundraising, and outreach
- Mothers who may be interested in leadership
- Working with Leader Applicants and/or concerns about mothers interested in leadership

NOTE: Some of these topics would also be discussed with Group workers; the Leaders Meeting discussions might be preliminary or complementary to the involvement of Group workers.

Co-Leader Communication
Diversity among Leaders

As an accredited Leader, you understand and are able to both present and represent LLL philosophy. There are many ways to put the philosophy into practice. Diversity strengthens LLL, making our message and help available to many different mothers. This diversity helps you relate to more mothers because they see that there is no one way to breastfeed, parent, or represent LLL and its philosophy as a Leader. However, diversity can also occasionally lead to disagreement or conflict.

Working through disagreements by keeping LLL goals foremost

When you and a co-Leader disagree, keeping your common goal in mind can help you resolve conflicts. You can explore options and possible solutions from the basis of your mutual interest as Leaders in helping mothers to breastfeed.

Approach differences and disagreements constructively—as an opportunity for learning.

- Give the disagreement or conflict immediate attention; postponement can intensify negative feelings.
- Handle any disagreement in a direct manner. Discuss it only with those involved, not with other Leaders or Group members.
- Listen carefully and consider other viewpoints. Avoid assumptions; inquire for further understanding.
- Use respectful dialogue, avoiding accusations. Use "I" messages ("I feel…when…") to explain your understanding and viewpoint. Be open and willing to change your mind if you receive new/different information.
- Together look for solutions that will enable you to satisfy your individual and mutual goals.
- When a conflict is resolved, put it in the past and move on.

If you need help resolving difficulties, you can discuss the situation with your support Leader, who may refer you to the resources and information available through the Communication Skills/Human Relations Enrichment program. (See **Communication Skills/Human Relations Enrichment Sessions,** pages 156 & 171.)

You may or may not be interested in developing friendships with Group workers and other Leaders. Keep in mind that women with different lifestyles, values and expectations can work productively together to help other mothers; friendship is not necessary to a respectful, effective working relationship.

Group Jobs

Sharing LLL work has many advantages. When members help with Group tasks, you can concentrate more time and energy on Leader responsibilities. Members often have useful ideas to contribute. In addition, members gain opportunities to learn more about LLL and feel satisfaction in contributing to its success.

MANAGING GROUP

Diversity strengthens LLL, making our message and help available to many different mothers.

> When members help with Group tasks, you can concentrate more time and energy on Leader responsibilities.

Leader-Only Jobs

A few Group responsibilities are for Leaders only:

- Leading Series Meetings,
- Providing one-to-one breastfeeding help as an LLL representative, by telephone, email (or other written communication), or in person,
- Taking responsibility for how Group funds will be used (see **Appropriate Use of Group Funds,** page 106.),
- Helping mothers prepare for LLL leadership, and
- Speaking as a representative of/on behalf of LLL.

ASKING MOTHERS FOR HELP WITH GROUP WORK

Why Mothers May Want to Help LLL

People volunteer for many reasons: out of gratitude for the information and encouragement they receive from LLL, because they want to help a worthwhile cause, for the personal benefits gained from involvement, and so many other reasons.

Benefits of helping with Group work include:

- Rewarding working relationships,
- Satisfaction of helping others,
- Learning new skills and developing others, and
- Child-friendly atmosphere.

On a deeper level, many mothers say that working with LLL gives them a sense of renewal and affirms their values. As one mother put it, "In our complicated society with its fluctuating values, it is refreshing to belong to an organization dedicated to the ideals of breastfeeding and mothering. I want to be part of that organization . . . to help it grow."

Approaching Mothers about Group Jobs

To find volunteers for Group jobs, the Leader can ask mothers individually or can make a general announcement about the need for help. A mother may feel more comfortable asking questions about the responsibilities one-to-one. Some people attach greater importance to the request if they are approached personally.

With the announcement approach, a mother has time to consider the responsibilities of the job and how it fits with her skills, interests, and other commitments. If more than one job is available, she can decide which one matches her available time, her interests, and her skills.

Many Leaders announce the need for help to the whole Group and, if there's no positive response, follow up by asking individual mothers. Similarly, you may encourage an individual mother to consider a particular job even though you are announcing the job's availability to the Group.

Matching an Individual with a Job

You may find the following "Window of Work" exercise useful in matching people and jobs. You could ask Group members to complete the exercise to help in identifying their interests and skills.

Window of Work

Divide a piece of paper into three columns. Label the columns with these headings:

Specific things you like to do or do fairly well
Specific things you would like to learn or are interested in
Specific things you do not like or want to do

MANAGING GROUP

When the exercise is complete, the first column will include talents, skills, hobbies, or activities a mother does well and enjoys doing; these may be of benefit to the Group and the mother may be most comfortable in jobs that highlight them. The second column will include interests and new things the mother would like to learn. As you talk together, you can see which Group jobs fit with her interests and can contribute to her learning. The third column includes information you might not otherwise know and the mother might not otherwise mention. An appropriate Group job will include some aspects of the first two columns and probably none from the third. If it is necessary to ask a mother to do something she prefers not to do, you can acknowledge this. Perhaps you and she might find ways, considering the mother's skills and interests, to make the job more acceptable.

The "Window of Work" can be re-evaluated from time to time. It may help you and the mother to identify changing interests. Opportunities to use and develop skills, to learn and broaden interests while supporting other breastfeeding mothers can help sustain a mother's involvement in the Group.

> A job description that lists regular and optional tasks and time frames makes a handy reference for both worker and you.

Helping Group Workers Get Started

Suggest a time period of commitment

Initially, a mother may be more willing to make a short-term rather than a long-term commitment. You might agree to a few months or a series of four meetings, with the possibility of continuing if the work is satisfying and going well or changing if it is not. Other mothers may prefer, and some jobs are better served by, an initial commitment that is longer. In any case, schedule times when you will meet to evaluate and to consider factors that influence continuing or ending the commitment.

Provide a written job description

A written job description is helpful to both Leaders and mothers, because job expectations are spelled out. Some Groups use a simple list with a paragraph describing each job. Not all Groups will need every job; job responsibilities will vary in each Group.

Possible Group Jobs

Treasurer
- Handles financial transactions including memberships and book sales at meetings
- Handles bank transactions and bookkeeping; completes financial reports

Librarian
- Maintains book collection
- Displays library at meetings; keeps track of book and pamphlet circulation
- May present a short book review at meetings

Greeter
- Welcomes mothers at the door and helps them with their belongings
- Introduces newcomers to Leaders
- Directs mothers to the Group Library and the meeting area
- Gives out nametags
- Maintains and gives out new mother packets

Refreshment Coordinator
- Arranges for a mother to bring refreshments each month
- Sets up the refreshment area at meetings
- Pours and serves refreshments

Publicity Coordinator
- Distributes meeting notices in the community
- Contacts newspapers about Series Meetings and special events
- Develops display of LLL materials for community events

Bulletin Board/Scrapbook Coordinator
- Coordinates library table/bulletin board display with Series Meeting topic
- Maintains a Group scrapbook and/or photo album
- Helps Publicity Coordinator with community displays

Hostess
- Offers her home for a series of meetings
- Stores Group Library during the series
- Provides a beverage, cups, and napkins for refreshments at meetings. (See **Sample Letter to a Hostess** in Chapter 2 page 55.)
- Arrives at the public meeting place in time to make sure it is open, checks for cleanliness and child-proofing, and arranges the seating

Fundraising Coordinator
- Plans and coordinates Group fundraising efforts, World Breastfeeding Week/World Walk for Breastfeeding events, etc.

Secretary
- Keeps track of meeting attendance
- Handles Group mailings
- Reminds mothers about meetings
- Takes and distributes minutes of Evaluation Meetings

Group Newsletter Editor
- Gathers LLL information and Group news
- Works with Leaders to develop and distribute newsletter to Group members

Some Groups keep a sheet describing the specific responsibilities of each worker with the file, notebook, or supply box for that job. Some Groups find it helpful to photocopy the pages of THE LEADERS' HANDBOOK related to each Group job. These pages can also be kept in the file or notebook along with the Group worker's job description. All the job descriptions can be compiled into a booklet; you and your co-Leaders each keep a copy, and one copy is kept in the Group Library.

A job description that lists regular and optional tasks and time frames makes a handy reference for both worker and you.

Group Librarian

- Transports books to meeting location for each meeting or at the beginning of each series of meetings.
- Arrives in plenty of time before Series Meetings to set up Library (if there's room, displays sale books and books from the Group Library pertaining to the meeting topic).
- Checks in returned books and reminds mothers about overdue books.
- Might make a brief announcement about the Group Library during the Series Meeting and/or highlight a new book or one pertaining to the meeting topic.
- Helps mothers find books as needed.
- Makes sure mothers know the sign-out procedure and offers to help a mother complete the information if she is holding her baby.
- Puts Library away at the end of the meeting.
- Reminds mothers about overdue books several days before the next meeting. Follow-up on overdue books is very important!
- Regularly (perhaps at the end of a series) checks the book collection, repairing and making recommendations for replacement when necessary.
- Covers new books as they are acquired. Inserts new issues of member publications and new or revised pamphlets in proper binders.
- Keeps Group Library supplies and inventory up-to-date.
- Could bring a small selection of books to special meetings as requested by Leaders.
- Attends Group Evaluation Meetings.
- Keeps in touch with Group Leader(s).

(See **Group Libraries,** page 117.)

Encourage Freedom and Decision Making

People are more likely to find satisfaction in jobs in which they develop their ideas and carry out responsibilities in their own way. Just as Groups benefit from several Leader styles, they benefit from the variety of approaches members bring to their Group jobs.

Evaluation Meetings are a great time to brainstorm ideas related to the Group and to appreciate the ideas, energy, and accomplishments of Leaders and Group workers. Attendance at Evaluation Meetings can be part of Group worker job descriptions.

When there are a number of Leaders and workers, Leaders and Group workers can pair up for reporting and support purposes. Then, although all Leaders and workers work together in the Group, Group workers always know which Leader to contact for help.

Periodically reevaluate the written job descriptions. Incorporate new ideas as Group workers who are doing them help assess the job and make suggestions.

Building a Team of Group Workers

A team of dedicated, enthusiastic mothers can be the key to a thriving LLL Group. Some of these suggestions may help:

> A team of dedicated, enthusiastic mothers can be the key to a thriving LLL Group.

- Keep a positive attitude. Expect mothers to want to participate. Enthusiasm is contagious.
- Offer a job to every mother who attends a full series of meetings, so she can become involved while her interest in the Group is high. Mothers can share jobs—for example, co-Librarians, Treasurer and Membership Treasurer, more than one Greeter for the busy pre-meeting time, rotating fundraising organizers.
- Work with individuals to match jobs with their interests, needs, and strengths.
- Hold regular Evaluation Meetings. Discuss Group management responsibilities and how to accomplish the work most efficiently and effectively.
- Emphasize the fun of working together. Plan time for refreshments and socializing.
- Listen to Group workers. They provide different views of Group needs and expectations. As often as possible, include workers in Group decisions.
- Let Group workers know they are appreciated. Say thank you with specific praise. Remember: thank the volunteer; praise her job.
- Encourage communication. Encourage Group workers to regularly attend Series and Evaluation Meetings.
- Take minutes of the Evaluation Meetings and distribute these to all Leaders and Group workers.

Common Reasons Volunteers Quit

Notice that "not enough time" is not on the list. Although volunteers sometimes give this as a reason, it is not the real reason. Their day did not get shorter; they just made other things their priority.

- **Too much too soon.** Work with the volunteers to decide how much responsibility they can cope with. Try not to prejudge their availability; let them know that you are happy for them to offer to do the amount that they can manage.
- **Feeling excluded.** People who know each other naturally interact together at gatherings. You may need to remind mothers to be friendly to newcomers to help them feel part of the Group.
- **Desperate need.** No one likes to feel trapped. Try to project your invitation as an opportunity to help with the Group, rather than desperation. Let the mother control the commitment, and respect the limits she sets.
- **Impossible goals.** Together, set goals that are achievable, worth achieving, and to which the individual believes she can contribute significantly. Define short-term objectives, encourage long-term visions, and recognise each stage of a project as it is completed.
- **No opportunity for growth.** Volunteer work should be interesting, provide variety, and offer a chance for developing skills and interests. Some routine work always needs to be done; try to make it fun and alternate it with interesting work. Some volunteers prefer to do tasks they are skilled at; others enjoy the challenge of something new.

- **Not enough appreciation.** Remember to say "please" and "thank you" often. An important aspect of appreciation is common courtesy, such as taking the time to return phone calls, answer notes, pass along information, etc. Consider giving a certificate or a small gift from time to time to recognize volunteer efforts.
- **Family/Friend conflict.** Family and friends may look at volunteer work as time away from them. They might appreciate being included in activities such as picnics, fundraising events, and special meetings, or when appropriate, in the work itself.
- **Conflict in the Group.** Even though women in LLL share many values, they will not always agree. Unresolved conflict can drain or deplete energy and enthusiasm.
- **Policy disagreements.** Volunteers who quit over disagreement with policy often state that the majority did not understand their position. Listen carefully and summarize all viewpoints accurately and respectfully. Solve problems together.
- **Not enough fun.** There is always plenty of work to be done; be sure to make time for fun, too.

Edited and excerpted with permission from an article by Paul C. Christian, *The Skywalker;* September/October 1987.

MANAGING GROUP

Remember that we can discourage potential volunteers by not asking for help. The opposite of asking people to take on too many responsibilities is not asking them to help: "No one told me they needed me." Keep in touch with mothers, and if they miss a meeting, touch base with them so the lack of contact does not become a reason to miss the next meeting. Then find out what responsibilities they might like to take on.

Adjusting the Workload to Group Circumstances
When there are many helping hands

The more people participating, the more the Group can accomplish. Consider subdividing the three basic areas of Group management—keeping track of people, money, and materials—to share the workload and create opportunities for people to get involved.

> Mothers who attend regularly and do not want to take on specific jobs can help the Group in many ways.

When simplicity is necessary

Groups with one or two Leaders and few mothers might need to keep to the basics. Small and new Groups often start with the jobs of Treasurer and Librarian.

Mothers who attend regularly and do not want to take on specific Group jobs can help the Group in many ways. For instance, you might suggest they:

- Greet newcomers and help mothers with their belongings when they arrive,
- Sit next to newcomers and talk with them before and after the meeting,
- Help keep the meeting discussion on topic,
- Allow newcomers a chance to talk and ask questions,
- Consider the impression careless remarks may have on mothers new to LLL,
- Encourage membership and sales so LLL will be there for mothers in the future,
- Support a mother with a fussy baby by empathizing with her feelings and affirming her efforts to calm her baby,

- Invite newcomers to the snack table and include them in conversations there,
- Show newcomers the Group Library; help them find and check out books as needed.

As they help more and more in these unofficial ways, you might encourage some participants to take on official Group jobs.

KEEPING TRACK OF PEOPLE

Keeping Track of Mothers Who Attend Meetings

Informing mothers about future meetings, special functions, or emergency changes in meeting locations can maintain and increase attendance.

- Keeping in contact with mothers between meetings, perhaps to follow up on a conversation started at the meeting or to help a newcomer feel welcome, can also influence attendance positively.
- The mothers with whom you keep in contact can be part of a database of individuals you might invite to help LLL financially.

Meeting attendance records

Many Groups pass an attendance sheet or notebook around the meeting circle. Some Groups ask mothers to sign in as they enter the meeting place. You can take care of attendance yourself or delegate the job to a Greeter or Secretary.

Attendance sheets might include:

- The meeting date,
- Series Meeting name and number,
- Names of the Leader(s) at the meeting and the hostess,
- A section for totalling the number of Leaders, new mothers, members, repeaters, and children,
- Space for each mother to write her name, address, email address, telephone number, due date, children and their ages, and membership status,
- As needed: columns asking if the mother is willing to bring refreshments, serve as hostess, or help the Group in some other capacity.

You might keep attendance sheets in a separate notebook/file or in the Group notebook/file along with a copy of the completed monthly report.

(See **Appendix 4** for a **Sample Sign in Sheet.**)

Caution: An attendance sheet is for LLL use only and is not used for other purposes.

New mother cards

Many Groups use Newcomer or New Mother Survey Cards to keep a master file of names. These cards are available from LLLI and may be available from your Affiliate or Area. Ask a newcomer to fill one out at her first meeting. Some Groups make a copy of the card for each Leader. (See **Appendix 3** for some samples of these cards and the information they request.)

> Informing mothers about future meetings, special functions, or emergency changes in meeting locations can maintain and increase attendance.

· ·

If you design your own card or form, you can add or adapt the information to suit the Group. In college towns, for example, it might be helpful to know if the mother is a student. Previous job experience might be of interest, especially when help is needed for a special Group job.

Master Address List

Most Groups find it helpful to keep a master list of mothers indicating those who are "active" and "inactive." Using cards or a computer database makes it easier to keep the list up to date and in alphabetical order.

Active list

The active list includes all paid members and women currently attending meetings. It might also include those who may no longer attend but who have expressed an interest in being informed about LLL activities and who may refer friends to LLL. It can also include all mothers who have called a Leader or attended at least one meeting during the previous series. Mothers on the active list would receive all meeting notices. The active list can be used to record when dues are paid, providing a reminder to send a renewal notice before the membership expires.

Inactive list

An inactive list might include former members and mothers who have attended meetings or contacted a Leader by phone or email in the past but did not pay membership. You may occasionally want to contact these mothers about special events or fundraisers.

PUBLICITY—HELPING OTHERS KEEP TRACK OF LLL

Although publicity is not listed as a basic Leader responsibility, promoting LLL is something every Leader does, sometimes without even specifically thinking about it. When a mother calls for breastfeeding help, you can mention Series Meetings and send a meeting notice. When you hear that a neighbor is expecting a baby, you invite her to a meeting. When you share your enthusiasm for LLL work with people you know, you stimulate their interest. All of these increase awareness of La Leche League and the LLL Group.

In some Groups, a Publicity Coordinator, with your guidance, takes responsibility for increasing the visibility of LLL in the community.

Check with your support Leader about review procedures before printing and distributing all new notices, cards, or news releases. She may have ideas that can help you.

Mother-to-mother is the best publicity

The phenomenal growth of LLL in its early years was based mainly on mother-to-mother contact. Happy mothers sharing their joy with friends continue to spread enthusiasm about LLL and breastfeeding. Many mothers attend their first meeting because an acquaintance invited them or told them about LLL. Mother-to-mother publicity can't be beat, but additional outreach can help. Here's how.

LLL's phenomenal growth in the early years was based mainly on mother-to-mother contact.

Meeting notices

There are several possibilities for announcing meetings:

- Mail or distribute Meeting Reminder Cards (available from LLLI or through your LLL Office). These can be mailed or distributed at the beginning of each series. Groups can design their own reminder cards as well. (See **Appendix 3.**)
- Produce a Series Meeting notice, such as the one in Appendix 4, which combines Series Meeting dates with information about LLL. Groups can also design their own meeting notices.
- Design a yearly notice that could use alternate titles for Series Meetings so that each is different. A notice covering 12 months can save time and money for a Group that meets in one location for the entire year.

No matter which option you choose, consider:

Accuracy. Always proofread, double-checking the time, location, dates, and topics of the meetings, and other information you offer; double-check spelling and grammar. Pay special attention to the spelling of names and the accuracy of telephone numbers and addresses (postal or email). If possible, have your partner or a co-Leader proofread the information as well. Put it aside and read it again the next day before making copies for distribution.

Image. A professional-looking presentation is important. Check to be sure the information is clear and the image is positive

Visual appeal. A good-looking meeting announcement is more likely to be read. Artistic training is not necessary to ensure a neat and clean announcement with plenty of white space and clear type in straight alignment. If you use the LLL logo, be sure the reproduction is clear and sharp. A hand-drawn version is not acceptable. Please refer to **Appendix 1** for the LLL logo policy.

Tone. Try to project a positive tone and respect for all individuals and their choices. Any appearance of judgment of bottle-feeding, separation, the medical community, or birthing options is damaging to the image of LLL.

Audience. The content and presentation of the notice will depend on the audience: LLL members only? Group attendees? Expectant or new mothers? Employed women? Health care providers? General public? For example, a meeting notice intended for health care providers may be formal and business-like. If the meeting notice will be distributed only to mothers who have been attending meetings, it can be tailored to the Group with information about special events, new babies, and new members. Obtain permission from mothers before printing any personal information including memberships and births.

Distribution. To save money and add a personal touch, prepare your notices in time to hand out at the last meeting of the series or the year. The rest of the notices can be mailed. Make extra copies available to participants to take home to friends. Some Groups include small LLL logo stickers to mark meeting dates on calendars.

It may not be practical to try to include everything on one meeting notice. You might want to consider making up more than one type of notice, for example posters, flyers, or bookmarks for public places and more detailed, specific meeting notices for Group members and health care providers.

Coordinating publicity efforts

Consider coordinating publicity efforts with one or more neighboring Groups. Chapter publicity that features more than one Group lets people know that Series Meetings (and all their benefits) are available at different times and places.

Displaying LLL materials in public places

An attractive meeting notice, poster, brochure, or bookmark displayed in a public place can highlight the local Group and increase community awareness of LLL services. Pamphlets or tear-off sheets stamped with the Group name and Leaders' names, telephone numbers and/or email addresses can also let people know what LLL has to offer. Some Groups use business cards in an attractive holder.

MANAGING GROUP

Meeting notices can also be posted in the community. Make the best use of time spent on publicity by choosing places where pregnant women and mothers of small children go, such as:

- Public libraries
- Children's shops
- Childbirth educators' offices
- Park district buildings
- Resale shops
- Preschools
- Laundromats
- Natural food stores
- Places of worship
- Hospitals and clinics
- Grocery stores
- Pharmacies
- Maternity shops
- Health care providers' offices
- Recreation centers

Make the best use of time spent on publicity by choosing places where pregnant women and mothers of small children go.

Be sure to get permission before posting a notice or displaying brochures. Remove dated material when it is no longer timely. To minimize nuisance calls, list only first names and telephone numbers of Leaders or only the Group name and one telephone number. For instance:

Call for directions:
Nancy 555-1234
Luann 555-4321
Lisa 555-1111
La Leche League of Anytown—call 555–5555

NOTE: When meetings are held in homes, check with the hostess before including her address on articles that are displayed in public places. It may not be prudent to include a private address on a public notice. It is better to have mothers contact a Leader for the address and directions to the meeting.

Today many mothers find
LLL by using the Internet.

Group Web pages

Today many mothers find LLL by using a computer and the Internet. The LLL Web site includes meeting and Leader information for Groups, Areas, and Affiliates.

A Group Web page is like a paper meeting notice and contains the same type of information mothers need to know about the Group and its meetings. To put your

Group information on the Web, contact the Internet administrator for your Area, country, Affiliate, or Division. Your support Leader can tell you who she is and how to contact her.

If your Area, country, Affiliate or Division doesn't maintain local Web pages, send a message to **groupweb@lalecheleague.org** (email). The instructions for getting a free Web page courtesy of LLLI and Prairienet, a service provider who has donated space to our Groups, will automatically be sent to you. This automated address will only send Group Web page instructions. If you do not receive a response within 24 hours, double-check the address and try again. (If the mail address is not typed exactly as shown, "reply" does not work.) To update the local Group's Prairienet page, email the new information to **webmaster@lalecheleague.org.**

If your Area, Affiliate, country, or Division maintains its own Group pages, send corrections to your Internet administrator.

Group Newsletters

Many Leaders and Groups find that newsletters are an effective way to keep mothers and participants up to date. A newsletter can save phone and meeting time by providing a hard copy of information such as the Series Meeting schedule, topics, directions to the meeting place, enrichment topics at Evaluation Meetings, and news of recent births (with permission).

Producing a Group newsletter is an optional activity. Sometimes a Group meeting notice develops over time into a newsletter. However, a Group newsletter is different from a meeting notice you might distribute to health care providers and others in the community. You could copy a one-page Group newsletter onto the back of meeting notices for members and meeting participants.

You might want to delegate the newsletter production job to a Group Newsletter Editor. You and the editor might plan each issue together. Contact your support Leader for additional ideas and review procedures, and remember to send a copy along with your meeting report. Here are some general suggestions to help get you started:

1. Identify the newsletter name, Group name, date, and page number on each page.
2. Use LLL sources for information and articles. Properly credit all sources. If you do use material from other sources, consider the following notes on copyrighted materials.

It is necessary to obtain permission to use more than a paragraph from published materials, including those produced by LLLI or an Affiliate. This credits and protects the work of the original author or publisher. All quotes need a reference to direct mothers to the original source for additional information.

To obtain permission to use more than a paragraph of material copyrighted by LLLI or an Affiliate, send your request to the Publications Director at LLLI or the appropriate Affiliate Publications Administrator.

Using Copyrighted Material

Include:

- Publication Number, title, pages, and paragraphs of the publication you wish to use
- How the material will be used
  - Name of the publication or handout, issue, date (if applicable)
  - Type of publication or handout
  - Intended audience of the publication or handout
- Number of copies to be printed
- Whether your publication or handout will be sold or given away

MANAGING GROUP

Permission to use copyrighted material as outlined above is granted to LLL _____(Area, Group, or Leader's name)

_____(address) _____ (fax) _____ (phone)

signed_____

(LLLI Publications Director or Affiliate Administrator)

If permission is granted, your letter will be returned, signed, by mail or fax.

Use this copyright statement (or the appropriate Affiliate copyright statement) after the quoted material in your publication or handout:

© Year, La Leche League International, reprinted with permission. Title, author, LLLI, Schaumburg, Illinois, USA.

(See **Copyrighted Materials, Appendix 1.**)

3. Review a draft of the newsletter, checking for accuracy, clarity, positive and respectful tone, and image and visual appeal. Check with your support Leader about review procedures for Group newsletters. She can help with proofreading as well as offer suggestions for content and appearance.

4. For your protection, use only first names and telephone numbers for Leader contact information.

5. For clear and consistent presentation, use the accepted style sheet for your Area/Affiliate/Division. (See Appendix 4.)

6. Respecting mothers' preferences for privacy, newsletters might include:
   - Series Meeting schedule,
   - Notices for special meetings (Toddler, Couples, etc.),
   - Directions to meeting place (with the hostess's permission),
   - Leaders' first names and telephone numbers,
   - Welcome to new mothers and new Leaders,
   - Births,

- Membership promotion,
- Thank you to new and renewing members,
- New Group Library books,
- LLL books for sale at meetings,
- Fundraiser dates and information,
- Recipes from LLL cookbooks (each is considered a paragraph for copyright purposes), and
- Short quotes (a paragraph or less) from Group Library books, your LLL member publication, or Leader publication.

7. In keeping with their purpose to provide LLL information relevant to meeting attendees newsletters do not include:
- Leader Applicants identified as Applicants,
- Information about organizations other than LLL,
- Articles from non-LLL sources,
- Copyrighted cartoons, drawings, and poems, or
- Newspaper clippings

8. Keep the audience in mind when compiling the newsletter. Remember that readers may be more or less familiar with LLL ideas.

News Releases

A news release can reach a large number of people with a small investment of time and effort. It can be a simple meeting notice or an article covering an aspect of breastfeeding and/or highlighting the LLL Group. Ideas/information you might include:

> A news release can reach a large number of people with a small investment of time and effort.

Aspects of breastfeeding
- Benefits to baby, mother, father, family
- Breastfeeding facts (from *Facts about Breastfeeding*, published annually by LLLI),
- Helpful hints

What LLL offers
- LLL Group meetings
- Telephone help
- Group Library
- Books for sale, LLL pamphlets and tear-off sheets

Special Group projects or events
- World Breastfeeding Week/World Walk for Breastfeeding
- Donation of a book or books to public library, clinic, etc.
- Display in your community
- Participation in a community event
- Work with other community groups

Milestones

- Anniversary of Group/Area/Affiliate, or the LLL founding
- Number of mothers served
- Accreditation of a new Leader

Leader or member participation in a relevant event

- Area/Division/Affiliate/LLLI conference
- Breastfeeding task force or other cooperative action

(See **Appendix 5** for Sample News Releases.)

From time to time, LLLI or your Division, Affiliate or Area may send Leaders easy-to-use news releases on current breastfeeding topics and events. You or the Group's Publicity Coordinator need only complete the heading and add local Group information to the blank spaces or ending paragraph. Consider retyping the news release in double-spaced format with contact information and local information filled in for a professional-looking presentation. For original news releases written by you or the Publicity Coordinator, check with your support Leader about review procedures before they are submitted to the newspaper. She may have suggestions for content, format, or tone.

Before sending in a news release, phone the newspaper to get the name of the editor or reporter responsible for community news. Then, send the news release directly to that person, keeping a copy for yourself. Always include a return address on the envelope in case your release does not reach its destination.

If the Group plans to send meeting notices to the newspaper on a regular basis, introduce yourself to the editor or reporter who will be handling them, so that you can build a positive relationship.

Be sure to include the name, address, and telephone number of the contact person at the top of the news release, so the editor can reach that person for further details. It is not necessary to include a cover letter with a news release. The fewer sheets of paper the better; use only one side of each sheet of paper. Some newspaper editors will accept news releases sent by email. Check with them first. This saves the editor having to retype it, which may increase its chances of being used and will reduce the chances of errors from retyping.

A news release is more likely to be published if it:

- Grabs the reader's attention with an interesting opening,
- Is brief, factual, and to the point (an editor who needs more detail will get in touch with the contact person for further information),
- Follows standard news release format (see box),
- Is addressed to the reporter or editor responsible for community news, and
- Is sent well in advance of the newspaper's deadline

Elements of a news release:

- **Contact**—name, address, and phone number of the person who can be contacted for further details;
- **Release date**—date that the article can be used, "For immediate release" or "For publication week of _____;"

- **Headline**—title or subject of the article; editors usually rewrite to fit the space in the newspaper; and
- **Lead**—opening paragraph, tells who, what, when, where, and why (the 5 Ws).

A news release is written in inverted pyramid style. Information is arranged in order of importance.

The News Release

1. Lead: indispensable facts (the 5 Ws)
2. Supporting facts
3. Secondary data
   - Double space the type.
   - Use one side of the paper only.
   - Leave wide margins on all sides.
   - End each page with a complete paragraph.
   - Use "-MORE-" at the bottom of the page to indicate that the article is continued.
   - Begin each additional page with "La Leche League (the country/Area)" and a page number.
   - Use "###" to signify the end.

If an article needs to be edited to fit the space on a newspaper page, information is cut from the bottom up. For this reason, you may want to put your Group's contact information in the first paragraph.

Photos

Photos are eye-catching and can say a lot. Pictures showing activity, such as photos from a recent fundraiser or World Walk for Breastfeeding are more likely to be published than those showing a group of people lined up in a row. Include a short paragraph of information from which the caption can be written.

It is necessary to obtain written permission to print the photo from all adults and a parent's written permission for all children in a photo.

Newspapers sometimes arrange to cover events with their own photographer. Check with the editor or photo editor to see what their policy is. Remember that photo events must often be scheduled weeks in advance and sometimes are pre-empted by breaking news.

Other Publicity Ideas

- **Cable television, public or school-affiliated radio or television stations**— Many cable, community, public access, or educational television and radio stations have a community bulletin board that is read or shown periodically. Send a postcard or email message with meeting information. (See **Appendix 5** for Sample Radio Announcements.)

- **Telephone listing**—Some telephone companies offer special rates to non-profit organizations; others require a more expensive business listing. In some communities, independent telephone directories offer reasonably priced listings. Some telephone directories have a community resource section that lists local services such as support groups. Some directories offer a listing of LLLI's 1-800 number (in the USA) for a very low monthly fee.
- **Community service directory**—Many communities publish a directory of public service organizations with a description of the work they do. Check with the local Chamber of Commerce, Red Cross, public health department, telephone company, community help hotline, or public library. This service is usually free.
- **Public library**—Librarians are usually happy to meet local LLL Leaders, especially if they bring along a copy of THE WOMANLY ART OF BREASTFEEDING to donate. An enthusiastic librarian can refer women to LLL when they ask for information about babies. Some libraries have a pamphlet section where you can place LLL publications stamped with Group contact information.
- **Community bulletin boards**—Look for these in shopping centers and laundromats. Small cards or posters are appropriate in these places. Check often to see that they are still there, intact and clean, and that the information is current.
- **Others**—Both community service groups and for-profit businesses that visit new residents and parents may be happy to distribute LLL brochures in their packets. Some set up tables of literature at fairs and conferences in the community.
- **Sometimes you may participate directly by helping to staff a stall or booth at a fair or conference.**
  NOTE: Check to be sure that the companies or service groups you ask to distribute information or for whom you help to staff a stall are not funded or otherwise supported by manufacturers of artificial baby milk. If you have questions or concerns about a company or service group, consult your support Leader.
- **Childbirth classes**—Classes or clinics that discuss childbirth and/or baby care may be willing to distribute LLL brochures and refer mothers to LLL. Check with both hospital-related and independent services.
- **Public service announcements**—Radio and television stations often feature these short announcements as a service to their community. (See **Appendix 5** for samples.)

MANAGING GROUP

KEEPING TRACK OF MONEY— THE GROUP TREASURY

Developing a Sound Financial Policy

While money may seem to have little to do with our purpose of helping mothers to breastfeed their babies, our financial resources affect our ability to carry out this purpose. Groups, Areas, Affiliates, Divisions and the larger body of LLLI need money to function. We all need to raise funds and spend wisely as we work together to fulfill our common goals.

Groups, Areas, Affiliates, Divisions, and the larger body of LLLI need money to function and to fulfill our common goals.

Fortunately, we can raise the money necessary to run a Group in ways that also promote LLL's basic purpose. LLL membership dues, sales of THE WOMANLY ART OF BREASTFEEDING and other LLLI-published books, and the annual World Walk for Breastfeeding enable Groups to raise money while providing mothers with breastfeeding help.

Consider this guide to setting priorities on items to sell in the Group:

- THE WOMANLY ART OF BREASTFEEDING
- LLL memberships
- LLL-published books
- LLL pamphlets and booklets
- Other books and products sold through LLLI, the LLLI Web site, or your Affiliate or Area.

Consult your support Leader about any other items a Group wants to sell or any other fundraising projects.

The Group Treasurer should be aware of local sales tax regulations and keep a record of the taxable items sold. The Area or Affiliate Treasurer or Area Financial Coordinator can provide information on local tax requirements.

Appropriate Use of Group Funds

Group funds need to be used for regular LLL activities that benefit mothers and babies. A Group's assets do not belong to the Leaders or members but to La Leche League. Money should be used to carry out LLL's purpose. Group expenses may include:

> If your Group has extra money after its bills have been paid, please consider donations to help more mothers breastfeed.

- Books and pamphlets for the Group Library
- Books and pamphlets for resale
- Pamphlets and tear-off sheets for new mother packs or to give or send to mothers
- Group supplies from LLL (New Mother Cards, etc.)
- Postage
- Telephone charges
- Copy services
- Leader dues (subscriptions)
- Help with Leader Applicant fees/materials if necessary
- Leader registration fees for workshops and conferences
- Group affiliation fees

You and your co-Leaders will jointly make decisions regarding the appropriate use of Group funds. Leader Applicants, Group workers, and members can offer suggestions (Evaluation Meetings are a good setting for this discussion) and may be major participants in helping the Group earn its money, but managing Group funds is a Leader responsibility. Consult your support Leader if there are questions or problems.

If the Group has extra money after its bills have been paid, please consider donations to new or needy Groups in your Area or to your Area/Division/Affiliate or to LLLI. These are always appreciated and keep LLL money in circulation to help more mothers to breastfeed. Or you might like to help a Group in another Area or make a donation to a special project such as translating and printing LLL materials in new languages. Contact your support Leader or LLL Office for more information about these and other opportunities to help LLL and breastfeeding mothers around the world.

The Group Treasurer

Every Group, large or small, has bills to pay, membership fees to collect, books to order and records to keep. It is absolutely essential that the Group's financial records be kept accurately. Although the Leader is ultimately responsible for any money paid into or out of the Group, it is a wise investment of time to find a trustworthy, reliable mother to handle the Group's financial transactions and record keeping.

If you cannot find a mother to act as Group Treasurer, you or a co-Leader will need to handle this responsibility. However, it is worthwhile asking a mother to act as Assistant Treasurer to handle financial transactions at meetings. This allows you to talk to mothers at meetings without being interrupted by money matters.

A Group Treasurer needs to be accurate and willing to give attention to detail. A financial background or bookkeeping experience is helpful but not necessary. Basic duties can include:

- Attending all meetings to sell and issue receipts for memberships, books, and other items, and to accept donations, or if unable to attend, arranging for a Leader or another member to do so,
- Keeping an up-to-date, accurate record of all financial transactions,
- Attending Evaluation Meetings and providing financial information for the monthly Group report,
- Depositing all money in the bank as soon after the meeting as possible,
- Keeping a record of memberships paid; sending remittances and member information to your Area and LLL Office,
- Writing checks to pay bills,
- Keeping a file of paid and unpaid bills, including bank statements and invoices,
- Keeping an inventory of materials for sale by the Group,
- Preparing Group orders (signed by a Leader),
- Paying Leader dues and Group affiliation fees as requested annually by your Area and LLL Office,
- Preparing and submitting annual financial reports as soon as possible after the end of the fiscal year as set by your Area and LLL Office, and
- Retaining Group financial records for the required length of time (usually seven years).

Group Budget

Most Groups project their income and expenses for a year.

Once a series or at least every six months, you and the Group Treasurer should compare the Group's financial situation and the budget. Such a review should include:

- Cash assets: checking, savings, and petty cash
- Memberships
- Bills due, including Area and any other LLLI/Affiliate/Divisional/National fees
- Inventory of books, pamphlets, and other items for sale
- Need for a fundraising project to be proposed to the Group.

> It is absolutely essential that the Group's financial records be kept accurately.

MANAGING GROUP

Regular review of Group finances allows you and the Group to make needed and timely adjustments. For example, if memberships are low, the discussion at an Evaluation Meeting could focus on membership promotion. If bills are overdue, the Group might plan a fundraising project to raise money. If inventory is high, you might talk about how to increase sales before ordering more. (See also **Appendix 2.**)

Fundraising Activities

As the Group becomes established and Group workers can help, you may want to consider fundraising.

While Groups can often meet their expenses through memberships and book sales, they sometimes decide to undertake special projects that require raising funds. Leaders experienced with Group fundraising find that it is important that Group workers and members understand and agree with how the funds they earn are going to be spent. A Group may want to purchase a large quantity of LLL pamphlets to stock their table at a health fair, or the Group may want to sponsor a Leader's continuing education by paying a portion of her conference expenses. The Group might want to increase publicity by informing community health care providers about the services LLL provides; this could involve the costs of buying brochures or leaflets, duplicating a cover letter, and postage. It might be appropriate to apply to local organizations for grants for specific purposes. Check with your support Leader for information.

Look in your Leader publication for helpful suggestions for fundraising.

LLLI publishes a useful resource called *The Funding Handbook,* and a brochure called *Helping Mothers around the World,* which are available through the LLL Web site. They may also be available through your ordering system.

A Group considering a fundraising project needs to think about the kind of activity, the likely financial gain compared to cost, and the time and effort required.

> Fundraising projects can be fun and give Group members and Leaders more opportunities to get to know each other.

Fundraising projects can be fun and give Group members and Leaders more opportunities to get to know each other. As the Group works together, mothers develop networks and strengthen their connection with La Leche League, and some may become interested in LLL leadership or in helping in other ways. So, fundraising projects not only generate funds, they also increase opportunities to achieve our goals.

A System for Keeping Financial Records
Organizing Group Treasury materials

The Group Treasurer's materials can be kept together in a notebook with pocket folders or in a portable file box.

- Zippered bag, flat pencil case, or envelope for money collected at meetings
- Receipt book with carbons for all transactions, whether in cash or check
- Current La Leche League order form and catalogue
- Current membership forms, cards or blank index cards to send to your Area and LLL office with the new member's contact details
- Income and expense sheets or ledger
- Inventory sheets or a list of sale items and their prices.
- Group budget
- Checkbook and deposit slips/book
- Bank statements

- Photocopy of the "Group Treasury" section of THE LEADER'S HANDBOOK and any other pertinent information from your Area and LLL office
- Pens
- Stamps
- Petty cash
- Envelopes

The Treasurer needs to bring her notebook or file to every meeting. If she is unable to attend, she can make arrangements to have it taken to the meeting so someone else can use the organizer to collect and process dues and money for items sold.

Group checking account

As a Leader, you need to protect yourself and LLL by not putting LLL funds into your own or anyone else's personal bank account. The Leaders of a Group open a separate account in the Group's name; they have all checks made payable to LLL of Group (name), not to LLL or an individual. The monthly statement the bank sends the Group provides a double-check of its financial transactions.

Banks sometimes provide free checking accounts (no monthly service fee and no minimum balance) to nonprofit organizations. If you are starting a new Group or if you need to change banks, go to the bank and explain the services offered by LLL and its charitable status. Open the account in the name of the Group, for example, "La Leche League of (Anytown)," not "La Leche League" or "La Leche League (Country/State)." Make sure the bank statement is sent to a Leader. This could be the Leader who is Treasurer or the Leader who serves as liaison with the member who is Treasurer.

If a bank requires a minimum balance in the account or deducts a service charge each month, you may want to consider another bank or other possibilities. For example, if the Group writes few checks, consider opening a savings account instead of a checking account. A bank check or money order could be written from the account when necessary. You may be able to use other types of banking facilities such as postal or email banking.

Whenever possible set up your bank account so that three people have signing authority and two people, one of whom is a Leader, are required to sign each check or withdrawal slip if using a savings account. If you are a sole Leader and the Group Treasurer, ask a member of your Group or your support Leader to be the second person. In some countries, it is a legal requirement for charitable organizations to have two signatories for a withdrawal. Remember that new signature cards must be signed for the bank whenever these authorized signatures change.

Record each check in the check register when it is written and each deposit when it is made. It is easy to forget to record a transaction if you postpone it. The record in the check register of money paid out and deposits made provides a double-check for the Group's income and expense record sheets. It is wise and responsible to balance the bank statement as soon as you receive it.

Group savings account

Some Groups may want to open a savings account in addition to a checking account. For example, a Group may want to save money for a long-range goal, such as sending representatives to a workshop or a conference. The Group may want to keep this money separate from the regular funds and to accumulate interest on the money.

Transfer funds to or from the savings account through the checking account, so there will be a record of the transaction. For example, if $10 is to be added to the savings account, deposit it in the checking account and write a check for $10 payable to the savings account. In this way, a record of all the Group money will be available in the checking account records.

If the Group has a savings account, the Treasurer needs to report this total on the annual financial report.

Income and expense record sheets

Income and expense record sheets provide a breakdown of all the money the Group receives and pays out each month. You and the Treasurer can then see the Group's overall financial picture at a glance and can recognize trends when they occur.

You can use accounting paper found at stores selling office supplies, paper with lines drawn to divide it into columns, or the sample income and expense sheets in Appendix 2. You may instead prefer to use a ledger or a computer program (printing a copy for your records). The column headings on the income/expense record sheets correspond to the entries on the annual financial report form.

(See **Appendix 2** for sample **Income and Expense Record Sheets.**)

Keeping Track of Group Income

> All money collected by the Group should be receipted, recorded, and deposited n the Group account as soon as possible.

Whenever the Treasurer receives income as cash or check, she writes out a receipt, using the carbon paper in the receipt book to make a copy. The carbon copies provide the Treasurer with an important permanent record. If Leaders have books or other items on hand to sell between meetings, be sure everyone has a receipt book, so that each sale is recorded. Include the date, the person's name and telephone number, the amount received, whether it was cash or check, the check number, and what was purchased.

As a safe accounting practice, have two people, one a Leader, count together cash income from a fundraising event. Write down the total cash amount, using a receipt form, and have both sign the form. The Treasurer then has a record of the amount raised that she can check against the amount banked.

Deposit all money collected by the Group in the Group checking account as soon as possible. Keep the deposit receipt with a full explanation of the money being deposited. Enter the deposit in the checkbook register.

Enter all income on the income record sheet: date of transaction, total amount of money received, and the name of the person from whom it was received. In the appropriate column to the right of the double vertical line, enter the amounts for each item sold, sales tax collected, or miscellaneous money received. Use a new line for each transaction, not for each item. If a Group must collect sales tax on items sold, record it in a column separate from the item sold, to make totalling easier when taxes are due to the government.

If money is needed from a savings account to pay for a special project, transfer it immediately into the checking account and write a check for the amount needed. Record this amount under the "savings account" column of the income record sheet. For every deposit the Treasurer should have a double record: a notation in the checkbook register and an entry on the income record sheet listing what each deposit was for.

Keeping Track of Group Expenses

Before writing a check be sure that there is sufficient money in the account. Service charges are payable on checks that are returned for any reason.

When you write the check, remember to:

- Make the check payable to the correct name.
- Avoid post-dating the check unless this is common business practice in your country.
- Be sure the Group name, Group bank account number, and invoice numbers are on the check.
- Write the names of members on the memo line or on the back of the check if the check is for membership.
- Be sure the check is signed by two people, one of whom is a Leader.

After a check is written, enter it in the checkbook register and on the expense record sheet. If the item being paid for is not in a category listed on the sheet, note it under "miscellaneous." If it falls into a category already listed, record it under the appropriate heading. If the check pays for an invoice that includes several different items, list each item in its appropriate category across the same line of the sheet. When paying an invoice, record the invoice number in the "paid to" column.

When all the columns are added up, the sheet will provide a record of how much the Group spends in each category.

For every check written, the Treasurer should have a double record: a notation in the checkbook register and an entry on the expense record sheet listing what was purchased. The Group Treasurer should also keep copies of paid invoices.

Pay all bills within 30 days. Write the Group name and account number and the invoice number or members' names on all checks to your Area, your Affiliate, or LLLI. If you wish to make several payments on one check, please indicate on the check or a separate sheet of paper what the check is for. When the bank statement arrives each month, compare the cancelled checks or list of checks to the expense record sheet and balance the bank statement.

Once a month, draw a horizontal line across the page under the last transaction in both the income and expense record sheets. Some Groups use the last day of the calendar month, others use the date of the Series or Evaluation Meeting. Total all columns to find the income and expenses for the month. The amount in the "total" column (to the left of the double vertical line) should equal the total of the amounts of all columns to the right of the double vertical line. Use a separate sheet each month for easier, more simplified bookkeeping.

Check with the Area or Affiliate Treasurer or Financial Coordinator about any sales tax requirements and when reports are due.

Annual Financial Report

An Annual Financial Report is required for each Group and is easier to do if accounts have been kept up-to-date each month.

An Annual Financial Report is required for each Group. (See **Appendix 2** for a sample form.) To complete the report, at the end of the fiscal year, go back to the totals for each month on the income and expense sheets and add all twelve numbers together for the appropriate entry on the Annual Financial Report. For example, the twelve monthly totals in the membership column, added together, give an annual total for membership income. In addition to income and expenses, the Treasurer will be asked to list several other aspects of Group finances, including unpaid bills, inventory, savings account balance, and Group assets.

Keep one copy of your Annual Financial Report in the permanent Group records and provide copies for your support Leader and your Area, your LLL Office, and LLLI, if applicable.

Handling Petty Cash

To avoid writing checks for small expenses, some Groups keep petty cash on hand. Petty cash can be extremely difficult to account for, so keep amounts low and use a separate accurate recording system. The Group Treasurer writes a check to "cash" and keeps the money in an envelope marked "Petty Cash." Keep petty cash separate from income received at the meeting and from the Treasurer's personal money.

For easier bookkeeping, keep petty cash at a set amount, such as $10. If there is $10 at the beginning, the receipts for expenses plus the money left in the envelope should always equal $10.

Keep all petty cash receipts and record them under the proper heading (postage, supplies, etc.) on the expense record sheet for the Annual Financial Report.

Keeping an Inventory Record

An inventory helps the Group determine what materials need to be ordered and shows what items the Group uses most frequently. If someone other than the Treasurer keeps the inventory, she will need to consult with the Treasurer each month to determine what was sold. (See **Appendix 2** for a **Sample Inventory Record.**)

To use the inventory record, fill in the names of items the Group normally has on hand in the left-hand column. Fill in the quantity of each item on hand at the beginning of the month (equal to the balance at the end of the previous month). Record the number of items sold during the month and the number the Group purchased. Calculate the balance on hand at the end of the month (stock – sold + purchased = balance) and the date. Every few months, check the inventory record against the actual number of items the Group has on hand to be sure the record is accurate.

Processing Membership Dues

1. Give the mother a subscription/membership form or card and receipt. If the mother is not attending meetings, the Treasurer can mail these items to her.
2. Send the new member's details; (name, mailing address, telephone number, category of membership) and "new" or "renew" on the appropriate form or card to your Area or Affiliate along with the payment, according to the dues breakdown or process used in your Area/Affiliate/Division. (See **Appendix 3.**)

3. Send memberships in promptly. Remember, new members are waiting to receive their member publication.

4. Enter new members on your master address/active list or database, the checkbook register, the income record sheet, and on the Group monthly report form.

5. Although members are responsible for notifying LLL of any change of mailing address, you may want to remind members to do this.

Promoting Membership at Meetings

Promoting membership makes good sense, both for mothers and for La Leche League. As a member, a mother receives the benefit of ongoing contact with LLL. Even if she no longer attends Series Meetings, she may receive a member publication, which will continue to offer her information and encouragement.

Members may also receive a catalogue and may be able to order publications at a discount. Income received from membership fees is vital to the future of the Area, the Group, the Division/Affiliate, and LLLI.

Be positive. Let participants know that there are expenses involved in running a Group and that their memberships are necessary to meet those expenses.

Give people something tangible to take home. Many Groups give out newcomer packets with special materials for participants who are attending their first meeting and a member's packet when a member pays her dues. Some Groups give coupons for book purchases from the Group.

Highlight member publications. Pass copies around during the meeting so people can see what they will get when they become members. The Librarian or other members could mention articles or columns they enjoy. Some Groups offer a past issue as part of the new member packet. Back issues may be available on request from your LLL office, with a book order at no charge or for the cost of shipping and handling.

Give mothers a written list of the benefits of membership. Put information about membership into every newcomer packet. Explain the benefits of membership.

Discuss membership and/or make a poster listing membership benefits. Let participants know that, if they are not ready to pay at the meeting, they can mail their checks to the Leader or Treasurer any time during the month. Keep self-addressed return envelopes on hand for this purpose. Some Groups' bank accounts may allow them to accept credit card payments for membership.

Recognize new members. Some Groups present membership cards/or small gifts to mothers who paid the previous month. This thanks new members and shows newcomers that most mothers who attend meetings are members. (See **Appendix 3.**)

Give member discounts as an incentive. Your LLL office may offer discounts to members when they order books directly. Many Groups offer this as well. Some Groups set a special member's price for THE WOMANLY ART OF BREASTFEEDING.

Draw attention to the Group Treasurer. Introduce her at the beginning of the meeting and offer a reminder at the end of the meeting. The Treasurer can station herself in a conspicuous, convenient spot after the meeting so participants can find her and see others buying books and paying memberships. Identify the Treasurer with a special nametag, so people will know who she is.

MANAGING GROUP

Promoting membership makes good sense for mothers and for La Leche League and gives mothers the benefit of ongoing contact with LLL.

Remind people about renewing their memberships. Put a reminder on a mother's meeting notice when it's time to renew, or send a separate renewal notice.

Mention that Leaders are volunteers and pay dues as well. Compare the cost of membership to other costs. For example:

> *"Feeding artificial baby milk for one week costs $_____ while membership in LLL for an entire year costs only $_____."*

> *"A one year LLL membership costs only $___ per month."*

Explain tangible ways the Group benefits from paid memberships. For example,

> *"We would like to thank those of you who paid membership. Thanks to your support, we have added these books to the Group Library: (name books)."*

> *"La Leche League services are free, but it costs money to deliver them to you. Your membership and donations help make LLL support and information available throughout the world every day of the year."*

Emphasize that membership ensures the future of LLL. Remind mothers that LLL is there to answer questions and provide information when they need breastfeeding help. By paying dues, they are helping to ensure that LLL will continue to be available to future generations of mothers.

(See **Appendix 3** for more information about encouraging memberships.)

KEEPING TRACK OF MATERIALS
Organizing Leader Materials

Each Leader organizes her materials to fit her personal style and the space available to her. Easy access needs to be a top priority.

Since a Leader's office is her home and most LLL work is accomplished in the course of daily activities, some Leaders keep materials where the family congregates. Others prefer to keep telephone helping materials near the telephone and other materials where they are out of sight until needed.

Leader materials

You might organize your Leader materials in five major categories corresponding to the basic responsibilities of leadership:

One-to-one helping materials

- LLL Leader's Log
- Meeting notices
- Supply of pamphlets and tear-off sheets for mothers

Meeting materials

- Series Meeting ideas
- Outlines or ideas for special meetings
- Enrichment topic ideas

Group management materials

- Catalogue and Leader order form

> Since a Leader's "office" is her home some Leaders keep materials in the kitchen or where the family congregates.

- Financial records, annual financial report
- Group Workers' names and phone numbers
- Group job descriptions
- Monthly Report Forms
- Membership list
- Support Leader correspondence

References

- THE WOMANLY ART OF BREASTFEEDING
- THE LEADER'S HANDBOOK
- THE BREASTFEEDING ANSWER BOOK
- Pamphlets and tear-off sheets
- Leader and Member publications
- Local Directory and other directories as applicable
- Articles filed by topic

MANAGING GROUP

Leader applicant materials

- *Becoming a La Leche League Leader*
- Leader Application Packet (current)
- Leader Accreditation Department representative correspondence
- Articles from LLL publications

Systems of Organization

Most Leaders find that their system evolves along with their involvement in LLL. Consider the advantages of these organizers:

- **Bookshelf**—a place you can keep references handy.
- **File cabinet**—files can be labeled and kept in alphabetical order.
- **File box**—takes up only a small space; can be carried by handles; additional boxes can be added.
- **Periodical file box**—keeps issues in order vertically; each periodical can be filed in its own box.
- **Ring binder**—materials can be rearranged and added to easily; portable.
- **Pocket folders**—inexpensive; portable.
- **File basket**—handy for to do and/or to read materials.
- **Tote bag**—can be packed and ready to go.

Tips for Organizing Selected LLL Materials:

1. **Leader and member publications—try storing these in ring binders or vertical file boxes.** Some publications have an annual index (often in the December issue) that is handy to photocopy and store in front as a cumulative index.
2. **Pamphlets and tear-off sheets**—these can be sorted numerically using the catalogue, alphabetically by title, or according to topics. They can be stored in portable file boxes, plastic sleeves, ring binders, or individual envelopes.

    In some Groups, a Group member, Secretary, or Librarian, keeps the pamphlets, and Leaders phone her when something needs to be mailed out to a mother. Or a Chapter may decide that one person will handle mailing for all the Groups. This job does not have to be done by a Leader.

3. **Leader's Log**—LLL Leaders may be required to use standard Leader's log systems provided by their National/Affiliate/Divisional/International organization. The sheets come punched so they can be kept indefinitely in chronological order in a binder. Others use their own system of record keeping using a notebook or exercise book. Whatever you use, it needs to be a permanent, accurate record of your helping contacts, and it needs to be easily accessible whenever the telephone rings.
(See **Chapter 1,** page 17 and **Appendix 4** for a sample log sheet.

4. **Meeting ideas**—Some Leaders like to keep two sets of files for each of the four meetings. In the first set of files they keep ideas from workshops and LLL publications that they plan to try. In the second set they keep the outlines, cards, visuals, etc., that they have used at meetings and that they might use again. Many Leaders keep additional files for special meeting ideas (Toddler, Couples, Teen, Employed Mothers) as well as enrichment topics.

5. **Handouts, outlines, articles**—Filing information by topic can make retrieval easier. For example, you might want to keep a photocopy of an article on jaundice in a file together with other articles and conference handouts on the subject. Make a new file for a topic that doesn't fit perfectly with the files already established. For example, it may be easier to find "crank calls" in a file of its own, rather than in the "telephone helping" file.

6. **Reports, correspondence**—You may also find it helpful to have separate files for Group business such as monthly Group report forms, correspondence with support or resource Leaders, completed financial reports, etc. Remember to print hard copies for your files if you use email to communicate.

7. **Directories and contact lists**—You might want to keep the Area directory, national directory, Group membership list, Group worker list, and other contact information all in one file.

8. **Forms, notices, lists**—Some Leaders keep multiple copies of forms and notices together in labeled files: monthly meeting report, income and expense sheets, Annual Financial Report forms, current meeting notice, hostess letter, Group job descriptions, etc.

9. **Ordering information**—This file might contain a current catalogue with potential purchases noted, Leader Order Forms, copies of previous orders, Group Library inventory. (See **Appendix 2** for ordering information.)

10. **Leader applicant materials**—Many Leaders keep a supply of LLL publications on hand for mothers interested in leadership, as well as articles and checklists for working with Leader Applicants. A separate file for each Applicant can hold correspondence to and from the Leader Accreditation Department representative.

Handling information

Here are some suggestions for managing the information that you handle on a regular basis, for instance Series Meeting materials, monthly meeting reports, and LLL publications.

- **Sooner is better than later**—Try to take care of things while your memory is fresh and before small piles become big stacks. Continually strive to move things toward their final place in your filing system.
- **Have a plan**—Develop a sorting system. One possibility could be to have a to do and/or a to read basket. You could keep a tote bag filled and ready to go; some Leaders have separate tote bags for Group, Chapter, and Area work. Some Leaders find that sticking to a routine keeps them on top of responsibilities. Many Leaders like to jot down notes for the Evaluation Meeting as soon as they return from the Series Meetings.
- **Keep reminders in view**—It can help to make lists and prioritize things according to when they need to be completed (today, this week, this month) or use a ranking system (must do, should do, could do) as headings. Some people find it helps to leave things in sight—but not allow piles to accumulate—until they are completed.

For example, keep the Group order on the kitchen counter until it is filled out and sent in. (See **Appendix 2**.)

Group Libraries

LLLI-published books and other selections from the Group Library reinforce the information and support Leaders offer and can help a mother explore many facets of breastfeeding, childbirth, nutrition, and parenting. Each LLL Group provides a lending library of books approved for this purpose. (See **Appendix 1—Bibliography: LLLI**.)

The Group Librarian

The job of Group Librarian has many benefits and satisfactions. The Librarian has access to all the books and back issues of member publications that the Group has on hand. She also has an opportunity to recommend new books that might interest mothers. At Series Meetings, the Librarian has a chance to meet the newcomers and help them find books to meet their needs.

The Group Librarian usually:

- Sets up the Group Library for display at Series Meetings
- Helps mothers find and check out books at meetings
- Keeps track of book circulation: replaces the sign-out card when books are returned, follows up on overdue books
- Can give a brief presentation at meetings on a new book or a book pertaining to the discussion topic
- Keeps a card catalogue or inventory list of all books that belong to the Group
- Prepares new books for the Library: adds a protective cover, affixes LLL reviews or qualifying statements inside, installs a pocket for the sign-out card, adds new book information to the inventory list

MANAGING GROUP

Each LLL Group provides a lending library of books to reinforce the information and support the Leaders provide to mothers.

- Buys library supplies when needed in consultation with a Group Leader; submits receipts to the Group Treasurer for reimbursement
- Repairs worn books and circulation pockets
- Attends Evaluation Meetings

Group Library supplies

Librarian's notebook or file

- Photocopy of this section of THE LEADER'S HANDBOOK
- Catalogue and order form. (See **Appendix 2** for information about ordering)
- Group Library inventory list or card catalogue
- List of books the Group would like to order when money is available

Supply box

- Book cover material
- Book pockets and index cards for making sign-out cards
- Index cards for catalogue or inventory notebook
- Tape for repairing books and pockets
- Magazine holders for the member publication, ring binder
- Copies of book reviews (from Leader or member publications) and summaries and qualifying statements from LLL Bibliographies
- Group identification stickers or rubber stamp with Leaders' phone numbers

Selecting books for the Group Library

Start with the basics. Each Group Library should contain at least one copy of the latest edition of THE WOMANLY ART OF BREASTFEEDING in one or more languages suitable to the Leaders and mothers of that Group. Also include a nutrition-oriented book such as WHOLE FOODS FOR THE WHOLE FAMILY .

Each Group library should contain at least one copy of THE WOMANLY ART OF BREASTFEEDING and if possible a nutrition book, a parenting book and a book on childbirth.

A book that presents an overview of childbirth and a book on parenting that supports the LLLI concept of loving guidance complete the basic Group Library.

Next consider LLLI-published books. These books are identified in the catalogue and listed separately on the Leader Order Form. Watch your Leader and member publications and the LLLI Web site for announcements of new books published by LLLI.

LLL-published books most fully reflect LLL philosophy; they are the only books recommended by LLL without reservation. Choose additional books from those that have been reviewed and approved for the LLL Bibliographies. (See **LLL Bibliographies,** page 163.)

Reviewers consider a book's content and presentation in light of LLL philosophy and information.

- How does this book agree with and reinforce La Leche League's purpose, philosophy, and mission?
- How does this book provide new information that supports or broadens the reader's understanding of LLL's purpose, philosophy, or mission? How does it compare with other books on the subject?
- Does it promote a cause in a way that would detract from LLL's basic focus on mothering through breastfeeding?

- Does the book conflict with LLL's purpose, philosophy, and mission?
- What makes this an outstanding book for LLL?

More information about the book evaluation process is available on the LLLI Web site or from your support Leader.

Book summaries are included in the LLLI Bibliography (available on the LLLI Web site) or in Affiliate/ID bibliographies. You can use the LLL Bibliographies to select titles that best suit the needs and interests of mothers who attend Group meetings. Not every book will be appropriate for every LLL Group worldwide, and some books on the LLLI Bibliography have not been approved for use in Affiliates or the International Division. Check your order form; if a book is not carried at your National/Affiliate/Divisional office, contact your support Leader or the Publications Administrator to see if the book is approved for use in Group Libraries. The Bibliography summaries also include disclaimer statements pointing out areas where books depart significantly from LLLI philosophy or approach. Placing copies of the disclaimers on the inside cover of all books that are accepted with qualifications will help clarify LLL information and philosophy for readers.

Many otherwise excellent books have some information that is outdated or not in accord with LLL information. Here is a qualifying statement you can use:

> *Please be aware that the author(s) may present ideas that are different from those you will find in La Leche League publications or that La Leche League supports.*

You might want to post a general statement like this beside the library books. Or you may be able to order pre-printed labels from your LLL office for no charge or make you own. You can decide whether a qualifying statement would be helpful in general or only necessary in specific instances.

Every so often a mother will offer to donate a book. Quite naturally, she may not know about our policy regarding Group Library books. If the book is recently published and one that might be of interest to Leaders and mothers, you can contact your support Leader or Publications Department representative, who can recommend evaluation of the book. The evaluation committee will need review copies from the publisher or individual who wants the book considered.

Funding additions to the Group Library

Groups can add to their library collections in many ways:

- Set aside money in the Group Treasury from membership and book sales for book purchases. Some Groups set a goal of adding one new book to the collection per series of meetings. The Librarian can keep a list of books the Group is interested in purchasing.
- Rather than using money from the Group's general fund, some Groups designate the profits of a particular fundraiser for library books.
- Many Groups place book orders with a neighboring Group or through a Chapter to qualify for quantity discounts and share shipping costs.
- Some Groups make a "wish list" of books they would like to add to their Libraries. The Librarian can talk briefly about a book or two during the business portion of the Series Meeting. A mother or several mothers might

want to contribute to the Group by helping to purchase a book they are interested in. You can acknowledge their sponsorship with a special bookplate.

- Some Groups have found success with an appeal letter to local businesses. They send a letter explaining the lending library service that the Group provides as well as a book wish list to businesses that serve parents. Businesses choose the book they would like to donate and you can acknowledge their sponsorship with a special bookplate.
NOTE: Be sure that the businesses you approach are those from which LLL can accept goods and services. If you have any questions or concerns about a business, consult your support Leader.

- Purchasing a library book is one way to use an honorarium received for an outside speaking engagement by a Leader or a mother's offer of payment for a Leader's services. As volunteers, Leaders do not accept payment for the help they provide.

Preparing a new book for the Group Library

When you receive a new book for the Group Library:

- Prepare the book for borrowing by filling out a sign-out card or a lending card with columns for the title, author, book number if used, date, borrower's name and phone number.
- Attach LLL Group identification. Some Groups print or type on the book pocket; some use labels or a rubber stamp. Include Group name, Leader name(s) and phone number(s), length of time the book may be borrowed, any special information, such as book number. Use a system that can be updated easily, because Leaders and telephone numbers may change over time.
- Affix an LLL book summary, review, or qualifying statement inside the front cover.
- List the book in the Group Library inventory or add to the card catalogue. An inventory helps Groups keep track of the Group Library collection. It can be kept on paper, on cards, or on a computer. The permanent record should include title, author, publisher, copyright date, book number/code (if the Group owns more than one copy of a title), date added to library, purchase price, donor(s).
- Protect the book with a permanent cover.

Identifying books to encourage returns

Mark each book with the Group's name, a phone number and address for easy return.

In addition to marking each book with the Group name and Leader name(s) and phone number(s), here are some suggestions to consider as you prepare books for the Group Library:

- Include a special message. Some Groups add a message on the inside cover:

  "We are delighted to share our books with you. Since other mothers look forward to reading them too, we would appreciate your cooperation in returning this book after one month. Thank you."

- Using a marking pen, print "LLL" across page edges on all three sides of the closed book. The writing is very noticeable and a reminder to the borrower each time she sees it that the book needs to be returned.

- Put a strip of colored tape across the bottom of the book spine. The Group Library book will stand out from her own if the borrower puts it in her bookshelf at home.
- Include a mailing label or envelope addressed to Group name, Leader or Librarian. Mark it book or library rate if a cheaper rate is available for this service. Groups in areas where mothers travel long distances to meetings might find this method helpful.

Following up on overdue books

Although it is the responsibility of the mother who borrows a book to see that it gets back to the Group Library, you or the Librarian may need to call a mother to remind her or even go to her home on occasion to retrieve the book.

Before and after meetings, you or the librarian can check the sign-out system to see if the book should have been returned at that meeting; if so, make a note about it.

A book that is not returned in one month is not alarming, especially if the mother was not able to attend the meeting. A few days before the next meeting, when a book would be a month overdue, the Group Librarian can give the borrower a reminder call or send a written reminder note. If the mother is not able to attend that meeting, she might be able to give the book to someone who will.

If the borrower moves out of town, the Group Librarian or Leader can write to tell her that others are waiting to read the book. Ask her to wrap it well and send it back.

As a last resort, if reminder efforts fail to bring a book back, a form letter detailing the cost of replacing the book may be necessary.

Displaying books at meetings

An attractive and organized Group Library display draws people to the table and helps them locate books of interest. Select from these ideas to make your Library inviting:

- Place books face up so the covers are easy to see. This can be a good way to display THE WOMANLY ART OF BREASTFEEDING, the books pertaining to the meeting topic, new books, and frequently borrowed titles.
- Set books up on end, spine facing out, with bookends to hold them together. Soft fabric glued to the bottom of the bookends will protect the tabletop. A piece of rubber-like material, cut the same shape as the bottom of the bookends, can prevent sliding. With two different bottom linings, bookends can be used on a variety of surfaces.
- A collapsible bookrack offers an advantage over bookends, because books are less likely to slide when one is removed.
- Cardboard or plastic crates save set-up time. Place books in the crates so the titles on the spines can be read and carry them to and from meetings right in the crates. Paint or cover a cardboard box with colorful paper to hide any printed advertising. A crate system easily expands as a Group Library collection expands.

MANAGING GROUP

Remind mothers about overdue books on a regular basis.

An attractive and organized Group Library display helps people locate books of interest.

Sample Overdue Book Letter

LLL of Anytown_____

Address_____

Date_____

Mother's name_____

Address _____

Dear _____

Our records show that you borrowed the LLL of (Group Name)'s copy of (book title) on (date borrowed). It is ____ months overdue. We will appreciate your taking time to return the book so it can be available for other mothers who may need the information in it.

If you are not able to bring the book to the next meeting on (date), please call (Librarian) at (phone number) or (Leader) at (phone number) to make other arrangements. Or mail the book to (Librarian), (address) or (Leader), (address).

If the book is lost or you would like to keep it, please send $_____ to cover the cost of replacing it. Thank you.

Sincerely,

Leader's signature

Book title: _____

LLL Catalogue price $_____

Shipping and handling $_____

Library supplies $_____

Total $_____

Encouraging Group Library use

Categorize the Group Library

LLL materials generally fall into these main categories: breastfeeding, childbirth, nutrition, and parenting. Children's books might be another possible category. Categorizing books makes it easier for both mothers and Leaders to find what they're looking for.

Categorizing can be as simple as putting books on the same topic next to each other between bookends or using four crates or boxes to separate books into the four topics. Some Groups add colored tape or dot labels to the book spines to signify one of the four categories, and display a small card or sign showing the color key.

Highlight individual books

Another way to encourage Library use is to feature one or more books at each meeting. Basic books, new books, books that pertain to the meeting topic, favorite books, books that haven't been taken out in a while all can be highlighted by displaying them in a special way on the library table or by mentioning them during the meeting.

> If your Group Library becomes large, you may need to highlight the basic books

Consider these ideas:

If the Group Library is set up using bookends, a bookrack, or crates, you can display several books face up in front of the others to catch attention. You can display featured books on top of colorful background paper or placemats or use small easels or stands to prop them up. If you have a bulletin or display board, you might post quotes from specific books.

You or the Librarian could talk about a featured book during the announcement portion of the meeting or at the end of the meeting as you remind participants to stop by the library table. Consider reading a quote from the book with a brief review.

Many Leaders note on their meeting outline which Group Library books to mention. Hold up one or two books and pass them around the room at appropriate points in the discussion. Encourage Group members to mention books they have read and found helpful.

If the Group Library collection becomes large, you may need to highlight the basic books so newcomers are aware of them and do not overlook them. Mention THE WOMANLY ART OF BREASTFEEDING, WHOLE FOODS FOR THE WHOLE FAMILY and basic books on childbirth and parenting

Display your LLL member publication. The Listed Leader of each Group receives the Group Library copy of the member publication. Highlight the current issue at Series Meetings, perhaps pointing out an article, a book review or a new breastfeeding research report. Point out that receiving this kind of information on a regular basis can be a significant benefit of LLL membership.

Placing the Group Library copies in a ring binder makes it easier for the collection to circulate like a book. Plastic magazine holders eliminate hole punching and make issues easy to page through. Some Groups keep the current year's issues in one binder and the previous year's in another.

LLLI Pamphlets, Brochures, and Tear-Off Sheets

Currrent LLL pamphlets, brochures, and tear-off sheets are listed numerically on the Leader Order Form.

LLL pamphlets and tear-off sheets cover common concerns or special circumstances and provide an easy and concise way to offer specific information. As new information becomes available, publications are added, discontinued, or revised. Check your current catalogue or Leader publication for updated information on these.

Other LLL publications include promotional brochures, flyers, directories, and catalogues. Many of these are available free or for the cost of shipping and handling.

Introductory packets of information

One way to introduce women to the wide variety of information available from LLL is give each person a welcome packet at her first meeting. You can fill a folder, envelope, or small bag with publications such as:

- A catalogue
- An introductory brochure about LLL
- An introductory pamphlet about the benefits of membership

MANAGING GROUP

One way to introduce women to the wide variety of information available from LLL is to give out welcome packets.

- Basic pamphlets and tear-off sheets pertaining to the needs of new breastfeeding mothers
- A Group Series Meeting notice
- A sample of your LLL member publication

Be sure to stamp or write the name and telephone number of the Group Leader(s) on each piece of information.

Some Groups vary the contents of the welcome packet, giving different information to pregnant newcomers and those with older babies.

Include only LLL materials in these packets.

Ideas for Organizing and Displaying LLL Pamphlets, Brochures and Tear-Off Sheets at Series Meetings

1. Place pamphlets and tear-off sheets in ring binders, individual envelopes, or plastic pockets.
2. Divide the materials to suit Series Meeting topics or helping topics.
3. Display them in the pockets on a bulletin/display board.

Fee or free?

Because of their cost and sturdiness, books and booklets belong in the Group Library. You might also want to offer selected, popular titles for sale.

A new Group or one with limited income may ask mothers to pay for pamphlets. Some mothers may find it more economical to buy a copy of THE WOMANLY ART OF BREASTFEEDING than to purchase individual publications.

LLL offers such a wide variety of pamphlets that it may not be practical or affordable to display them all or give them all away. A Group may want to keep one of each in the Group Library and sell or give away only those with widest appeal.

Leader use of pamphlets and tear-off sheets

Many Leaders keep a supply of basic LLL publications on hand

- for reference as they are planning Series Meetings,
- to send to mothers who call with questions, to reinforce or add to the information and suggestions they cover during the telephone helping calls, usually with a Series Meeting notice and membership information, and
- for use at a Series Meeting, to refer a mother to an answer to a question on a specific breastfeeding situation, especially if it is not related to the meeting topic.

Ordering pamphlets, brochures, and tear-off sheets

It can be helpful if one Group worker or Leader is responsible for keeping track of the LLL publications the Group has and uses.

Keep only a few of the less-requested sheets in stock to reduce the chances of ending up with outdated publications.

- Check Library and welcome packet supplies after each meeting; check with each Leader about her phone-helping supply at the Evaluation Meeting. Reorder as needed.

- Check supplies at the end of each series; reorder in bulk quantities. Neighboring Groups or Groups in a Chapter might want to combine orders to save time and money.
- Order popular publications in bulk and those in less demand individually. Since publications are revised often, keep only a few of the less-requested sheets in stock to reduce the chances of ending up with outdated publications.

SPECIAL GROUP SITUATIONS

Starting a new Group

The Area Coordinator of Leaders is responsible for the inauguration of all Groups in the Area.

MANAGING GROUP

New Groups can be formed in several ways:

- A new Leader starts a new Group when she is accredited.
- A Leader who moves may decide to start a new Group in her new community if it doesn't have one or if travel to meetings of her original Group is difficult.
- A large Group splits into two Groups or a Leader starts a new Group in a neighboring community.

If a Leader Applicant plans to start a new Group, she informs the Leader Accreditation Department representative while they are corresponding during the application for leadership. When she is accredited, the new Leader's support person in the Leader Department helps her with her plans for starting and leading a new Group.

A welcome from the Area

Your support Leader will welcome you as a Leader. From this point on, you can turn to your support Leader for help getting started. Many Areas send "New Group Kits" that include a directory of Groups, Leaders, Area resource Leaders, and the forms used by Groups in the Area.

Naming a new Group

It is important to consult with your support Leader before deciding on a name for a new Group. In some cases, certain formats are needed for insurance purposes. For mothers seeking a Group, it is helpful if the Group name reflects your geographical location.

For mothers seeking a Group, it is helpful if your Group name reflects your geographical location.

Support for new Groups

Some financial help and other assistance may be given to new Groups, such as:

- A listing in the LLLI, Area and Affiliate/National directory of Groups;
- A certificate of affiliation for its first year;
- Group ordering information from LLLI or the appropriate LLL office;
- A subscription to the member publication sent to the Listed Leader for the new Group Library;

- A "New Group Kit" which contains pamphlets and tear-off sheets that have been found to be especially helpful when starting a Group; and
- Help from a sister Group program that operates in some Areas or Divisions.

A new LLL Group may be able to have some of its setting up expenses charged on account. Before buying books for the Group Library check with the Area. Many Areas lend or give new Groups a starter library of basic books. An established Group or Chapter may also be willing to "adopt" a new Group while it is starting out. Check with the Area Coordinator of Leaders.

Each Group pays a yearly Group affiliation fee to LLL. A new Group, however, is excused from the Group affiliation dues for the year in which it is formed. After the first year, the new Group will be charged the annual Group affiliation fee for the upcoming calendar year.

New Group Treasury

Open a checking account in the Group's name as soon as possible, so that Group funds will be kept separate from your personal funds.

As funds accumulate, you will want to buy more books for the Library and add to the supply of LLL pamphlets. Whenever possible, send full payment with each order. (See **Keeping Track of Money—The Group Treasury,** pages 105-114 for other financial essentials.)

New Group Library

Keep it simple. Check with the Area about the availability of a starter collection of basic Group Library books. At first, you may want to include some of your personal copies of LLL books in the Group Library. You can clearly mark these and replace them with books purchased for the Library as Group funds become available.

Display samples of pamphlets and a catalogue in a prominent place so meeting participants can see that additional books and other publications and products are available from LLL.

A new Group's introductory packets

Initially, you may want to use low-cost items such as copies of the catalogue, membership information, and perhaps some tear-off sheets to make up welcome packets for mothers attending their first meeting.

New Group publicity

You might let women know there's a new LLL Group in the community in the following ways:

- Invite friends and acquaintances to get together.
- Announce the formation of the Group in the newspaper. Include an invitation for interested mothers to call you for more information.
- Distribute LLL posters and meeting notices to locations in the community.
- Distribute meeting notices and/or LLL brochures to health care providers.

- If the Area Coordinator of Leaders or your support Leader knows of people in the area who have requested LLL literature or indicated an interest in LLL, send a meeting notice letting them know that a Group is forming.

(See **Publicity—Helping Others Keep Track of LLL,** pages 97-105 for more on publicity.)

The first meeting

For the first meeting, it can be helpful to meet in someone else's home or a public place, so that you do not have to both lead the discussion and act as hostess. Aim for a central location to draw women from different areas.

Welcome each person at the door. No matter how many or how few mothers attend, your warmth and interest are important.

Begin on time and allow plenty of time for introductions. Tell something about yourself, the local Group, and LLL. Invite participants to tell about themselves, their families, whether they've breastfed a baby and mention what interests or questions bring them to a La Leche League meeting.

You may need to provide some simple, nutritious refreshments for the first meeting. After that, ask for volunteers.

End the meeting on time and remind mothers about purchasing memberships and THE WOMANLY ART OF BREASTFEEDING. Invite all to come to the next meeting and bring friends.

Monthly Group report

As soon after the meeting as possible, complete the Group Report and send it to your support Leader, who as an experienced Leader with wide knowledge of many Groups, can give you support and guidance. When the Group has one or two workers, you may decide to write the Group report together at the Evaluation Meeting.

The goal of La Leche League is to help each mother achieve a happy breastfeeding experience. Whether a mother is one of many at a meeting, or the only one to attend, she and her baby are important. If just one mother breastfeeds her baby because of the new Group, your efforts have been worthwhile. Your enthusiasm and attention can help the Group grow, one mother at a time.

Lone Leadership

Many Leaders around the world lead LLL Groups alone and some lone Leaders enjoy the challenge and the often hidden advantages.

- Lone leading gives you a chance to develop your own leading style.
- Lone leading is an opportunity to develop a consistent meeting atmosphere.
- Decision-making is simplified. You do not have other Leaders to confer with.

It is helpful to meet in someone else's home or a public place, so that you do not have to both lead the discussion and act as hostess.

MANAGING GROUP

If just one mother breastfeeds her baby because of the new Group, your efforts have been worthwhile.

Make the most of regular attendees

- Make finding and working with Group workers a top priority. Look for potential and interest in leadership.
- Schedule regular Evaluation Meetings. They can provide support and encouragement in planning and problem solving. Seek opinions from Group workers and encourage them to offer ideas for how the Group can be improved.

Streamline Group work

Here are some suggestions to help keep your work mother-sized:

- Concentrate on basic responsibilities.
- Keep meeting plans and preparations simple.
- Avoid procrastination; spread your LLL work throughout the month rather than trying to do everything just before the meeting.
- Schedule the Evaluation Meeting and finish the Group report while the meeting is fresh in your memory.
- Try combining Evaluation Meetings with fun activities such as a picnic or trip to the park. It may take longer to get the business done, but you will evaluate the meeting, make plans for the next one, and complete the Group report as you socialize, and everyone participates in an activity with their children.
- Handle phone calls efficiently, sending an LLL pamphlet or catalogue as follow-up to save time.

Use LLL resources

Use your printed and people resources to learn more, maintain your energy and enthusiasm, and to stimulate your creativity.

Keep in close contact with your support Leader, ask for help with difficulties, and let her know your needs.

Use your Leader publications as a source of inspiration, encouragement, and connection with other Leaders.

- Try to obtain new books and LLL publications. If cost is prohibitive, see if the local library will order books on request.
- Review the basics in THE LEADER'S HANDBOOK.
- Attend Chapter meetings, if available, to network with other Leaders. (See **Chapter Meetings** in Chapter 6, page 167.)
- Attend LLL workshops and conferences to keep up on meeting ideas, breastfeeding research, and current LLL information. (See **Continuing Education Events for Leaders** in Chapter 6, page 166.)
- Visit another Group, if possible, to give you new perspectives and ideas.
- Remember lone leadership is usually temporary. The Leader Accreditation Department representative can offer ideas and information for helping mothers find out about leadership and prepare to become LLL Leaders.

Keep careful track of money

As a lone Leader, you are responsible for all financial aspects of the Group. Though you might consult with Group members regarding decisions related to spending money, the ultimate responsibility for fulfilling the financial requirements falls on you. Be thoroughly familiar with the information in the section, **Keeping Track of Money—The Group Treasury,** pages 105-114.

Plan ahead so you will have money to pay Group bills. Keep accurate records and record all transactions promptly. Consult your support Leader or Area/Affiliate Treasurer or Financial Coordinator if you have questions or need ideas.

Keep expectations realistic

- Set realistic goals according to the basic responsibilities of leadership. As a lone Leader you can accomplish only so much; too high expectations may result in frustration.
- Concentrate on the positive, long-term effects of the Group. Feel good about the individual help you offer one-to-one and at Series Meetings.

Remember that there really is no such thing as a lone Leader. There are thousands of Leaders all over the world. Some Leader somewhere is leading a meeting at the same time as you are. Write, call, meet, or email other Leaders and share with each other your challenges, ideas, and successes. Support from other Leaders enhances your ability to give support to breastfeeding mothers.

When a Leader Moves to a New Group

If a Leader moves to your community, welcome her to the Group. In addition to the many tasks of settling her family, the Leader may be handling unsettled feelings. She may mourn the loss of relationships in her former community including her "old" Group and co-Leaders. Be understanding of her need for time to adjust. Before her first Series Meeting, she may appreciate an opportunity to get acquainted with you, the other Leaders, Leader Applicants, and Group workers. To provide her with background and a brief overview, you and Group members might give a brief history of the Group and general information about the mothers the Group serves; you might talk about how you currently divide responsibilities. Your Chapter might plan an informal "get acquainted" meeting for the new Leader to help her feel welcomed and comfortable.

When you move to a new community, inform the Area and your LLL office by completing the appropriate form. Ask your former support Leader to give you some contact information about Groups in your new locality or check the Group information on the Group Web site. If there is more than one Group in the area, you may want to attend a number of meetings to get a feel for the dynamics and style of each Group. As a move-in Leader, you may want to get involved with the new Group right away, leading meetings, helping by phone, and assuming Group management tasks. On the other hand, you might prefer to wait until you are settled in your new home before gradually assuming Leader responsibilities.

Communicating and adjusting to change

Integrating individual leading styles and routines can be a challenge. A new Leader may introduce a flurry of ideas and feel hurt if these ideas are dismissed; established Leaders may feel that the suggestions are criticisms of the Group. Here are some ideas that may help:

MANAGING GROUP

As a lone Leader, feel good about the help you offer one-to-one and at Series Meetings.

- Remember that everybody wants to be appreciated for her time and effort.
- Set up times after Series Meetings to compare notes and evaluate together. Exchanging feelings and opinions openly and honestly will help you to solve differences. (See **Evaluation Meetings** pages 81-85 and **Shared Leadership** pages 86-90.)
- If you are new to the Group, learn as much as you can about the Group before making suggestions.
- Be open to suggestions; after all, a new approach may work just fine.
- At Series Meetings, include the new Leader by redirecting questions or concerns to her.
- List the new Leader's telephone number first in publicity.

Splitting a Group

Providing mother-to-mother support is the essence of LLL help. Sometimes the best way to serve mothers in the community is to split the Group. Think of a Group as a temporary structure that changes over time and can multiply.

Reasons Groups split

> Varied locations and meeting times offer more chances for mothers to attend meetings.

- **High attendance**—When more than 15 mothers regularly attend meetings, it may be difficult for each to have the opportunity to ask questions and contribute to the meeting discussion.
- **Wider geographic interest**—When several mothers travel to meetings from another area, it might be helpful to start a new Group there.
- **Varied schedules**—More mothers in a community might be able to attend Series Meetings if there is more than one Group, with more than one meeting time (one day and another evening, on different days of the week, at different times of the month).
- **Many Leaders in a Group**—A split gives Leaders more opportunities to lead and help more mothers.

How to split a Group

- When Leaders decide that a Group is ready to split, contact your support Leader for the procedure to follow.
- Keep communication lines open; this can be a vulnerable time for friendships and feelings. Be sure to discuss:
    - Which Leaders will go with each Group
    - How to divide the Group assets: Treasury, Library, inventory
    - How to handle joint projects such as publicity and fundraising
- Notify your support Leader and LLL Office of the Listed Leader for each Group. Fill out and submit a **Leader Change of Address/Status Form** (see sample in **Appendix 4**) so the proper changes can be made regarding the Listed Leader, Group directory listing, and Group Account Number.

Meet as co-Leaders to discuss the timetable for the split, the division of Group materials and money, as well as the potential changes to the support network for Group workers. Talk about the split with Group members and invite their questions and concerns. Approach the change with the knowledge that a split is a positive event for LLL in the community.

A lone Leader in a Group in which there is consistently high attendance may consider a split because she believes she can meet the needs of the participants more effectively in two smaller Groups. Responsibility for two Groups and two Series Meetings each month is a lot of work. With this workload, it may be especially important to share the management tasks with Group workers, to let mothers know about leadership, and to keep in contact with your support Leader.

Change of Leader status or address

Whenever a Leader moves or changes her status she needs to complete the appropriate form. These forms are available from your support Leader, on the LLLI Web site, or may be requested from your LLL Office. Send the completed form to your support Leader or to the person named on the form. See **Sample Forms** in Appendix 4.

MANAGING GROUP

Reactivating

If a Leader who has been retired wishes to return to active status, she should contact the Area Coordinator of Leaders for specific requirements. She will usually be asked to:

- Attend Series Meetings, where available,
- Be thoroughly familiar with the latest editions available in her language of THE WOMANLY ART OF BREASTFEEDING, THE BREASTFEEDING ANSWER BOOK, and THE LEADERS' HANDBOOK,
- Become familiar with the latest LLL pamphlets and tear-off sheets available in her language that are part of the Applicant Reading Set and with the information contained in the Breastfeeding Resource Guide or its approved counterpart,
- Read the past year's issues of Area Newsletters and member publications,
- Participate in Evaluation Meetings and Chapter Meetings, if possible,
- Attend a workshop or conference, where available,
- Correspond with the Area Coordinator of Leaders concerning her plans for leadership, and
- Re-sign the Letter of Commitment.

Group at a Standstill

When a Group is thriving with consistent or rising attendance at each meeting, Leaders feel they are doing a good job. But suddenly there may be few, if any, new faces at meetings and total attendance drops off. Instead of growing, the Group seems to be standing still.

Every Group has its ups and downs in attendance, no matter how long it has been established. The time of year can play a part. Attendance often decreases during holiday seasons and months of extreme temperatures; pleasant weather may bring an increase. You may attribute the lack of new mothers or falling attendance to your leadership skills. Although this is possible, it is usually not the case.

> Every Group has its ups and downs in attendance, no matter how long it has been established.

Bringing a Group out of a slump

Set meeting goals to ensure that meetings use time efficiently and help mothers feel welcomed and valued.

- Start the meeting on time.
- Welcome participants.
- Encourage mothers to talk; ask experienced mothers to encourage newcomers to participate.
- Come well prepared for the topic and make sure that you cover the basics and answer questions.
- Be sensitive to image and the impressions the Group leaves with a newcomer.
- End the meeting on time.

Hold a special Evaluation Meeting. Offer a general invitation to everyone at the Series Meeting. At the Evaluation Meeting, talk about the tone of the meeting and the format. Invite participants to say what makes them feel comfortable, what they need, the kind of discussion they enjoy and learn best with. Invite them to help you develop meeting plans that may be attractive to more women.

Keep in touch with mothers between meetings. Letting a mother know you care and are thinking of her might encourage her to return to the next meeting, read a little more, or call with a question.

Invite mothers who call to come to meetings. Let mothers know that their babies are welcome, too.

Call mothers or send reminder notes after the meeting. A short call or simple note can remind women of the meeting date and place and what the Group has to offer. For example:

> Dear Lina,
>
> We were so happy to talk with you at the meeting last Wednesday and hope you had some questions answered. If questions or problems arise before our next meeting, feel free to call. Hope to see you next month.

Follow up if a mother comes to several meetings and then misses one:

> Dear Iris,
>
> We missed you at the meeting last week. We discussed "The Art of Breastfeeding and Avoiding Difficulties." If you have any questions, feel free to call, and we hope to see you at the Public Library meeting room on Wednesday, June 18 at 10 AM.

Give each pregnant woman a stamped, self-addressed postcard to mail to you when her baby is born. Follow up with a congratulatory call or note a few days after you receive the card.

Use stickers or cards with Leader name(s), telephone number(s), and email address(es) on them. Whenever you send or give printed information to a mother you can include a sticker or card.

Let participants know how significant they are to the Group's success. Tell them how important their contributions to the meeting discussion are; offer them Group jobs so they will know that LLL needs them. Suggest mothers share their enthusiasm about the Group and the information and support LLL can offer; word-of-mouth is excellent publicity!

Try new publicity ideas. Discuss ideas at an Evaluation Meeting. (See **Publicity— Helping Others Keep Track of LLL,** pages 97-105.)

Consider inviting fathers. Inviting fathers to attend a complete series might bring a Group out of an attendance slump. Over the course of the series, you can decide whether to continue as a Couples Group or to invite fathers to attend occasional meetings. (See **Fathers** in Chapter 2, page 52.)

Continue to do the best job possible. Maintain a regular meeting schedule. Meeting on a regular basis is vital to mothers finding LLL. If there are no new participants, take advantage of the opportunity to discuss subjects in depth.

MANAGING GROUP

Disbanding a Group

Disbanding a Group is a difficult decision.

Groups consider disbanding for several reasons:

- The Leader moves, takes a Leave of Absence (for six months or more) or retires.
- A lone Leader is no longer willing or able to continue handling the Group on her own; there is no Leader Applicant and mothers are unwilling or unable to accept responsibility for the Group jobs.

> If even a few women are attending meetings, there is a need for LLL and LLL information in that community.

Alternatives to disbanding a Group

Before disbanding, consider potential alternatives. If even a few women are attending meetings, there is a need for LLL and LLL information in that community.

Is there a potential Leader Applicant in the Group? Perhaps holding an Evaluation Meeting and frankly discussing the Group's situation will bring forth someone willing to continue the Group.

Is there a clinic, agency, or health care professional in the community who might be interested in forming a Professional Breastfeeding Resource Center? (See **Professional Breastfeeding Resource Center Memberships** in Chapter 8 for more information.)

Have you exhausted all means of and places for publicity? Consider some new ideas or approaches.

Could the Group merge with another nearby Group? Some women, accustomed to travelling long distances, may be willing to attend Group meetings farther away. If necessary, the merged Group might need to reconsider meeting times and places to meet the needs of the travelling mothers.

Is another Leader available? She might be willing to lead the Group for a few months, possibly until an Applicant is accredited. Contact nearby Groups to explore this possibility. Because of the amount of work involved in keeping two separate Groups going, it is wise to plan carefully and clarify at the outset so everyone knows exactly how many months she will be able to assist and what each person needs to plan to do following this deadline.

How to disband a Group

If an LLL Group has no alternative but to disband:

1. Notify your support Leader.
2. Decide on a closing date for the Group.
3. Pay all unpaid bills.
4. Let mothers know that the Group will disband. Announce the Group's closing throughout the last series of meetings, so that mothers can plan to attend another Group, form a non-LLL breastfeeding support group, etc. Encourage mothers to continue as members of LLL.
5. Remove posters and meeting notices from places in the community. Thank people for their support and let them know that the Group could form again when an accredited Leader is available.
6. Arrange for Group information to be removed from the LLLI Web site and your Area/Affiliate/country/Division Web site, and other Web sites such as those of community resource centers that may have been publicizing the Group's meetings. (See **Group Web Pages,** page 100.)
7. Turn over the Group Library and all Group supplies to your support Leader or the Area Coordinator of Leaders. Books and supplies purchased with LLL funds belong to LLL, not the Leader.
8. Make sure treasury records are up-to-date and turn over all money to the Area Coordinator of Leaders. Close all bank accounts and complete a financial report for the year-to-date.

CHAPTER FIVE

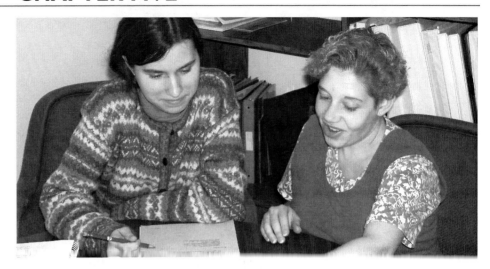

Helping Mothers Become Leaders

AN IMPORTANT RESPONSIBILITY

Leaders have a tremendous influence in shaping the future of La Leche League. Most women who apply for accreditation as LLL Leaders do so with the help and encouragement of their local Group Leaders.

How do you as a Leader fulfill the responsibility to take an active interest in helping other mothers find out about leadership and help them prepare to become LLL Leaders? You begin as you demonstrate the LLL leadership role in the normal course of leading meetings and managing the Group.

Our goal is to accredit Leaders who have the experience, knowledge, and skills they will need to do their job with confidence and pleasure. Leader Applicant, Leader, and Leader Accreditation Department (LAD) representative work together throughout the application so the Applicant will:

- Understand the Leader's role and responsibilities;
- Appreciate how personal breastfeeding and mothering experience forms a basis for both the Leader's and LLL's credibility; and
- Develop the knowledge and skills necessary to help mothers as an LLL Leader.

This chapter provides a general overview of your role related to Leader accreditation. For detailed information on all topics relevant to accreditation, contact your LAD representative. She can answer specific questions as well as provide written resources and outlines for workshops. Read and keep on hand relevant articles from Leader publications. These resources—your LAD representative and your file of articles—will provide you with up-to-date information to turn to when you want to review how to attract, encourage, and assist Leader Applicants.

> Our goal is to accredit Leaders who have the experience, knowledge, and skills they will need to do their job with confidence and pleasure.

Just as women learn about breastfeeding and mothering by observing and interacting with breastfeeding mothers, women learn about LLL and leadership by observing and interacting with Leaders. From the time a mother attends her first Series Meeting, she begins building her knowledge base about breastfeeding, LLL philosophy, and LLL as an organization. As a Leader, you give concrete meaning to "LLL" and "LLL leadership." When a mother goes on to explore, apply, and prepare to be a Leader, you represent LLLI as both model and mentor.

Make Leadership Attractive and Accessible

Because LLL uses a mother-to-mother approach, all women who take an active part in Series Meetings do, at one time or another, take on a leadership role. Some mothers may want to take on the responsibilities of accredited LLL Leaders. As you lead Series and Evaluation Meetings and encourage participation in the Group, you encourage leadership. Your enjoyment of your work and the information you offer about La Leche League and your responsibilities encourage others to become interested in LLL leadership.

Evaluation Meetings Are Key

Evaluation Meetings can be powerful opportunities for members to learn about La Leche League, Group work, and the role of a Leader when they include:

Assessment of the recent Series Meeting and planning for the next, including:
- Group dynamics and the flow of the meeting
- Keeping discussion focused
- Creating a respectful, accepting atmosphere
- Ensuring that questions are answered and resources are suggested.

Enrichment beyond the basic Series Meeting topics:
- LLLI as an organization
- Mother-to-mother help.

Encouragement for each participant's "leadership" through:
- Fulfilling a specific Group responsibility
- Providing relevant, helpful information at Series Meetings
- Helping mothers feel welcome at meetings.

Management of Group tasks, including:
- Ongoing Group jobs
- Special activities.

You make LLL leadership attractive when you:

- Show that you enjoy being a Leader and talk about the benefits and satisfactions of leadership.
- Provide opportunities for ongoing learning about breastfeeding and LLL by referring to THE WOMANLY ART OF BREASTFEEDING, Group Library books, and other LLL publications.
- Acknowledge mothers' contributions to the meeting discussion.
- Listen and respond to questions about LLL and LLL leadership.

- Invite participation in Evaluation Meetings.
- Invite participation in Group management through Group jobs.
- Encourage attendance at workshops and conferences.

You make LLL leadership accessible when you:

- Show where you get information including:
  - Written resources (THE WOMANLY ART OF BREASTFEEDING, THE LEADER'S HANDBOOK, THE BREASTFEEDING ANSWER BOOK, LLL pamphlets and information sheets, Internet resources)
  - The LLL support system (other Leaders, Area/Division/National/ Affiliate/ LLLI resource and support Leaders)
- Discuss *Becoming a La Leche League Leader* with interested mothers.
- Hold workshops for women who want to know more about LLL leadership.

Workshops for Interested Mothers

A workshop for interested mothers can be simple or elaborate. You might want to contact your LAD representative for suggestions. Be sure to refer to and answer questions about:

1. The prerequisites to applying for LLL leadership (see a current Leader Application Packet);
2. LLL philosophy (the ten concepts);
3. The basic responsibilities of an LLL Leader; and
4. The requirements and preparation for LLL leadership.

If possible, give each participant a copy of *Becoming a La Leche League Leader* and copies of relevant material (e.g., *Overview of Training Curriculum for Leader Accreditation*) from the Leader Application Packet.

How Willing? How Able?

Allow time—at least one full series of meetings—for you to get to know a mother and for her to get to know LLL. Consider the prerequisites to applying for leadership and the qualities that are important to the work of an LLL Leader.

Breastfeeding and mothering experience—A Leader needs firsthand knowledge of breastfeeding and mothering. Be certain the mother you are considering has the basic experience described in the prerequisites (see a current Leader Application Packet).

Personal traits—In order to facilitate effective discussions and help other women breastfeed, as well as present and represent LLL appropriately, a Leader needs to relate respectfully to others, communicate effectively, provide appropriate assistance, and give generously (and realistically) of her time and attention. Be certain the mother you are considering has these abilities or is willing to develop them.

Command of language—One of a Leader's basic responsibilities is to keep up-to-date with information; another is to report regularly on her work to LLL. A Leader needs adequate language ability to complete her initial training, maintain her knowledge base, communicate effectively with mothers at meetings and one-to-one, and report her needs and accomplishments to the organization.

> Consider the prerequisites to applying for leadership and the qualities that are important to the work of an LLL Leader.

Interest in the Group and LLL—A candidate for leadership shows sustained interest in LLL by becoming a member, fulfilling Group responsibilities, and (if available) attending Series and Evaluation Meetings regularly.

Knowledge base—A candidate for LLL leadership has read the most recent edition of The Womanly Art of Breastfeeding available in her language, reads her member publication, and is interested in reading other publications that will help her learn more about breastfeeding and LLL's purpose, philosophy, and mission. If some of these materials are not available in her language, the Leader and/or LAD representative will provide necessary information/resources.

(See **Appendix 1: Leader Accreditation.**)

Consult With Co-Leaders: Do You Agree?

> All the Leaders in the Group should be able to support the application and share their knowledge and experience with the Applicant.

Although one Leader in the Group sometimes takes on the responsibility of working with the Leader Applicant, all the Leaders should be able to support the application and share their knowledge and experience with the Applicant. If a Leader has a concern or question about a mother's readiness to submit an application for LLL leadership, she needs to discuss it with the other Leaders in the Group. If any Leader in the Group disagrees about the appropriateness of an application, explore the issues together.

Define the problem or concern. Does it relate to an experience or personal traits prerequisite? If it relates to experience, is there a way for the mother to meet the prerequisite? For instance, if she does not meet the organizational experience prerequisite, she may just need to become an LLL member or need to acquire and read The Womanly Art of Breastfeeding.

If the concern is about one of the personal traits, identify the trait. Is there a skill (such as communicating acceptance and respect, listening, or projecting a positive attitude) that the mother needs to improve? If so, consider how, when, and where you might help her work on it? You might begin by saying something like, "Jane, I have some questions about a comment you made at the last meeting. Can we talk about it?" Your approach focuses on providing information about LLL's expectations for Leaders, problem solving, and communication skills. You respectfully present objective standards, explore possible solutions with her, and invite her (if she is interested) to find one that will work for both her and LLL. Although the Leader Applicant will work on many skills during her application, you will want to have reasonable expectation that she can and is willing to develop the skills necessary to represent LLL as a Leader. If you are uncertain, consult with a LAD representative and/or the mother. You may decide to initiate this work before beginning an application.

On the other hand, after talking together you and your co-Leaders may discover that the concern relates to personal preference or style. In this case you can proceed with the confidence that Leaders are a diverse group of women bound together by our common philosophy and mother-to-mother approach. Or you may decide that you need more information about the mother's experience, beliefs, and interests.

BEFORE THE APPLICATION

Your discussions with the potential Leader Applicant will help her decide if she wants to apply for LLL leadership and will help you confirm whether you can support an application with your written recommendation. Begin by reviewing the contents of the Leader Application Packet. With your printed Leader resources at hand, meet with the prospective Applicant to discuss the prerequisites to applying, the criteria for accreditation, LLL philosophy, basic Leader responsibilities, and the application requirements. It may take several meetings to thoroughly cover all of these topics.

Prerequisites to applying for leadership and criteria for Leader accreditation

Before meeting with the mother to discuss the prerequisites and criteria for accreditation, review "Applying for Leadership" (See **Appendix 18 of the Policies and Standing Rules Notebook** in Appendix 1). When you get together, invite the mother to tell you about her experiences that relate to each of the experience prerequisites. If you have questions or concerns, consult "LLLI Prerequisites to Applying for Leadership—Guidelines for Leaders" (part of Appendix 18) and/or a LAD representative. It is important that both you and the Leader Accreditation Department feel confident that the mother meets the prerequisites before proceeding with an application.

Talk about the personal traits a Leader needs and how she demonstrates them. Ask the mother how she sees herself incorporating these traits in her current interactions with other mothers. Explain the criteria for Leader accreditation, and invite the mother's questions.

LEADER ACCREDITATION

If, in your discussions, the mother's point of view seems to differ from LLL's, explore the differences with her before you proceed.

LLL philosophy—the concepts

The concepts are the essence of LLL philosophy. Even if you have discussed the concepts on other occasions and are sure the mother understands them, be sure to discuss them with her one by one before she applies for leadership. This can help assure both of you that she understands, agrees with, and can provide a personal example of LLL philosophy in action. It might be helpful for the mother interested in leadership to think about how she would explain a concept to someone else—someone new to La Leche League.

As you discuss LLL philosophy, include these aspects:

- Understanding each concept individually,
- How the concepts relate to one another,
- Mothering through breastfeeding as a practical philosophy,
- How the concepts are revealed in Leaders' and mothers' experiences, and
- How we present LLL philosophy while respecting other choices.

(See **Appendix 1: Policy Statements: Concepts.**)

Here are the concepts along with some sample questions and chapter references for THE WOMANLY ART OF BREASTFEEDING that may be helpful to your discussion. One question or statement may be all you need to open the door to discussion. You might want to develop your own discussion starters as well or instead.

Mothering through breastfeeding is the most natural and effective way of understanding and satisfying the needs of the baby.

What are some of the ways breastfeeding helps a mother better understand and meet her baby's needs? (THE WOMANLY ART OF BREASTFEEDING, "Why Choose Breastfeeding?")

Mother and baby need to be together early and often to establish a satisfying relationship and an adequate milk supply.

What were your first weeks of breastfeeding and mothering like? How is "early and often" a help in getting breastfeeding off to a good start? (THE WOMANLY ART OF BREASTFEEDING, "Your Baby Arrives")

In the early years, the baby has an intense need to be with his mother which is as basic as his need for food.

How did you learn to recognize your baby's need to be with you? How do you see yourself using your experience to help another mother understand her baby's needs in balance with her own needs and those of her family? (THE WOMANLY ART OF BREASTFEEDING, "Making a Choice")

Breast milk is the superior infant food.

How would you explain the benefits of human milk? (THE WOMANLY ART OF BREASTFEEDING, "The Superior Infant Food")

For the healthy, full-term baby, breast milk is the only food necessary until the baby shows signs of needing solids, about the middle of the first year after birth.

What signs of readiness for solids did you see in your baby? Why wait until about the middle of the first year to introduce food other than human milk? (THE WOMANLY ART OF BREASTFEEDING, "Ready for Solids")

Ideally, the breastfeeding relationship will continue until the baby outgrows the need.

What does "outgrowing the need to breastfeed" mean to you? (THE WOMANLY ART OF BREASTFEEDING, "Weaning Gradually, with Love")

Alert and active participation by the mother in childbirth is a help in getting breastfeeding off to a good start.

In what ways can the childbirth experience affect how a mother and baby get started breastfeeding? Why discuss childbirth at a La Leche League meeting? (THE WOMANLY ART OF BREASTFEEDING, "Plans Are Underway")

Breastfeeding is enhanced and the nursing couple sustained by the loving support, help, and companionship of the baby's father. A father's unique relationship with his baby is an important element in the child's development from early infancy.

What kinds of support help to enhance and sustain breastfeeding? How is the mother-baby relationship different from a baby's relationship with father or other important persons in a baby's life? (THE WOMANLY ART OF BREASTFEEDING, "The Manly Art of Fathering")

Good nutrition means eating a well-balanced and varied diet of foods in as close to their natural state as possible.

How have you found the nutrition portion of THE WOMANLY ART OF BREASTFEEDING helpful for you and your family? (THE WOMANLY ART OF BREASTFEEDING, "Nutritional Know-How")

From infancy on, children need loving guidance which reflects acceptance of their capabilities and sensitivity to their feelings.

What does the term "loving guidance" mean to you? How do you see loving guidance develop as part of your interaction with your child from infancy on? (THE WOMANLY ART OF BREASTFEEDING, "Discipline Is Loving Guidance")

If there are differences

If, in your discussions, the mother's point of view seems to differ from LLL's, explore the differences with her before you proceed. Suppose, for example, your discussions with the mother lead you to believe she disagrees with an aspect of LLL philosophy. As you talk about the relevant concepts, explain that Leaders present and represent LLL philosophy. If the mother voices disagreement or her actions seem to conflict with the philosophy, you can explain that LLL asks that Leaders, as its representatives, agree with and provide examples in action of LLL philosophy. With that explanation, a mother might be able to say, "I just can't agree" or "I'm not sure if I agree" or "I think you've misunderstood."

In the first instance ("I just can't agree"), the mother herself will most likely decide not to apply.

In the second ("I'm not sure if I agree") you have the opportunity to help the mother learn more about LLL philosophy. Offer her relevant reading material (e.g., sections of THE WOMANLY ART OF BREASTFEEDING, THE LEADER'S HANDBOOK, your Leader publication, and/or LLL-approved books) and a chance to discuss it. Consult your LAD representative for more specific suggestions. Reading and reflection can give the mother a chance to form her own opinion. If the difference is something the mother cannot or will not work on, explore with her other ways she can achieve her goal of helping women breastfeed than as an LLL Leader.

The third instance ("I think you've misunderstood") calls for careful listening on your part. When you believe you have come to understand, ask for feedback to make sure. Continue to clarify and offer more information on LLL philosophy. Clear communication can help the mother reach her own decision.

Basic Leader Responsibilities

Most Leaders begin with the basic Leader responsibilities. After a period of time some Leaders replace one or more of the basic responsibilities with work for the Area, Division/Affiliate, or LLLI.

LEADER ACCREDITATION

Basic responsibilities of an LLL Leader

An LLL Leader:

- Helps mothers one-to-one, by telephone or in person, keeping accurate records of these helping situations;
- Plans and leads monthly Series Meetings;
- Supervises the management of the Group, including membership, finances, Group workers, Group Library, and materials for sale; informs the Area Coordinator of Leaders (usually through the District Advisor/Coordinator) about her LLL activities through written monthly reports;
- Keeps up-to-date on all important breastfeeding information, taking advantage of opportunities provided through LLL for continuing education through publications, meetings, correspondence, and the network of resource Leaders; and
- Takes an active interest in helping other mothers find out about leadership and helps them prepare to become LLL Leaders.

As you discuss Leader responsibilities, include these aspects:

- **Accountability**—what is expected of a Leader and what a Leader can expect; the importance of reporting and consultation.
- **Resources**—printed resources and a Leader's support network.
- **Mother-to-mother help**—LLL's approach to supporting breastfeeding mothers.
- **Confidentiality**—how and why Leaders keep mothers' personal and identifying information private.
- **Commitment**—how Leaders balance LLL work and family needs.

If the mother is unwilling or unable to fulfill basic Leader responsibilities, talk with her further before you proceed. What does she want to accomplish as a Leader? You might like to use the "Window of Work" exercise (see page 91), which asks for a list of skills, aspirations, and dislikes. Let her know that, as a basis for any work a Leader will do for LLL, the leadership application focuses on developing the knowledge, attitudes, skills, and approaches necessary to fulfill basic responsibilities. Explore with the mother how her goals will fulfill LLL's mission. With your mutual agreement that the mother's goals are compatible with LLL's and that she is willing and able to keep her fees current, keep up-to-date with Leader education, communicate with the organization, and do the application work, you can proceed with an application.

The Application Work

Most Leaders begin with the basic Leader responsibilities.

Using the *Overview of Training Curriculum for Leader Accreditation* from the Leader Application Packet, talk with the mother about the parts of the application and their purposes. Show her what reading is required and the checklist of topics you will discuss together (see pages 150-152). If you have copies of the *Breastfeeding Resource Guide* and *A Preview of Mothers' Questions/Problems and Group Dynamics/Management* handy, you could show her these too. Explain the application procedures and how she will work with the Leader Accreditation Department representative. Assure her that both you and the LAD representative will be available to offer guidance and suggestions and to help as appropriate. Let her know that, with input from you and the LAD representative, the Leader Applicant develops a flexible plan to learn all she needs to know while continuing to meet the needs of her family.

APPLYING FOR LLL LEADERSHIP

As a Group Leader, you are responsible for discussing leadership with the mother, telling her honestly if you cannot recommend her, and giving her information about appealing any decision to not recommend. (See **Leader Accreditation Appeals** in Appendix 1.) Remember that the LAD representative is available to help with possible approaches and to suggest relevant articles.

If, after your discussions, the member is ready to apply for LLL leadership and you are ready to support her application, use the forms in the Leader Application Packet. Your recommendation includes important information for the LAD representative. Answering the questions completely and offering relevant examples, where appropriate, will aid her in providing effective help. When the LAD representative has received the application form, the application fee, and at least one Leader's recommendation, and when she feels confident to proceed, a candidate for LLL leadership is considered a Leader Applicant.

Keep in mind that prior to accreditation, the Applicant is not a representative of La Leche League and is not covered by LLLI liability insurance. She cannot act in the name of LLL by leading a Series Meeting, helping mothers one-to-one, or speaking to outside groups. An Applicant should not be put in a position where she might appear to represent LLL, even if a Leader is not available. To avoid confusion, we ask that mothers do not introduce themselves as Applicants in public settings, such as Series Meetings or Internet chat lists.

Use your creativity to think of ways to offer the Applicant opportunities to practice one-to-one helping (for example, role-play) and leading meetings (she can lead a mock meeting or help to lead Evaluation, Enrichment, or Chapter Meetings) without putting her in the position of representing LLL before she is prepared and authorized to do so.

> Preparation for LLL leadership focuses on developing experience, knowledge, and skills to perform basic Leader responsibilities.

LEADER ACCREDITATION

DURING THE APPLICATION— LEARNING, PRACTICE, AND DIALOGUE

Preparation for LLL leadership focuses on developing experience, knowledge, and skills to perform basic Leader responsibilities. The Leader Applicant will work on her own and in collaboration with you and her LAD representative. The application includes:

- **Learning opportunities,** where the Leader Applicant will develop her information base, skills, and knowledge about LLL leadership responsibilities.
- **Practice opportunities,** where she will practice one-to-one helping, handling situations that can arise at meetings, and other aspects of basic Leader responsibilities. (You can use the *Preview of Mothers' Questions/Problems and Group Dynamics/Management* at any time during the application.)
- **Written and oral exchanges,** which will give her feedback and support.

Some Applicants may want to do all the reading and discussing first and then practice skills; others may want to practice as they go. Many Applicants choose to have a formal practice session at the end of the application to bring together what they have learned and confirm that they are ready to represent LLL as accredited Leaders.

With input and suggestions from you and the LAD representative, the Leader Applicant designs her application work to incorporate requirements, such as completing specific reading and the *Breastfeeding Resource Guide* (or its approved counterpart), with supplementary reading, activities, and/or exercises of her choice to help her feel competent and confident to represent LLL as a Leader. The Applicant works on her own at a pace and in a manner that takes into account her learning and work styles and her commitments to her family. While an average application takes about a year, many Applicants find that they can complete it in significantly less time.

Leader Applicant and LAD representative work together

Leader Applicant, LAD representative, and Leader all work together, keeping in touch as the Applicant prepares for leadership.

During her application, the Leader Applicant writes her personal history of breast-feeding and mothering and sends it to her LAD representative. Her work related to her personal history offers a variety of learning opportunities and forms the basis for dialogues (written "conversations") with the LAD representative about topics relevant to accreditation as a Leader. Dialogue letters build on what the Applicant writes, relating her personal experience, knowledge, impressions from her reading, and attitudes to the work of an LLL Leader. Dialogues, on one topic or a variety, can include one or several interchanges.

Leader Applicant and Leader work together

You and the Leader Applicant will meet regularly to focus on the Applicant's preparation for LLL leadership. Together, set out a plan that will help the Applicant:

- Increase her breastfeeding knowledge base.
- Learn where to find information, develop her resource library, and organize materials.
- Learn about managing Leader responsibilities.
- Balance LLL and family responsibilities.

Design the particulars of the work plan to suit the information and experience the Applicant brings to the application as well as her learning style. Draw from both your experience and LLL resource materials (LEADER'S HANDBOOK, THE WOMANLY ART OF BREASTFEEDING, the *Breastfeeding Resource Guide*, LEAVEN and/or other Leader publications, THE BREASTFEEDING ANSWER BOOK, LLL pamphlets and tear-off sheets). Explore, discuss, and practice the topics on "A Checklist of Topics to Discuss in Preparation for LLL Leadership" on pages 150-152.

Be sure to discuss how each topic relates to the basic Leader responsibilities. Make them concrete by:

- Planning Series Meetings together, and
- Role-playing one-to-one helping and Series Meeting situations (such as the situations in the Preview).

Planning a Series Meeting together

After the Leader Applicant has read and you both have discussed the relevant chapters of THE LEADER'S HANDBOOK, meet to plan the next Series Meeting. One or more Leaders and Applicants can plan the meeting at an Evaluation Meeting or at another time.

1. Explore the appropriate Series Meeting guide.
2. Look over other meeting outlines and/or brainstorm new ideas.
3. Discuss a variety of approaches the Leader might take.
4. Select and develop a meeting plan.

Benefits to the Applicant, Leader, and Group:

- The Applicant usually offers new ideas.
- She knows the objectives of the meeting and can help keep it on topic.
- The Applicant sees plans become reality, including:
    - How a Leader adapts a meeting plan to meet the needs of the participants.
    - How a Leader keeps the topic focused.
    - How discussion techniques are used.
    - How visual aids affect participation.
    - Why a Leader might have more than one meeting plan.
- The Applicant can build a folder of meeting ideas annotated with references and evaluations.

LEADER ACCREDITATION

Practicing one-to-one helping

Leaders help mothers one-to-one in person and over the telephone; some may also help via email. Early in the application, suggest that the Applicant read Chapter 1, "Mother-to-Mother Help," in THE LEADER'S HANDBOOK. You might also give her copies of articles that you've found helpful.

When you meet to discuss her application or discuss topics from the checklist, also talk about and practice one-to-one helping. You can use situations you make up, those from the Preview, or questions/problems from your Leader log or online sources (be sure to remove all identifying information about real mothers first).

Some topics you might include are:

- Keeping information handy and up-to-date.
- Using a Leader's Log.
- Active listening, offering appropriate information, recapping, and review.
- Fitting telephone helping into our day.
- Keeping children happy while helping mothers.
- Responding to common concerns.
- When and how to contact resource Leaders.

Use role-play to practice one-to-one helping. The Applicant will:

- Discover how she can most effectively organize information and keep it handy.
- Develop her ability to listen effectively and elicit and provide relevant information in the context of telephone helping, without the advantages of in-person communication.
- Prepare to start her work as an LLL Leader with confidence and proficiency.

After the role-play, together assess the exercise honestly:

- What went well,
- What could be improved, and
- What resources would help.

The Breastfeeding Resource Guide

The Leader Applicant may choose to complete *The Breastfeeding Resource Guide* on her own, or she may ask you to work with her on some or all of it. If you work together, consider how she likes to learn and what format will be most practical for her. For example, you and she might:

- Look up answers together, making pertinent notes.
- Use the questions as a basis for role-play.
- Use the questions to tab Leader resources or make a set of phone-helping cards.
- Work with other Applicants and/or Leaders in an informal or workshop setting.

Leader Applicant Workshops

- Are planned by Leaders; the LAD representative can help.
- Can be formal or informal and include one or many sessions.
- Give the Leader Applicant a broader view of La Leche League.
- Help an Applicant gather ideas from her peers.
- Can be part of developing a local support system.

Leader Applicant, LAD Representative, and Leader Work Together

Leader Applicant, LAD representative, and Leader all work together, keeping in touch as the Applicant prepares for leadership.

The LAD representative complements and supports the work of the Applicant and Leader by:

- Discussing topics from a broader (perhaps Area, National/Affiliate/Division, or LLLI) point of view.
- Suggesting alternative focuses.
- Covering additional topics.
- Finding resources or letting you know about new ones being developed.
- Answering questions and helping to resolve difficulties.

With the goal of orienting the Applicant to the work of an LLL Leader, the Applicant, Leader, and LAD representative work together to ensure that the Applicant has the required:

- Breastfeeding and mothering experience.
- Personal qualities.
- Breastfeeding knowledge base and awareness of resources.
- Leadership skills.
- Understanding of LLL philosophy.

Successful completion of the *Preview of Mothers' Questions/Problems and Group Dynamics/Management* provides confirmation that accreditation is appropriate.

WHEN THERE ARE DOUBTS ABOUT THE APPLICATION

The Leader Applicant, Leader, and LAD representative work together—each with her responsibilities, knowledge, experience, and focus—to determine whether accreditation is appropriate. From time to time, we find that accreditation as an LLL Leader would not be an appropriate outcome.

The Applicant, considering events in her life and what she is learning about the responsibilities of leadership, might decide she does not have time for or does not want to do the work of a Leader. The LAD representative or Leader, considering the development of the Applicant's skills, attitude, and knowledge base, might decide that she could not represent LLL or effectively help breastfeeding women as a Leader.

To help avoid this disappointing situation:

- Be sure to cover all the necessary information prior to an application.
- Help maintain the Applicant's learning and interest by meeting with her often to explore, discuss, and practice what she needs to prepare for LLL leadership.
- Invite questions: work with doubts and concerns before they become impediments.
- Problem-solve where necessary—for example, if the Applicant finds it difficult to fit more LLL time into her schedule or to develop certain skills or traits.
- Be open to exploring ideas—for example, related to organization (time/materials), loving guidance, or ways to learn and practice skills.
- Keep in contact with the LAD representative to ensure that you are working together to provide information, support, and encouragement to the Applicant. The LAD representative can also help you work through concerns and doubts and can suggest additional resources and ideas.

If, from your observations and discussions, you have doubts about proceeding with the application:

Define your concern. Is your concern about philosophy, a specific behavior or personal trait, the development of an adequate information base, or communication skills?

Do a reality check. If your concern stems from something the Applicant said, check it with her. If it's a behavior you have observed, ask her about it.

Communicate your concern. If the source of the concern is relevant to accreditation, point it out to the Applicant and discuss whether it is something she can and is willing to work on.

Consult with the LAD representative and, together with the Applicant, decide on a plan of action that includes specific things to do, a time frame, and how you will evaluate progress.

Remember that problem-solving and conflict resolution skills can be important parts of preparation for LLL leadership. By addressing problems as they arise, you contribute to development of these skills.

If, from your observations and discussions, you have doubts about proceeding with the application, define your concern, do a reality check, and communicate your concern.

LEADER ACCREDITATION

A PREVIEW OF MOTHERS' QUESTIONS/ PROBLEMS AND GROUP DYNAMICS/ MANAGEMENT

The *Preview* provides an opportunity for practice and assessment of the Leader Applicant's readiness to assume basic Leader responsibilities.

The exercises from the *Preview* can be done:

- Throughout the application, as part of your regular meetings with the Applicant to discuss topics and practice skills.
- At the end of the application, as a review and formal practice of skills.
- In combination, with some during the application and some at the end.

> The Preview assures everyone that the Applicant has the basic information and skills to begin working as a Leader.

The *Preview* brings together what the Applicant has learned, identifies areas that would benefit from more work, and assures everyone that she has the basic information and skills to begin working as a Leader.

The *Preview* exercises cover:

- One-to-one helping situations.
- Group situations, including facilitating discussion, challenges to leading a discussion, responding to criticism, helping mothers prepare for leadership.
- Attention to skills such as offering information and listening, as well as organizing and retrieving information.

Although the LAD representative will make general suggestions about completing the *Preview*, the Leader and Applicant will design the exercise themselves. Keep these suggestions in mind:

1. Use as many of the situations as possible, varying them creatively from your actual Leader experience.
2. Add helping situations you or the Applicant think she needs practice with, whether or not they are suggested by the LAD representative.
3. Role-play as many helping situations as possible; follow with discussion and evaluation.
4. If possible, complete at least two helping situations over the telephone, one scheduled and the other unscheduled.
5. Practice using printed Leader resources.
6. Assess the practice exercises honestly.
7. Plan for ongoing education.

Both Applicant and Leader send their assessment of the Preview exercise(s) to the LAD representative. Dialogue letters may cover additional needs.

THE STATEMENT OF COMMITMENT

The LAD representative sends the Leader Applicant the Statement of Commitment. She signs and returns it, along with her accreditation fee. The LAD representative also signs the Statement of Commitment, forwards it and the fee to the appropriate LLL Area, Division, or Affiliate, and lets the Applicant and her new co-Leaders know that she is an accredited LLL Leader.

Welcoming the New Leader

- Remember that you are now co-Leaders.
- Together, plan who will lead the next meeting or series of meetings. Talk about how you will support each other's role at meetings.
- At Series Meetings, help focus participants' attention on the new Leader.
- Meet to redistribute Group responsibilities. For example, decide together who will complete the meeting report, who will order books and materials, who will work with each Group worker.
- Bring the new Leader's talents and areas of expertise to the attention of Area administrators so she can be invited to help with work in the Area or at the Area Conference.

WHEN THERE'S NO LEADER APPLICANT IN SIGHT

Certain situations can contribute to a lack of Leader Applicants in a Group. These suggestions can help.

New or rejuvenating Group—Be patient. During the first year or so attendance may be low. The Leader may be the only one in the Group who has experienced breastfeeding as presented in THE WOMANLY ART OF BREASTFEEDING. As soon as possible, invite women who attend Series Meetings regularly to attend Evaluation Meetings and take Group jobs.

"I could never be like you or do what you do."—Encourage the mother's self-confidence. Thank her for specific contributions to the meeting discussion or Group management. Communicate your enjoyment of LLL leadership. Reassure her that Leaders are not "perfect" and continue to learn about many aspects of breastfeeding, helping, and parenting; that it is possible to strike a balance between LLL commitments and family needs; that Leaders share the workload. Encourage her to visit other Groups and see that Leaders have different experiences and use different leading styles.

Leader's expectations are too high—Look for mothers who enjoy breastfeeding and mothering, find LLL ideas workable, attend meetings regularly, and help out in the Group. Notice when a mother begins to make suggestions to the Group from her experiences and reading.

Leader is looking for someone like herself—Let LLL philosophy and goals be the common ground. Focus on the Group member. Can she do the job of an LLL Leader? Leaders don't have to be good friends in order to work together respectfully and effectively. Differences in Leaders' personalities and interests often mean helping a wider range of mothers.

Leader thinks she is too busy to work with an Applicant—Hold regular Evaluation Meetings. Encourage members who show an interest in leadership to read appropriate LLL materials. Invite them to LLL conferences and workshops. Don't wait too long to approach an interested mother about leadership.

Leader is a one-woman show—Recognize this trait and invite participation in the Group. Involve members in Group jobs and Evaluation Meetings.

Lone Leader—Use suggestions in this chapter to make LLL leadership attractive, available, and attainable.

Many Leaders in the Group—Meet with mothers interested in leadership to discuss what the Group can accomplish with additional Leaders.

LEADER ACCREDITATION

Look for mothers who enjoy breastfeeding and mothering, find LLL ideas workable, attend meetings regularly, and take Group jobs.

A CHECKLIST OF TOPICS TO DISCUSS IN PREPARATION FOR LLL LEADERSHIP

Use your experience and Leader resources (THE LEADER'S HANDBOOK, THE WOMANLY ART OF BREASTFEEDING, THE BREASTFEEDING ANSWER BOOK, pamphlets and tear-off sheets, the material in the Leader Application Packet, your Leader publications) to explore, discuss, and/or practice the following topics and skills, relating each to the Leader Applicant's preparation to fulfill the responsibilities of an LLL Leader. Add topics and themes you think would be helpful, and contact your LAD representative for additional suggestions.

Topic	Dates	Resources	Comment

Breastfeeding management
  selected topics from the *Breastfeeding Resource Guide*
  when to consult or refer; where to get help
  relevant LLL philosophy
  published resources (LLL's, how to assess other information)
  how we keep up–to-date
  providing information rather than advice			

Child development/parenting
  common parenting concerns
  solids, infant and toddler nutrition
  weaning
  loving guidance
  relevant LLL philosophy
  separating LLL philosophy from apparently related ideas
  incorporating information in Series Meeting and one-to-one helping
  published resources			

Communication/helping skills
  helping as an informed peer
  the art of listening
  gathering information
  selecting and communicating information
  confidentiality
  working with personal biases
  identifying and overcoming obstacles to communication
  respect for the experience and information each individual brings to a discussion or question			

One-to-one helping/Leader's log
  organizing materials for telephone helping
  telephone helping with young children present
  maintaining a log of one-to-one helping
  Group dynamics/ facilitating discussion
  balancing discussion
    ensuring LLL information is presented
    creating a welcoming atmosphere (to questions, ideas)
    respectful disagreement (with information)			

Topic	Dates	Resources	Comment
Series Meetings planning Leader's, Applicant's, Group workers' roles promoting membership mixing causes toddlers at meetings			
Evaluation Meetings how to evaluate a meeting the importance of reporting evaluation and follow-up on Group jobs appropriate enrichment topics			
Group Treasury record keeping memberships sales fundraising			
Group Library LLL bibliographies keeping the library up to date recommending books to mothers keeping track of books how to order library materials critical reading			
Publicity meeting notices, announcements			
Working with others (co-Leaders, Group workers) shared leadership combining different approaches and work styles building agreement accountability and autonomy			
Organizing materials forms Leader resources meeting ideas			
Time management balancing LLL responsibilities with family needs basic Leader responsibilities and other activities delegating			
Image first impressions Leader's role in the community			

Topic	Dates	Resources	Comment
Accountability			
the purpose of			
our accountability to LLL and mothers			
LLL's accountability to us			
the Leader's Statement of Commitment			
Published resources			
THE WOMANLY ART OF BREASTFEEDING			
THE LEADER'S HANDBOOK			
THE BREASTFEEDING ANSWER BOOK			
LLL pamphlets and tear-off sheets			
Leader and member publications			
Area Library			
LLLI Web site			
Continuing education opportunities			
Chapter Meetings			
Workshops for Leaders and Leader Applicants			
Area/National/Affiliate/Regional Conferences			
LLLI Conferences			
LLLI			
Bylaws, policies			
purpose, philosophy, and mission			
LLL structure and support beyond the Group			
how a Leader accesses support			
whom to go to for what			
Chapter, District, Area, Region, Affiliate/Division, LLLI			
online support			
Leader Department; Leader support			
Professional Liaison Department			
Leader Accreditation Department			
Communication Skills/Human Relations Enrichment Dept.			
Conference/Events Department			
Finance Department			
Publications Department			
LLLI Board of Directors			
LLLI or National/Affiliate Office			

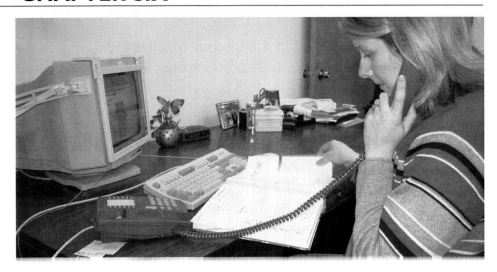

CHAPTER SIX

Keeping Up-to-Date

A Leader's work is central to the service LLL provides breastfeeding mothers and babies. Supporting this work—the Leader helping mothers—is a network of human and printed resources to help you keep up-to-date. When you need to know more or need encouragement for your endeavors, you can turn to LLL's network of support and resource Leaders, publications, meetings, workshops, conferences, and other continuing education opportunities.

LLL SUPPORT NETWORK

Just as LLL's breastfeeding help is based on mother-to-mother support, our network of support for Leaders is based on experienced Leaders providing support to other Leaders and Groups. The structure of this support network may vary throughout LLL worldwide.

Areas, Divisions, and Affiliates provide Leader support through departments and programs, helping Leaders keep up-to-date and carry out their work. Affiliates and Divisions, together with the LLLI Board of Directors, Executive Director, and staff at the LLLI Office in Schaumburg, Illinois, USA, make up La Leche League International.

Following is an overview of the LLL support network as it has developed to the date of this publication. Explorations by the organization could lead to different structures and support responsibilities.

LLL's network of support for Leaders is based on Leaders providing support to other Leaders.

LLLI Board of Directors

The LLLI Board of Directors establishes the policies that guide the organization. It determines new programs, oversees the business affairs of the organization, and hires an Executive Director, who implements the Board's policies and directs day-to-day operations. The Board's general powers include the responsibility to maintain the vitality of LLL as it pursues its purpose and mission.

LLLI Executive Director

The LLLI Executive Director is directly responsible to the LLLI Board of Directors and maintains regular, close communication with the Chairman of the LLLI Board. The LLLI Executive Director is responsible for furthering the LLLI mission and the effectiveness of LLLI's global operations.

LLL Affiliates

LLL Affiliates are autonomous entities, each bound to LLLI by the Agreement of International Principles of Cooperation, which they have signed with LLLI. Affiliates are Canada, Ligue La Leche (Canada Français), Deutschland, Great Britain, New Zealand, and Switzerland.

LLL Affiliates share the philosophy, purpose, and mission of La Leche League International and are committed to mutual support and communication.

Each Affiliate has its own governing body to meet the legal requirements of its country and direct the work of its Leaders. Each develops its own administrative structure, support and resource network, and job descriptions. All Affiliates are financially independent of LLLI. Affiliates pay an annual affiliation fee to LLLI based on the number of members and Leaders.

LLL Affiliates vary in size. Three Affiliates, Canada, Great Britain, and New Zealand, are English-speaking; Ligue La Leche is French-speaking; Deutschland works in German as well as English; Switzerland works in three languages, French, German, and Italian.

Each Affiliate produces its own publications that support and educate Leaders and mothers in the language and cultural context of the Affiliate. Five of the Affiliates publish their own member newsletter. Affiliates may provide—by purchasing for resale, reprinting, or translating—LLLI pamphlets and books, such as THE WOMANLY ART OF BREASTFEEDING and THE BREASTFEEDING ANSWER BOOK, or produce original pamphlets and books. Some Affiliates publish newsletters for health care providers and alumnae newsletters for Leaders and members.

LLL Divisions

There are three LLLI Divisions: Eastern United States Division (EUS), United States Western Division (USWD), and the International Division (ID). Divisions provide support and act as a resource for Areas and Area administrators, including orientation and ongoing training, written resources (such as handbooks and newsletters), workshops and meetings, and a network of support and resource Leaders.

Division structure and services may differ from one Division to another according to the needs of the Areas and the goal of keeping volunteer jobs manageable. Divisions and Areas are mutually accountable to each other and to Leaders. They are also accountable to LLLI and support its purpose, philosophy, and mission.

LLL Areas

LLL Areas are geographical units. Depending on circumstances, an LLL Area may consist of several countries, a single country, or a region of a country. An Area may be divided into Districts, each of which is made up of a number of Groups. The Area Council is the management team that handles the business of the Area, including setting goals, planning for Area and Leader needs, and providing support and resources to Area Leaders.

The Area organization serves as a link between Leaders and the Affiliate or Division. The Area is accountable to Leaders, LLLI, and the Affiliate/Division.

Areas provide information, resources, and support to Leaders within the scope of:

- Leader responsibilities and skills
- Leader accreditation
- Conferences and workshops
- Communication skills
- Publications
- Finances
- Medical and legal issues

The Area Council includes resource and support Leaders who have developed knowledge, experience, and skills in specific areas. Their responsibilities may vary according to the Area and the needs of Leaders and Groups. Some positions may be shared by more than one person; others may not exist in some Areas or may have different names.

Department names and division of responsibilities may also vary by Area, Affiliate, or Division. Your support Leader can give you specific information about the administrative structure and support and resource personnel for your Area and Affiliate/Division.

Leader Department

The Leader Department provides direct support to Leaders as they help mothers, lead Group meetings, or provide other service to the Area or larger organization. Members of the department correspond with Leaders and answer questions, offer suggestions, and provide information and resources such as newsletters and workshops. Department members are also available to help Leaders work through problems or difficulties.

Members of an Area Leader Department might include an Area Coordinator of Leaders, one or more Assistant Coordinators of Leaders or District Coordinators, and several District Advisors/Coordinators (depending on the Area or Affiliate/Division). Some Areas include other resource or administrative positions in this department, such as an Administrative Assistant, Area Secretary, Area Public Relations Coordinator, or Area Librarian.

Leader Accreditation Department

The Leader Accreditation Department (LAD) is an international department that works with and within LLL Affiliates, Divisions, Regions, Areas, and Districts. An international LAD helps maintain the integrity of La Leche League worldwide by accrediting Leaders according to universal LLLI accreditation criteria. (See **Chapter 5, Helping Mothers Become Leaders.**)

> The Area organization serves as a link between Leaders and the Affiliate or Division and includes resource and support Leaders who have knowledge, experience, and skills in specific areas.

KEEPING UP-TO-DATE

Members of the department answer questions about Leader accreditation, help Leaders as they work with mothers interested in leadership, and work with Leader Applicants and Leaders throughout the application. They might also help plan or participate in Leader Applicant workshops or sessions at workshops and conferences.

Area LAD personnel might include a Coordinator of Leader Accreditation and one or more Associate Coordinators of Leader Accreditation.

Conference/Events/Continuing Education Department

This department plans, coordinates, and carries out Area Conferences, workshops, or other events, including the program, facility, publicity, registration, finances, evaluation, and other details of the event. Department members may also be available to provide support and assistance to other Area resource and support Leaders planning Leader or Leader Applicant workshops or other events.

The department might include an Area Conference Supervisor or Area Coordinator of Events (or other position title, depending on the Area), a Local Conference Chairman, committee coordinators, members of the various committees, and other Area resource Leaders.

Communication Skills/Human Relations Enrichment

This department offers Communication Skills/Human Relations Enrichment (HRE) sessions and workshops for Leaders, Leader Applicants, Group members, parents, and health professionals. The sessions and workshops are presented by trained Communication Skills/HRE facilitators/instructors. Participants develop and practice skills in active listening, reflecting feelings, offering information, problem solving, conflict resolution, and other helping and communication skills. (See Communication Skills/Human Relations Enrichment Sessions in this chapter.)

An Area's Communication Skills/HRE Department might include one or more Communication Skills/HRE Facilitators or Instructors and perhaps a Communication Skills/HRE Facilitator/Instructor Trainer. (In some Affiliates/Divisions, the Trainer is part of the Affiliate/Division staff and is available to train Communication Skills/HRE facilitators/instructors anywhere in the Affiliate/Division.)

Publications

The Publications Department is responsible for written materials in the Area. This might include producing and distributing publications for Leaders (such as an Area Leaders' Letter or other Leader journal), LLL members (if they don't receive NEW BEGINNINGS as a benefit of membership), or health professionals. Several Areas and Affiliates also publish alumnae newsletters for Leaders and members.

Some Areas translate LLLI materials such as books, periodicals (LEAVEN, NEW BEGINNINGS, *LAD Lifeline*, BREASTFEEDING ABSTRACTS), pamphlets, and information sheets into their country's language(s), or they may create their own. If an Area has a Web site, this might also be part of the Publications Department.

Department members might include an Area Communications Coordinator, Publications Administrator or Coordinator; Area publication editors; pamphlet, translation, or distribution coordinators; and perhaps a Web site manager.

Finance

This department is responsible for the financial management of the Area, including the budget, financial transactions and records, tax and other legal requirements, and financial reporting to the Area, Affiliate/Division, and LLLI. The department may also offer support and resources to Group Leaders and Treasurers, including help with budgeting and other financial management concerns, fundraising, and information about country and local tax requirements.

Department members in an Area might include an Area Financial Coordinator or Administrator, Area Treasurer, Area Funding Development Coordinator, Area Walk Coordinator, and Area Fundraising, Marketing, or Sales Coordinators.

Professional Liaison Department

The Professional Liaison (PL) Department provides support and accurate, up-to-date information to Leaders helping mothers in medical, legal, or other complex or unusual situations. (See **Support for the Leader Dealing with Medically or Legally Related Issues**.)

Department members serve as a resource for Leaders with medically or legally related breastfeeding questions and assist Leaders with communicating and working with health care professionals. They have resources and outlines for presentations to medical professionals, and they may also be available to speak to medical professional audiences themselves. They help Leaders keep up-to-date on current breastfeeding information through articles in Area publications, correspondence, and conference/workshop sessions.

Area PL Department members might include the Area Professional Liaison and one or more Assistants or Associates.

KEEPING UP-TO-DATE

Professional Liaison Leaders serve as a resource for Leaders with medically or legally related breastfeeding questions.

SUPPORT FOR THE LEADER DEALING WITH MEDICALLY OR LEGALLY RELATED ISSUES

The Professional Liaison (PL) Leader provides the Group Leader with additional help when a mother needs information about a medically related breastfeeding situation or has a breastfeeding problem outside the scope of the Leader's knowledge. Like all LLL Leaders, the PL Leader does not give medical advice. She uses her reference collection as well as her experience to aid the Leader as she helps mothers and babies. The PL Leader can also provide information on some legal situations related to breastfeeding. (See also **Breastfeeding Questions and Possible Medical Implications,** in Chapter 1.)

Like all LLL Leaders, the Professional Liaison Leader does not give medical advice.

Before Contacting the Professional Liaison Leader

When faced with an unfamiliar situation or problem, look for information in your own collection of LLL-published materials. These might include:

- THE WOMANLY ART OF BREASTFEEDING, THE BREASTFEEDING ANSWER BOOK, other books published by LLL.
- LEAVEN, NEW BEGINNINGS, other LLL publications for Leaders or members.
- LLL pamphlets, leaflets, information and tear-off sheets.
- BREASTFEEDING ABSTRACTS or other LLL publications for health professionals.

- LLLI Web site, including online access to the Center for Breastfeeding Information and a collection of frequently asked Help Form questions (FAQs) and sample answers.

THE WOMANLY ART OF BREASTFEEDING And THE BREASTFEEDING ANSWER BOOK have indexes at the back. NEW BEGINNINGS, LEAVEN, and BREASTFEEDING ABSTRACTS have annual indexes. Other LLL books and periodicals may also have indexes you can check. Your LLL catalogue may include an index of book or other titles.

Many articles from back issues of LEAVEN, NEW BEGINNINGS, and BREASTFEEDING ABSTRACTS are available on the LLLI Web site. You can search for them by key words, topic, or publication date/issue.

Contacting the Professional Liaison Leader

If you are unable to find the information you need to help a mother, you may want to contact a PL Leader. You can then relay the information you obtain from the PL Leader back to the mother, rather than asking the mother to contact the PL Leader.

The PL Leader has a wider range of published materials at her disposal than most Leaders. She can also draw from the experience and knowledge of other PL Leaders. Since she is contacted frequently about unusual situations, she tends to have up-to-date information available on these subjects. She is familiar with medical resources and may have access to medical references on breastfeeding.

For unusual cases not covered in her references, the PL Leader can contact her Affiliate/Division PL resource Leader for additional input. The Affiliate/Division PL Leader may turn to the LLLI Center for Breastfeeding Information (CBI) for additional references and information. If necessary, the CBI Manager can refer the problem to members of the LLLI Health Advisory Council. (See **Center for Breastfeeding Information** and **LLLI Professional Advisory Board,** both in Chapter 8.)

Completing a Medical Questionnaire

Before contacting a PL Leader, fill out a Medical Questionnaire form (sample in **Appendix 4**). This form is a learning tool for Leaders as well as an aid to the PL Leader. It may be helpful to keep several blank Medical Questionnaire forms with your Leader's Logs.

The Medical Questionnaire is designed to help you define the problem and request appropriate information from the mother. Sometimes just filling out the form can help you answer a mother's question on your own. If you are still unsure, the completed Medical Questionnaire provides the PL Leader with the information she will need to research the problem.

When filling out the form, use descriptive terms that are as specific as possible. Too much information is better than too little.

You can mail, fax, or email the completed Medical Questionnaire or read it to the PL Leader over the telephone. If a mother needs help as soon as possible, complete the form and contact the PL Leader immediately.

Sometimes just filling out a Medical Questionnaire can help you answer a mother's question.

Online PL Support for LLL Leaders

The Online Professional Liaison Resource (OPLR) Leaders support all LLL Leaders in several ways. They are a resource for medical, legal, outreach, and professional activities for Leaders doing online Help Forms or LLL chats, as well as for those who need immediate assistance but can't contact their local PL Leaders. They redirect Leaders to their regular channels in the LLL chain of support for non-urgent questions.

OPLR Leaders are also available to assist Leaders in representing LLL to the professional community on the Internet. For example, Leaders need to remember the professional nature of some email lists and follow established guidelines when representing LLL online. (See **Representing La Leche League Online** in Chapter 1.)

Contacting the Online Professional Liaison Resource Leader

If you are helping a mother in a medically related breastfeeding situation and can't find the information you need in your own materials, you may want to contact a PL Leader. If the mother contacted you by telephone, in person, or postal mail, first check with your local PL Leaders.

If they are not available and you think the situation is urgent, or if you are a Leader who needs assistance in answering a mother's question in an Email Breastfeeding Help Form from the LLLI Web site, contact a member of the Online PL Resource Team. Complete an OPLR Leader Contact Form, which is located on the LLLI Web site at **http://www.lalecheleague.org/llleaderweb/FIN/oplr.html** (contact your support Leader for the username and password). Your form will be routed to one of the OPLR Leaders for research.

Completing an OPLR Leader Contact Form helps the OPLR Leaders keep their workloads manageable. When you take the time to complete a Contact Form (which is essentially the same as the Medical Questionnaire form found in Appendix 4), you may find that you are able to answer the mother's question with your own resources. If you still need PL resources, OPLR Leaders are able to help more quickly and effectively if the form is completed. They try to respond within a day or two in an emergency.

LLL PUBLICATIONS

LLL publications are a primary source of information for Leaders. While your personal breastfeeding experience provides insight and understanding, LLL publications support your experience with background information, research findings, and the accumulated knowledge of mothers over more than 45 years. LLL publications can help you keep up-to-date, prepare for and lead Series Meetings, and support mothers who call with breastfeeding concerns.

Online Professional Liaison Resource Leaders are available to assist Leaders in representing LLL to the professional community on the Internet.

KEEPING UP-TO-DATE

LLL publications support a Leader's experience with background information, research findings, and the accumulated knowledge of mothers over more than 45 years.

THE WOMANLY ART OF BREASTFEEDING

THE WOMANLY ART OF BREASTFEEDING is LLLI's classic guide to breastfeeding. It provides information and support, including breastfeeding facts and management techniques, along with affirmation and encouragement for the breastfeeding relationship. You need the most recent edition available in your language so you can refer to it often.

The book's index directs the reader to the information she needs. If you let a mother know that information or a suggestion was found in THE WOMANLY ART OF BREASTFEEDING, it's an easy transition to suggesting she might want to own a copy. When you refer to THE WOMANLY ART OF BREASTFEEDING during Series Meeting discussions, mothers see that this reference is one they can turn to again and again.

THE WOMANLY ART OF BREASTFEEDING is the most important book in a Group Library. Every Group needs one or more copies to lend to mothers. It is also the basic book for a Group to offer for sale. Profits from its sale provide a financial foundation for the Group Treasury, and mothers have a source of essential breastfeeding information and support.

If bookstores in your community sell THE WOMANLY ART OF BREASTFEEDING, you may want to offer a discount to members or mothers attending meetings. Purchased through an LLL Group, THE WOMANLY ART OF BREASTFEEDING comes "packaged" with LLL warmth and support.

> Purchased through an LLL Group, THE WOMANLY ART OF BREASTFEEDING comes "packaged" with LLL warmth and support.

THE BREASTFEEDING ANSWER BOOK

THE BREASTFEEDING ANSWER BOOK is a comprehensive, fully referenced guide to breastfeeding management. The easy-to-use format provides both basic information and in-depth material. The book is divided into chapters and organized by breastfeeding situation, problem, or concern. Each chapter has an extensive list of references. A thumbnail guide on the back cover helps direct the reader to the appropriate chapter. The detailed index helps you find specific information quickly, as well as locate multiple references to a particular breastfeeding situation.

As a comprehensive breastfeeding reference, THE BREASTFEEDING ANSWER BOOK includes many options that go beyond the normal course of breastfeeding. Not all options apply to every situation, and you would not need or want to mention every suggestion to every mother.

You are not expected to know all the detailed information on breastfeeding management included in the book, but it is important to have access to this valuable LLL resource if it's available in your language.

LLL Leader Journals

LLL Leader journals include LEAVEN (published in English by LLLI), Leader publications produced by Affiliates or Divisions, and Area publications for Leaders such as Area Leaders' Letters. (See **Materials in Languages Other Than English,** in this chapter.) Their purpose is to inform and inspire you, help you keep up-to-date on current breastfeeding and LLL information, and encourage you in performing basic Leader responsibilities.

Articles and columns focus on the basic responsibilities of LLL leadership, breastfeeding research, publications, funding development, and activities of Groups and Leaders in all parts of the Area, Affiliate/Division, or world. It's a good idea to keep back issues on file for reference.

LLL Member Journals

LLL member journals include NEW BEGINNINGS, LLLI's bimonthly publication for members, and member publications produced by Areas and Affiliates. (See **Materials in Languages Other Than English,** in this chapter.) Member publications provide information and inspiration to mothers and Leaders through articles, stories, poems, and photos. Features are often written with the first-time mother in mind, approximating what she might experience at an LLL Series Meeting.

You can use LLL member journals during Series Meetings and when helping mothers one-to-one. Narrative stories often contain inspirational passages that can be used as opening or closing comments at Series Meetings. One mother's story may offer information and encouragement to another mother facing a similar challenge. Informative features can help open the discussion topic or add supporting material. For example, the "Eating Wisely" column in NEW BEGINNINGS may provide part of the focus for Meeting 4. Question-and-answer columns may offer an interesting starting point for discussion at Evaluation or Enrichment Meetings. Book reviews can help you select books for the Group Library. Highlighting member publications at meetings can encourage mothers to become LLL members.

KEEPING UP-TO-DATE

LLL Pamphlets, Booklets, Brochures, Information and Tear-Off Sheets

Leaflets, pamphlets, booklets, information sheets, and tear-off sheets are topic-specific publications. They can be sold, offered in the Group Library, included in new mother packets, or used in educational and outreach settings in the community. You can also give or send them to mothers to help summarize and reinforce information. Brochures help promote LLL programs or events and inform others about the benefits of breastfeeding.

Health Care Professional Publications

BREASTFEEDING ABSTRACTS is published quarterly by LLLI for health care providers. Several Areas in the International Division and some Affiliates also produce newsletters for health care professionals. Many Leaders subscribe to these valuable resources as well. These publications may include abstracts or summaries of recent research articles on breastfeeding from the medical literature, a lead article that covers a topic of current interest in the field of lactation, and reviews of professional books. Your Professional Liaison Leader may have a file of back issues.

Materials in Languages Other than English

Through the efforts of volunteers all over the world, LLL breastfeeding information is available in more than 20 languages. Translations of LLLI publications, along with original pamphlets in various languages, are primarily published and distributed by International Division Areas and the Affiliates. Non-English publications available directly from LLLI are listed in the LLLI Catalogue (No. 401–20), the LLLI Spanish Catalogue (No. 421–20), the LLLI Translated Books Catalogue (No. 1113–20), and on the LLLI Web site.

Through the efforts of volunteers all over the world, LLL breastfeeding information is available in more than 20 languages.

Contacts for obtaining LLL publications in languages other than English are listed in the Global Publications Directory (No. 404–20) and the LLLI Translated Books Catalogue (No. 1113–20), both available from the LLLI Catalogue and on the LLLI Web site.

There are also a number of Leader and LLL member publications produced by International Division Areas and the Affiliates. Many are in languages other than English. To subscribe to one of these publications, contact the Area Coordinator of Leaders or Affiliate representative. Refer to the LLLI Personnel Directory (No. 405–13), the International Directory (No. 402–20), or the LLLI Web site for contact information.

Newsletters for Leaders
- Austria (German) – *Beraterinnen Rundbrief*
- Canada (English) – *Canadian Collage*
- Deutschland (German and English) – *Beraterinnen Brief / Allegro*
- Future Areas of Africa and the Middle East (English) – *ALL in the Family*
- Future Areas in Asia (English) – *ALL around Asia*
- Future Areas in Europe (English) – *Future Lives*
- France (French) – *La LLLettre*
- Great Britain (English) – *Feedback*
- Ireland (English) – *The Irish Leader*
- Israel (English and Hebrew) – *IsraeLL*
- Italy (Italian) – *Latte e Miele*
- Japan (English and Japanese) – *Nakama*
- Ligue La Leche (Canada Français; in French) – *La Berceuse*
- Mexico (Spanish) – *Déjame que te cuente LLLigueña*
- The Netherlands (Dutch) – *KringLLLoop Circle*
- New Zealand (English) – *Mosaic*
- South Africa (English) – *SunLLLight*
- Switzerland (German, French, and Italian) – *Beraterinnenbrief / Lettre aux Animatrices / Lettera alli Consulenti*

Newsletters for LLL members
- Austria (German) – *Infobrief*
- Belgium (French) – *LLLiaison*
- LLL of Maceio, Brazil (Portuguese) – *Bollletim Informativo*
- Colombia (Spanish) – *Nuevo Comienzo* (read by Spanish-speaking mothers and Leaders in Latin America and Spain; also available from LLLI)
- Deutschland (German) – *Mitglieder Brief*
- France (French) – *Allaiter Aujourd'hui*
- Future Areas in Asia (English) – *Close to the Heart*
- Great Britain (English) – *LLLGB News*
- Hungary (Hungarian) – *LLL Lapja*
- Italy (Italian) – *Da Mamma a Mamma*
- Ligue La Leche (Canada Français; in French) – *La Voie Lactee*
- The Netherlands (Dutch) – *Borstvoeding Vandaag*
- New Zealand (English) – *Aroha*
- Spain (Spanish) – *Informacion trimestral* (Catalonia, Madrid, and Andalucia)
- Switzerland (German) – *buLLLetin* (also read by mothers in Germany and Austria)

For information about non-English materials available on the LLLI Web site, see **Online Resources from LLLI** in Chapter 8.

LLL Bibliographies

LLLI publishes the LLLI Bibliography, which contains the titles of books that have been approved for use in Group Libraries. (See **Selecting Books for the Group Library** in Chapter 4.) To recommend a recently published book you think should be included in the LLLI Bibliography or to express concerns or other thoughts about books already approved for the LLLI Bibliography, contact any member of the LLLI Book Evaluation Committee. Committee members can be reached through the LLLI Publications Department or the LLLI Web site. (See **Book Evaluation Committee** in Chapter 8.)

Areas and Affiliates have the option to compile their own LLL bibliographies of books. Contact your support Leader to find out if your Area or Affiliate has its own list of books that are helpful to parents and supportive of the mission, purpose, and philosophy of LLLI.

You can find reviews of books in the LLL bibliographies in LEAVEN, NEW BEGINNINGS, or your Area/Division/Affiliate's Leader or member publications.

LLL INTERNET RESOURCES

Because the LLLI Web site is updated frequently with the latest information from LLLI, you can rely on it as your first choice for breastfeeding information on the Internet. Review non-LLL Internet resources on breastfeeding with the same "critical reading" standards you use for printed material. (See **Using Non-LLL Sources** in this chapter, and **Representing La Leche League Online** in Chapter 1.)

KEEPING UP-TO-DATE

You can rely on the LLLI Web site as your first choice of breastfeeding information on the Internet.

LLLI Web Site

The LLLI Web site at **http://www.lalecheleague.org** offers a variety of information for Leaders. Some of the Leader pages are password-protected; you can obtain the username and password from your support Leader or the LLLI webmaster.

The Leader area of the LLLI Web site includes:

- Hundreds of Leaven articles.
- Meeting ideas submitted by Leaders around the world.
- Sample answers to frequently asked questions (FAQs) on online Help Forms, which you can use and modify for the particular circumstances of the mothers you are helping.
- The OPLR Leader Contact Form, which you can send to a volunteer Online Professional Liaison Resource Leader if a Help Form question is outside the scope of your knowledge or resources (see **Contacting the Online Professional Liaison Resource Leader** in this chapter).
- LLLI Bibliography for a listing of books you can use in Group Libraries (check with your support Leader to see if specific listings are appropriate where you live).
- The complete text of the LLLI Policies and Standing Rules Notebook.
- Many Leader Accreditation Department (LAD) documents, including materials that are part of the Application Packet.
- Leader Specialty File—listings of Leaders with special areas of expertise.

The "public" area of the LLLI Web site includes an archive of NEW BEGINNINGS and BREASTFEEDING ABSTRACTS articles. You can search for LEAVEN, NEW BEGINNINGS, and BREASTFEEDING ABSTRACTS articles by key words, topic, or publication date/issue.

You can access the Center for Breastfeeding Information (CBI), LLLI's collection of professional research articles, through the LLLI Web site. If you are a first-time user, you'll be asked to register to receive your own personal username and password. You can then search the CBI database by key words, subject, title, author, or publication date/issue and receive a list of citations. Because of copyright regulations, you'll need to look up the articles in your local library or pay the CBI fees to receive copies. (See **Center for Breastfeeding Information** in Chapter 8.)

For more information about the LLLI Web site and the resources it provides to Leaders, members, and the general public, see **Online Resources from LLLI** in Chapter 8.

Other Online Resources for Leaders

Many Areas, Affiliates, and Divisions have Web sites with resources for Leaders. LLLI's Web site has links to other LLL Web sites, or you can contact your support Leader to find out if your Area or Affiliate/Division has a Web site and how to access it.

The LLLUSA Web site at **www.lllusa.org** has links to Area, Division, and department files and resources, as well as projects that LLL is engaged in within the United States. Leaders in the US can contact their support Leader or Area Coordinator of Leaders for the username and password.

Many Areas, Divisions, Affiliates, and LLL departments maintain email lists as a means to exchange ideas and information. Often documents are distributed this way, which saves postage and printing costs while still allowing documents to be distributed via postal mail to Leaders without email access. The publications chat list (ALLECats) is open to LLL editors and other publications people from all over the world. The LAD list (LADialogue) is open to LAD representatives from all over the world.

Some Leaders have joined informal, unofficial email discussion groups for Leaders such as TLC (The Leader Connection), enLLLace (a similar discussion group for Spanish-speaking Leaders), or other Leader discussion groups in their language, country, Area, Affiliate, or Division. These discussion groups do not represent LLL or its purpose and philosophy nor do they replace LLL's network of support and resource Leaders. (See also **Email Lists** in the next section.)

Leaders who participate in email discussion groups enjoy the opportunity to kindle friendships, share ideas and encouragement, and create Leader-to-Leader connections. For more information about joining an email discussion group, contact the list owner or a Leader who participates on the list.

If you're interested in creating your own email discussion group with other Leaders, please set it up as a "private" and "hidden" list so it can't be found by anyone typing "La Leche League" into a search engine.

USING NON-LLL SOURCES

Most situations and questions Leaders encounter when helping mothers and babies can be answered using LLL's people, published, and Internet resources. Not only are LLL resources extensive, credible, reliable, and consistent with LLLI recommendations, they also present information and suggestions in ways that let mothers decide for themselves what is best for their situation.

Leaders sometimes turn to non-LLL sources to find information for mothers in unusual situations. The amount of accurate breastfeeding literature has increased dramatically in recent years. However, before using non-LLL sources, whether published or on the Internet, you'll need to read them critically and carefully, evaluating them in light of LLL recommendations.

If you find information in a non-LLL source that might be pertinent to a mother you are helping, first determine whether that information conflicts with what you have read in LLL publications. If there is no conflict, you can offer the new information to the mother, providing the source so the mother and/or her doctor can refer to it directly.

If there is a conflict between the information you've found in another source and the usual LLL recommendations, consult a more experienced Leader or a Professional Liaison Leader before offering it to a mother. LLL recommendations have come about as the result of many years of experience on the part of mothers, researchers, and health care providers.

You can offer the mother information from various viewpoints, especially when sources disagree. It is always up to the mother in consultation with her health care provider to make her own decision about the course of action she chooses.

Critical Reading

Critical reading of breastfeeding information begins by comparing the information to documented research on the topic and by determining the type of information you are reading. The further removed the information is from the original research report, the more apt it may be to contain errors, omissions, misinterpretations, or oversimplifications of vital information.

Popular reports interpreting research for a wider audience are often published in magazines and newspapers or cited on radio and television. These reports may or may not accurately reflect the information in the original research article. They may not include information on how the research was conducted and won't usually explain the shortcomings or qualifications the researchers cite in the original article.

If you want to follow up on something you have read or heard, your local library is a good place to start. Often a librarian can help you get a copy of the original research study through the library's network of resources.

When you have a copy of a research study, you can look at it from several angles. Note what conditions were created by the researchers and evaluate how closely they correspond to those faced by the average mother. You can see how the researchers themselves described their findings. Were they seen as definitive or merely suggestive? Did they recommend further studies to confirm their conclusions? Consider the scope of the study. Conclusions based on findings taken from one individual would be less significant than a study using thousands of subjects. Another consideration

> LLL resources present information in ways that let mothers decide for themselves what is best for their situation.

KEEPING UP-TO-DATE

> By reading critically, you can decide if the information may be applicable to the mothers you help.

is how the study was funded. Work funded by a particular interest group or industry may be less objective than an independent study.

By reading critically, you can decide for yourself if the information may be applicable to the mothers you help. You can also contact your Professional Liaison Leader for help in evaluating and interpreting medical or technical information from any source.

Web Sites

Leaders also need to read and evaluate information from Web sites and email lists with a critical eye: Who is the author? What are his or her credentials? Who sponsors the Web site? Is the information backed by properly cited research studies?

Although excellent medical information generally can be obtained from college and major medical center Web sites, inaccurate and/or obsolete material can be found on even the most authoritative sites.

Email Lists

Although the exchange of thoughts and ideas on an email list or discussion group is usually informal, the communication is written. Messages posted to a list, however, are neither peer-reviewed nor edited. You may need to regard such text with caution, even if the writer is a recognized authority on the topic being discussed. Be careful when sharing non-referenced, anecdotal, or personal observations and/or opinions posted on these lists, and request permission from the original writer before you share such messages with others.

LactNet is an email list for specialists and professionals in the field of lactation. Leaders, as specialists in lactation, also subscribe to and participate in this email list. If you choose to participate in LactNet as a Leader, keep in mind that you are representing LLL to these health professionals and that everything you post affects the image of La Leche League. (See **Representing La Leche League Online** in Chapter 1.)

Rumors and hoaxes

Many widely circulating health-related email messages or warnings are mostly myths or hoaxes, often referred to as "urban legends." Please check the validity of these types of email messages before sharing them with others.

CONTINUING EDUCATION EVENTS FOR LEADERS

One of LLL's greatest strengths is our worldwide network of Leaders, who continually share and learn.

Getting together with other Leaders at meetings, in workshops, at conferences, and on the Internet can strengthen your knowledge and skills. Leaders inspire other Leaders with Series Meeting ideas, one-to-one helping techniques, fundraising projects, and tips for balancing LLL with family. This is one of LLL's greatest strengths—our worldwide network of Leaders who continually share and learn, enhancing the solid base of information and experience available to breastfeeding mothers.

Another area of learning and reinforcement takes place when Leaders get together: support and encouragement for the kind of mothering we want to give our children. Many Leaders find that they share a common bond in their parenting goals.

Even though this kind of interaction often takes place on an informal basis, there are many opportunities in La Leche League especially designed to provide Leader enrichment, education, and skill enhancement.

Chapter Meetings

An LLL Chapter is formed by Leaders, usually from neighboring Groups, who choose to meet regularly to discuss topics of mutual interest. Chapters may or may not follow District boundaries. Isolated Leaders may choose to meet on the Internet, getting together in person as time and finances permit.

Usually one person (or a small group of people) agrees to coordinate the Chapter for a period of time. She makes arrangements and notifies the others when and where the meeting will take place, who will provide refreshments, if any, and what will be covered during the meeting. She also reports to the Groups' support Leader(s) on the Chapter's activities.

Some Chapters decide on discussion topics meeting by meeting; others develop a yearly schedule of topics. Many Chapters set aside time for announcements of Group activities; some use part of the meeting to discuss challenging helping situations.

Chapters help Groups and Leaders to help each other. The networking is invaluable. Groups often collaborate on community activities and/or fundraisers. Groups can save money by ordering as a Chapter and taking advantage of quantity discounts.

LLL Workshops

A District Workshop is organized by (or with the assistance of) the support Leader for the Groups in the District. Sometimes the Leaders and Leader Applicants in several Districts get together, or an Area, Region, or Affiliate/Division might hold a larger workshop. Depending on travel distance, workshops might be held once or twice a year. A small registration fee may be charged to cover the cost of materials and other expenses. Your registration fee and travel expenses can be paid out of Group funds. Check with your support Leader about Area/Affiliate guidelines for using Group funds to pay registration fees or travel expenses for Leader Applicants.

Several topics are usually planned to meet the needs of the Leaders and Leader Applicants who attend. The topics may be presented by Area/Division/Affiliate resource and support Leaders or local Leaders.

Topics covered at workshops relate to the Leader role. For instance, they might include breastfeeding research and management, counseling and communication skills, organization tips, working with health care providers, Series Meeting ideas, and helping mothers prepare for leadership. Area/Affiliate personnel may use the opportunity to bring Leaders up-to-date on Area/Affiliate news, plans, procedures, and guidelines. Get-acquainted and personal enrichment topics are often included as well.

LLL workshops are a wonderful opportunity to network with neighboring Leaders as well as LLL resource and support Leaders. Both Leaders and Leader Applicants find the experience energizing.

Chapters help Groups and Leaders to help each other.

KEEPING UP-TO-DATE

LLL workshops are a wonderful opportunity to network with neighboring Leaders as well as LLL resource and support Leaders.

LLL Conferences

For many Leaders, attending an LLL Conference is a highlight of their years of involvement.

For many Leaders, attending an LLL conference is a highlight of their years of involvement. There are many opportunities to learn from speakers and informal chats with other Leaders. The opportunity to spend time in a totally supportive atmosphere, where breastfeeding and loving parenting are the norm, reinforces what Leaders believe.

Area, National, Regional, Division, Affiliate, and LLLI Conferences are usually announced in LEAVEN, NEW BEGINNINGS, Area and Affiliate/Division publications, and on the LLLI Web site well in advance, so everyone has plenty of time to make plans. LLL Groups, Chapters, Areas, Divisions, and Affiliates often sponsor special fundraising activities to enable Leaders to attend these events.

Area Conferences

An Area Conference is a one- or two-day event providing information on breastfeeding and parenting in a uniquely supportive environment. Leaders, parents, health care providers, and other specialists lead a variety of sessions throughout the conference. An Area Conference is open to all who are interested in learning about breastfeeding and related topics. There may be sessions scheduled specifically for Leaders and Leader Applicants as well as sessions on many aspects of parenting. Some Area Conferences offer continuing education credits for health care providers. (See **Continuing Medical and Health Education Activities** in Chapter 8.)

Areas usually schedule conferences on a regular basis, once a year or every other year. A central location may be chosen or the site may vary from year to year. Upcoming Area Conferences are listed in Leader and member publications and on the LLLI Web site. Your support Leader or an Area Council member can provide information about upcoming Area Conferences in your Area or neighboring ones.

Affiliate, National, Regional, or Division Conferences

Affiliate/National/Regional/Division conferences not only cover a wider geographic area but also cover an extensive selection of topics. Many combine support for Leaders and Area/Division/Affiliate personnel with opportunities to network with health care providers. Many also offer a wide variety of special LLL guests and professional speakers and provide continuing education credits for health care providers. (See **Continuing Medical and Health Education Activities** in Chapter 8.) Check Area/Division/Affiliate publications, LEAVEN, NEW BEGINNINGS, and the LLLI and Area/Division/Affiliate Web sites for announcements about these special learning opportunities.

LLLI Conferences

Once they have attended an LLLI Conference, many Leaders vow to attend as many future conferences as possible.

LLLI Conferences are usually held every other year in a major city that has an international airport and easy access by ground transportation. A hotel large enough to house the event under one roof is necessary, since several thousand adults and children attend the conference. Meetings, sessions, meals, and workshops are scheduled from morning to evening, providing topics of interest to everyone who attends.

Speakers include breastfeeding experts, health care providers, and well-known authors. A unique aspect of an LLLI Conference is the opportunity to hear experienced parents from all over the world discuss topics that are relevant to families. Once they have attended an LLLI Conference, many Leaders vow to attend as many future conferences as possible.

Communication Skills/Human Relations Enrichment Sessions

Communication Skills and Human Relations Enrichment (HRE) are programs designed to help participants develop and enhance communication skills. Trained Communication Skills/HRE facilitators/instructors offer a variety of workshops for Leaders, Leader Applicants, Group members, and other interested parties at stand-alone sessions or in conjunction with LLL workshops and conferences.

Communication Skills/HRE workshops provide opportunities to learn more about and practice basic communication skills, such as identifying feelings, empathetic listening skills, asking effective questions, presenting information, setting limits, and problem solving.

Many Areas and Affiliates offer additional Communication Skills/HRE sessions such as:

- Interactive Group Leading
- Conflict Resolution
- Assertion Powers
- Communicating with Children

The Communication Skills/HRE program has been developed over the years by experienced LLL Leaders. The program is based on approaches found in books that include *People Skills* (Bolton), *Getting to Yes* (Fisher and Ury), *Please Understand Me* (Keirsey and Bates), and *Difficult Conversations* (Stone, Patton, and Heen).

To find out more about communication skills sessions and workshops offered in your Area or Affiliate, contact your support Leader or a member of your Area/Affiliate's Communication Skills/HRE Department. (See **Communication Skills/Human Relations Enrichment** in the **LLL Areas** section of this chapter.)

Other Continuing Education Opportunities

Leaders seeking additional educational opportunities related to breastfeeding may be interested in becoming an LLLI Peer Counselor Program Administrator. LLLI offers Peer Counselor Program Administrator training workshops for Leaders and others wishing to start an LLLI Peer Counselor Program. (See **Breastfeeding Peer Counselor Program** in Chapter 7.)

For Leaders interested in becoming lactation consultants or maintaining their certification, LLLI's Lactation Specialist Workshops, designated LLLI Conference sessions, and LLLI Independent Study Modules offer continuing education credits for lactation consultants (CERPs) as well as other health care professionals. Area/Division/Affiliate conferences may offer continuing education credits also. (See **Leader/Lactation Consultant** in Chapter 7, and **Continuing Medical and Health Education Activities** in Chapter 8.)

Communication Skills/Human Relations Enrichment sessions help participants develop and enhance communication skills.

KEEPING UP-TO-DATE

Many Leaders enjoy attending health care provider conferences and workshops, including Area/Division/Affiliate-sponsored events and LLLI's Lactation Specialist Workshops and annual Seminars for Physicians. Others take college or university classes to explore new interests or complete a degree. Colleges and adult or business education organizations may offer courses and training workshops in specific areas such as grant writing, fundraising, nonprofit issues, writing, editing, Web site design, computer skills, and other areas of interest to LLL Leaders and administrators.

CHAPTER SEVEN

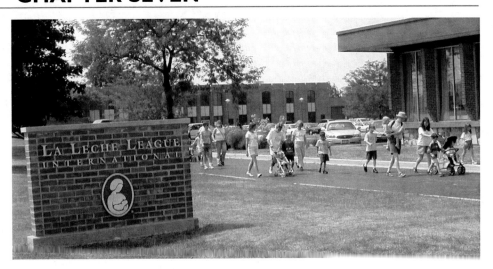

Additional Opportunities for Leaders

The definition of an active Leader in the LLLI Policies and Standing Rules (PSR) Notebook states: "An active LLL Leader pursues the La Leche League mission through basic Leader responsibilities as defined in the Policies and Standing Rules Notebook and/or other service to LLL. An active Leader's fees are current, she keeps up to date with Leader education, and she communicates regularly with the organization."

Leaders are often involved in service to LLL other than the basic Leader responsibilities defined in the PSR—helping mothers one-to-one and on the phone, leading monthly Series Meetings, managing the Group, keeping up-to-date on breastfeeding information, and helping other mothers find out about leadership and prepare to become LLL Leaders. Once a Leader has gained experience as a Group Leader, she sometimes takes on other responsibilities in addition to or instead of leading a Group, after consulting with her co-Leaders and support Leader.

Leaders add to their responsibilities as time, interest, and energy permit. Many Leaders see these additional responsibilities as opportunities for personal development and fulfillment while working to promote breastfeeding. No Leader is expected or required to extend herself beyond the basics. Neither is she restricted to these basics if she has the talents and desire to support LLL in some other vital way.

Some Leaders choose particular activities that meet a specific need of breastfeeding mothers in their community. For example, monthly meetings for employed breastfeeding mothers might complement the standard Series Meetings or an LLLI Breastfeeding Peer Counselor Program might be launched to better serve a particular community. Other Leaders promote LLL and breastfeeding at a booth at a health or community fair. Leaders are sometimes invited to speak to teens at a local school, to health care professionals or mothers at a local hospital, or to work with breastfeeding mothers at local health clinics. Work as an LLL representative on government committees and task forces or with Non-Governmental Organizations (NGOs), such as UNICEF or WABA provides still other opportunities to pursue the LLLI mission. Some Leaders have specialized skills, for example in marketing or public relations, that they choose to use for LLL, locally, nationally, or globally

> **Many Leaders see these additional responsibilities as opportunities for personal development and fulfillment while working to promote breastfeeding.**

A Leader balances her activity level from month to month and from year to year throughout her leadership career. When considering whether any of these options are viable for you or your community, think in terms of interested and affected parties in your community. Your Leader support network is your first source of information about participation in any activity. It is important to discuss your plans with your co-Leaders and to inform your support Leader as you expand or reduce your LLL volunteer work. The remainder of this chapter provides more information about:

- Planning and leading optional meetings
- Writing for LLL publications
- Opportunities in LLL administration—Area, Region, Division/Affiliate
- Special LLLI committees and work groups
- Answering the hotLLLine
- Peer counselor program
- Cooperative action with other organizations supporting breastfeeding
- World Walk for Breastfeeding
- Leader/lactation consultant
- LLL service online

For information on other activities that may be of interest to you, contact your support Leader.

PLANNING AND LEADING OPTIONAL MEETINGS

> **It is important to discuss your plans with your Co-Leaders and to inform your support Leader as you expand or reduce your LLL volunteer work.**

Depending on the needs of the community, the local Group may want to offer special meetings or a special series of meetings. Special meetings are optional. Generally, Leaders wait until they have a good background in leading Series Meetings before moving on to leading special meetings and classes. It is important to talk your plans over with your co-Leader(s) and your support Leader before organizing a special meeting or class.

In some areas, special meetings serve a group of mothers whom LLL would not ordinarily reach. Some of the special meetings offered by LLL Leaders are Enrichment Meetings, Toddler Meetings, Couples Meetings, Employed Breastfeeding Mother Meetings, Tandem Breastfeeding Meetings, Breastfeeding Twins Meetings, Breastfeeding Classes, and Breastfeeding Classes for Teens.

Chapter 2, "Planning and Leading a Series Meeting," includes general information that applies to leading LLL meetings of any type. In this chapter you'll find additional information about leading Enrichment Meetings, Toddler Meetings, Couples Meetings, Employed Breastfeeding Mothers Meetings, classes for teens, and breastfeeding classes. Your support Leader and the LLLI Web site at **www.lalecheleague.org** are two other sources for information and ideas about special meetings.

ENRICHMENT MEETINGS

Many Groups hold Enrichment Meetings in addition to Series Meetings. Enrichment Meetings focus on a topic in depth, and are usually attended by Group members, Group workers, Leader Applicants, and Leaders. A Leader can choose to hold an Enrichment Meeting any time she thinks it will meet the needs of the Group.

Meeting Format

An Enrichment Meeting is usually one of four types. Use any style that you think suits the Group, or try a combination.

- **Unstructured enrichment**—Leaders, Leader Applicants, and mothers spend time socializing. Mothers naturally bring up their experiences and concerns.
- **Leader-led enrichment**—The Leader guides a discussion on a selected topic.
- **Mother-led enrichment**—The Leader asks a Leader Applicant or Group member to prepare a topic for discussion.
- **Invited speaker or presentation**—The Leader invites an outside speaker to make a presentation or speak on a topic of interest to the mothers; consult with your support Leader on review procedures for speaker selection. When selecting a speaker, consider what the topic and/or speaker contributes to the purpose and mission of LLL, as well as the purpose of the meeting.

Many groups combine Evaluation Meetings with their Enrichment Meetings by spending 10 or 15 minutes critiquing the last Series Meeting and discussing Group business before moving on to an enrichment topic.

You may find that after posing an introductory opening question to make sure that everyone becomes acquainted, you only need one discussion topic question and the conversation flows from then on. Sometimes the most successful Enrichment Meetings are those where the discussion is kept informal.

Meeting Focus

In addition to the list below, good sources for topic ideas are mothers, workshops and conferences, the LLLI Web site, and Leader and member publications.

- Nurturing ourselves as mothers
- Maternal emotions and sexuality
- Nighttime parenting and sleeping arrangements
- Streamlining housework
- Organizational skills for families
- Living on less, saving money
- Fast, nutritious meals
- Toddler nutrition
- Loving guidance
- Creative play ideas
- Children's book favorites
- Sibling rivalry
- Parenting older children
- Traveling with children

> Sometimes the most successful Enrichment Meetings are those where the discussion is kept informal.

MORE OPPORTUNITIES

- Reducing holiday stress
- Specific aspects of LLLI philosophy
- Communicating with partners about LLL ideas
- History of LLL
- LLL's image—sharing first impressions
- Group Library book review
- Discussing an article from an LLL publication
- Learning about LLL leadership role
- Sharing LLL workshop or conference experiences
- Demonstrating food preparation or craft skills

Choose a time and location

Enrichment Meetings are held to meet the needs of Group members, Group workers, Leader Applicants and Leaders. Consider morning, lunch time, afternoon, dinner time, and evening when choosing a time for the meeting. Some Groups prefer a set time and location, while other Groups need more flexibility. Groups that hold their Series Meetings in a public place may find that Enrichment Meetings are a nice opportunity for Group members to become more involved by hosting a meeting. Others find a park or outdoor location keeps older children happy while mothers focus on the discussion.

Handouts, books, and items for sale

Handouts, books, and items for sale are often not needed at Enrichment Meetings. If you do want to offer a handout, check with your support Leader for handout review procedures. If it is convenient, it is nice to have the Group Library on hand. The low-key atmosphere gives mothers a chance to browse through the books at a more leisurely pace.

TODDLER MEETINGS

Many mothers continue to attend Series Meetings after their initial breastfeeding questions have been answered. They come to offer help to other mothers and to receive support themselves. Because discussions at LLL Series Meetings traditionally meet the needs of pregnant and new mothers first, a special meeting where mothers can thoroughly discuss the joys and challenges of extended breastfeeding can help meet the needs of mothers of older babies and toddlers.

> A special meeting where mothers can thoroughly discuss the joys and challenges of extended breastfeeding can help meet the needs of mothers of older babies and toddlers.

Some Groups hold a Toddler Meeting once a series; others hold monthly Toddler Meetings. Still other Groups have no set schedule for Toddler Meetings but plan one whenever the toddler population merits one. A Chapter might organize Toddler Meetings, giving mothers the opportunity to enlarge their support networks.

Choose a time and location

Some Groups hold Toddler Meetings during the day at a time when children are fresh and rested. At an informal meeting, everyone can sit among the little ones and playthings for a relaxed discussion. You can begin with discussion-starter questions (often the discussion starts on its own) and offer LLL information, suggestions, philosophy, and resources as needed.

Other Groups hold Toddler Meetings during the evening. Some mothers feel uncomfortable talking about their children while the children are listening. Perhaps an older toddler would be more comfortable staying home with father near bedtime. Some mothers may prefer to bring their breastfeeding toddler along to the evening meeting, dressed and ready for bed. You may want to discuss this with the mothers before deciding on a meeting time.

When choosing a location to meet, pay close attention to the area where toddlers will play and perhaps enjoy a snack. Toddlers are curious and love to explore. Make sure the meeting area is toddler-proof, both for the safety of the toddlers and the peace of mind of the hostess and mothers eager to participate in the meeting discussion. When planning for snacks/food, keep in mind possible spills and allergies. It is your responsibility to find out where the hostess or facility allows food and to inform everyone at the meeting. Leave the meeting space clean when you are finished. Clean-up time can be an extended opportunity for the mothers to socialize.

> Make sure the meeting area is toddler-proof, both for the safety of the toddlers and the peace of mind of the hostess and mothers eager to participate in the meeting discussion.

Meeting notices

Mothers may be unsure whether their child is welcome or expected at special meetings. Including a note like this may help: "As at all La Leche League functions, we welcome babies in arms and small children who would be unhappy away from their mothers." One Group that holds a monthly Toddler Meeting includes this note on their meeting notice: "Our Group is for mothers of toddlers, as well as for those interested in parenting a breastfed toddler. Your children are welcome at our meetings. Feel free to bring a snack for your child; because of possible food allergies we ask that you not share your snacks with other children without parental permission and that you help ensure that your own drink bottles, etc., are out of toddler reach." Check with your support Leader about review procedures for meeting notices before making copies to distribute; she can offer suggestions for content or appearance.

MORE OPPORTUNITIES

Handouts, books, items for sale

A handout can be helpful for the busy mother of a toddler; she can take it home to review the information and ideas she heard at the meeting. You can use articles in Leader and member publications and the LLLI Web site to collect information and materials to produce a printed sheet. Your support Leader can also provide handout ideas. Check with her about review procedures for handouts you wish to distribute.

You may want to have a selection of appropriate pamphlets and Group Library and sale books on hand. Consult the appropriate LLL Bibliography or current catalogue to see what books and pamphlets are available on the topics of weaning, toddler breastfeeding and nutrition, parenting, and loving guidance.

Loving Guidance

Look at the child (eye contact)
Offer choices—small ones for small people
Very quick distractions are helpful
Include your child in what you're doing
Need freedom within limits
Get your home safety-proofed

Get to the cause of temper tantrums or misbehavior
Unconditional love and focused attention
Interesting opportunities for activity
Don't ask (Would you like to go now?) State what you mean (It's time to go)

Attempt to child size a toddler's life to make it easy to "do myself"
Num nums please?—Your child needs you to receive him with joy and enthusiasm most of the time
Constant safety supervision
Expectations and Environment—Are they realistic and appropriate?

Meeting Format

Many Leaders find that an informal discussion with one or two broad topics and two or three discussion-starter questions for each topic works well. Mothers at Toddler Meetings are often moving about the room tending to their little ones, so it is helpful if the discussion is easy to follow. Some Leaders like to jot down topics as they come up on a large pad of paper or piece of cardboard. There are many meeting ideas available in Area publications and on the LLLI Web site (look for meeting ideas under Leader information or do a search on "toddler meetings").

> Another popular meeting idea is to locate passages in LLL resources and mark quotes for mothers to read and discuss.

Another popular meeting idea is to locate passages in LLL resources and mark quotes for mothers to read and discuss. This is a great way to bring out research on advantages of extended breastfeeding or suggestions for loving guidance. The questions posed in the "Toddler Tips" column of NEW BEGINNINGS (available on the LLLI Web site) or in similar columns in your member publication are also great questions to get discussions going, remind mothers of LLL resources, promote membership, and cover a variety of topics.

Thoughts for Mothers of Nursing Toddlers

- All children do eventually wean.
- Toddlers wean naturally at varying ages. Avoid comparing your child with another. Instead consider the needs of your child and your family when thinking about weaning.
- The span of time when you are the center of your child's existence is short when compared to a lifetime.
- The attention you pay to your toddler now is a good investment in his/her emotional future.
- Breastfeeding, like all relationships, has its ups and downs. Your feelings about your little breastfeeding person will vary. You will go through times when you are very accepting of your child's breastfeeding and times when you are not. This is normal.
- Having doubts? Look at your child. A happy, learning, secure child is evidence that you are doing a fine job parenting. Pat yourself on the back and feel proud.

Meeting Focus—Toddler Meetings

The focus of the meeting may depend on how often you hold Toddler Meetings. In a once-yearly meeting you may want to discuss many topics; in a monthly meeting you might prefer to focus in depth on just one topic. The following is a list of some general topics for Toddler Meetings, followed by areas to consider during the discussion.

- **Little breastfeeding persons:**
  - Need or habit
  - Increased breastfeeding
  - Breastfeeding in public
  - Limiting breastfeeding
  - Night-time breastfeeding
- **Your partner:**
  - Finding time for each other
  - Nighttime sleeping arrangements
  - Sex
  - Presenting benefits of toddler breastfeeding to fathers
  - Father's role in discipline
  - Coping together
- **Nighttime challenges:**
  - Getting to bed; going to sleep
  - Fear of darkness; nightmares
  - Night wakefulness
  - Coping with exhaustion
- **Coping with outside pressures:**
  - Criticism from relatives and friends
  - Differences of opinion with health care provider
- **Toddler behavior:**
  - Regression, clinginess
  - Children and television
  - Effect of nutrition and diet
  - Temper tantrums
  - Recognizing age-appropriate behavior
- **Growing up, growing family:**
  - Toilet learning
  - Preschool education
  - Spacing of children, fertility
  - Sibling rivalry (be sensitive to one-child families)
  - Travel with toddlers
  - Holiday/vacation weaning
- **Loving guidance:**
  - Discipline—teaching vs. punishing
  - Attitude—being your child's coach, instead of your child's adversary
  - Offering children choices
  - Avoiding problem situations
  - Distraction
  - Setting reasonable limits and enforcing them gently
  - Dealing with our anger
  - Acknowledging and accepting the child's feelings

Remind mothers at Toddler Meetings that most of the toddler behaviors that worry parents have nothing to do with breastfeeding.

MORE OPPORTUNITIES

Toddler Meetings are a time for sharing ideas, not necessarily solving individual problems.

Sample Discussion Plans

Following are three sample discussion plans for Toddler Meetings, ready to use as is, or just to give you ideas as you develop your own discussion plans. Remind mothers at Toddler Meetings that most of the toddler behaviors that worry parents have nothing to do with breastfeeding but are often age-appropriate behaviors that will disappear as their child matures. Toddler Meetings are a time for sharing ideas, not necessarily solving individual problems. Support for looking at the toddler years positively instead of negatively (such as the "terrible twos" attitude) can help mothers help themselves. Each mother knows her own child best.

If you expect a large meeting, where many of the mothers do not know each other, consider using an icebreaker question with the introductions. An icebreaker question gives each mother a chance to share a little about herself, but uses only a few minutes of the meeting. A few icebreaker questions are:

- What is your favorite park to visit with your child/children?
- What is a restaurant that you have found to be family friendly?
- What item do you always pack when traveling with your toddler?

It is important to include a qualifying statement at the beginning of the meeting. See Chapter 2 for some sample qualifying statements.

SAMPLE TODDLER MEETING DISCUSSION PLAN

Possible Title/Focus
Little Breastfeeding Persons

Opening Questions

1. Today we will be looking at life with a little breastfeeding person—what things you might expect and how to keep your breastfeeding relationship enjoyable. To begin, what was your child's breastfeeding pattern as an infant, and how has it changed?

   Listen for, and bring up if not mentioned:
   - Huge range of normal
   - Mothers' concerns
   - Mothers' satisfactions

2. What do you see as the benefits of breastfeeding through toddlerhood or beyond?

   Listen for, and bring up if not mentioned:
   - "Magic" way to calm a hurt or upset child
   - Peaceful way to reconnect after a hard day
   - Help during illness, can breastfeed through stomach upsets, avoids dehydration
   - Reduces illness and allergies
   - Gives mother a chance to sit down

3. As their babies grow into toddlers, some mothers find that they have mixed feelings about breastfeeding. What are you enjoying about your breastfeeding relationship, and what would you like to change?

Follow-Up Questions

1. As our children grow from infancy to toddlerhood, the saying "an infant's want is an infant's need" does not always apply. Instead mother and child work out a breastfeeding relationship that satisfies both mother and baby. At about what age could your child begin to accept limits on breastfeeding, and what approaches to limit-setting did you find successful?

2. It is easy for most mothers to understand the need an infant has to breast-feed on demand. As the infant grows into a toddler, some mothers feel they need to put some limits on breastfeeding. What are some gentle, effective ways you have found to keep your breastfeeding relationship in balance?

   Listen for, and bring up if not mentioned:
   - Limiting times and places to breastfeed, length of feedings
   - Remind mothers to be sensitive to how many limits the individual child can handle
   - Consider introducing only one limit at a time
   - Need vs. habit—radical changes in child's behavior; clinging, regression indicate need
   - Eliminating problems by changing attitude, avoid critical people
   - Welcoming child with open arms, benefits of one-to-one attention
   - Reducing activity level for both mother and child
   - Finding a breastfeeding buddy

3. What is one thing you do to help you and your child get some sleep?

   Listen for, and bring up if not mentioned:
   - Variety of sleeping arrangements, bedtime routines, earlier bedtimes
   - Napping together, okay to nap even if you don't have an infant

Possible Title/Focus

Coping with Outside Pressure

Opening Questions

1. While it is clear that breastfeeding a child beyond the first twelve months of life is something we have in common with the majority of mothers through-out history, in many cultures today we stand out as different. We may face crit-icism at times. How do you feel about this criticism? How do you deal with it?

2. In his book, *The Ultimate Breastfeeding Book of Answers*, Jack Newman says "I am an advocate of 'indiscreet' breastfeeding—the more that people see babies at the breast, the more 'normal' it will be." Yet many women are reluctant to set themselves apart as odd or different by breastfeeding a tod-dler in public. What is your comfort level with public breastfeeding? How do you handle situations where your toddler would like to breastfeed, but you feel uncomfortable?

3. A breastfeeding toddler may be aware that peers and/or adults disapprove of continued breastfeeding. How can we protect our children from social dis-approval and help them deal with the situation constructively?

4. How do you respond to pressure from friends or family members to leave your child before you are ready?

MORE OPPORTUNITIES

SAMPLE TODDLER MEETING DISCUSSION PLAN—

Possible Title/Focus

Breastfeeding Your Toddler or Writing the Book on Toddler Breastfeeding

Opening Questions

1. What is your biggest concern about breastfeeding your toddler?

Listen for, and bring up if not mentioned:

- Nighttime breastfeeding
- Asking to breastfeed at every possible opportunity—every time mother sits down or talks on the telephone—sign that child needs one-to-one attention
- Breastfeeding in public, choosing a code word for breastfeeding
- Biting
- Breastfeeding habits—e.g., tugging on the other nipple or mother's earlobe
- Weaning—what's "normal," how to
- Fertility
- Criticism from friends, relatives, spouse, health care provider

2. Pass around a basket with index cards and pencils. Ask the mothers to write a question or concern they have about breastfeeding a toddler. Collect the cards, mix them up, and redistribute. Now, going around the room, ask them to read out the concern on the card that they now have. Discuss each concern; point out that many of the women attending have the same concerns.

3. La Leche League is based on mother-to-mother sharing. If our Group were writing a book about breastfeeding toddlers, what chapters would our book include? Write down the ideas suggested on a large sheet of paper.

Listen for, and suggest as chapter titles if not mentioned:

- Nighttime parenting
- Weaning
- Criticism
- Benefits

Go through each chapter and ask mothers to write the book by offering tips from their experience. Using one large paper per chapter, write down their ideas. Ask for a volunteer to type up the suggestions later and send a copy to each attendees.

Follow-up questions

1. How do you find time to spend with your partner?
2. How do you find time for yourself?
3. What is your favorite tip for making travel with a toddler easier?
4. What is your child's normal eating pattern for solid foods?

Listen for and bring up if not mentioned:

- Toddlers eat less than infants do
- Toddlers like small, frequent meals, grazing
- Meals are balanced over a week, but not over a single day
- Your milk is the best food your child will ever eat
- Concentration of immune factors in milk increases as child gets older

COUPLES MEETINGS

A Couples Meeting can take many forms depending on the needs of the Group. The meeting can be a social gathering with no set discussion, or it can be a formal meeting. Some Groups schedule a Couples Meeting once a series; others hold a Couples Meeting when Group members request one. In some communities, Groups invite couples to attend regular Series Meetings instead of inviting mothers only. (See the section on **Fathers** in Chapter 2.) Another arrangement is to have an annual family picnic/Couples Meeting, held outside to accommodate all the children; that way there are no child care issues. Some Groups hold Couples Meetings together, for example a combined Couples Meeting can be held for a morning Group and an evening Group in the same town. Holding Couples Meetings is optional.

> Speak with confidence, avoiding nervous or apologetic laughter. LLL is offering parents something of great value – support for loving parenting.

Choose a Time and Location

Many Groups schedule Couples Meetings on a Friday night or weekend. For some families this is a more relaxed time than a weeknight. There may be more opportunities for the care of older children on weekends as well. Check with the mothers in the Group to choose a time that is best for most families.

When choosing a location remember to plan for twice as many people. Choose a public place or hostess's home with plenty of seating. It is a good idea to check ahead of time with those who plan to attend in order to get an idea of the number of children who may come as well as their ages. A note on the meeting notice, such as "As at all LLL functions, babies in arms and small children who would be unhappy away from their parents are welcome," may help couples decide whether or not to bring their children. Be sure your site can accommodate any plans to serve food.

MORE OPPORTUNITIES

Format

For a Couples Meeting, format choices range from an unstructured social event to a planned meeting, similar to a Series Meeting. Some Groups have been very successful with a more informal approach, creating a breastfeeding version of a popular board game or TV game show to warm people up, break the ice, and get the laughter flowing. For a more formal meeting, a Leader may find that topics involving general aspects of family life—e.g., communication, sleep, dealing with relatives, lifestyle decisions, child spacing, loving guidance—help the group warm up to the discussion. It's helpful to know the group and tailor the discussion to meet its needs. You can ask for discussion topic ideas from mothers at the Series Meeting before the Couples Meeting is scheduled or pass out index cards at the beginning of the meeting for anonymous questions.

Many Groups claim that the most popular Couples Meetings include food. Some Groups hold a Couples Meeting in conjunction with a potluck (bring and share) meal or picnic; some Groups plan a dessert buffet. A Couples Meeting can be a great way to introduce recipes from WHOLE FOODS FOR THE WHOLE FAMILY or other LLL cookbooks.

Special Considerations

Fathers need parenting support, yet may have a difficult time asking for it. Fathers gain support by listening to experiences and ideas at Couples Meetings and through the informal chatting—perhaps with a baby in their arms—before or after the meeting. Meeting and talking with other breastfeeding families can provide reassurance and help fathers look at things positively.

Some fathers are wary of LLL and don't quite understand why people would want to get together to talk about breastfeeding. Other fathers may disagree with information or ideas their partner heard at meetings. For these reasons it is important to make a good first impression. Your professional and level headed demeanor, as well as an introduction describing Leader accreditation, can help. Talking about LLLI and its global influence, LLL publications, the Professional Liaison resource network, and opportunities for continuing education all demonstrate our credibility. Speak with confidence avoiding nervous or apologetic laughter. LLL is offering parents something of great value—support for loving parenting.

Keep in mind that mixed groups communicate differently than women-only groups. Men often save their questions until the meeting is well underway; sometimes they say little until the trip home. The women in the Group may make heroic efforts not to participate, so as not to deprive the men of opportunities to contribute. Be prepared for this thoughtful silence when you ask a question and allow a lengthy pause for the Group to reflect on the question. Look around the group, inviting everyone to participate, before moving on with a follow-up question to a mother you know will be comfortable contributing.

> Be prepared for a thoughtful silence when you ask a question and allow a lengthy pause for the Group to reflect on the question.

You may be concerned about the role your partner plays at Couples Meetings. A frank discussion with your partner about your concerns might help you relax. It might also be good for the Group to see that even a Leader's family "takes what it needs and leaves the rest." You may be surprised at the amount of breastfeeding support and knowledge your partner can offer. He might be the best one to answer, "How can I be close to my baby if I can't feed him?" To a man's ears, another man's answer may mean more than a woman's answer.

Sometimes a Leader's partner may be unable or prefer not to attend a Couples Meeting at all. That may help mothers who come alone feel more at ease and encourage others to attend without partners.

Couples Meetings often attract regularly attending members who know each other well. Their partners may feel more at ease if they have an opportunity to get acquainted over refreshments before participating in the meeting discussion.

Handouts, books, and items for sale

You may want to display the Group Library and sale books for perusal. Select titles from LLL Bibliographies or the current catalogue on parenting and other topics that are specifically related to your discussion plans. Books about fathering tend to be popular at Couples Meetings.

Meeting Focus—Couples Meetings

The following list contains sample questions for several possible focuses for Couples Meetings. Consider using an icebreaker question if the attendees do not know each other well.

- **Nighttime needs, breastfeeding**
  - How do you respond to your child's nighttime needs and still meet yours?
  - What is one thing your family does to help everyone get a good night's sleep?
  - Which advantage of breastfeeding is most important to you?
  - What issues would you consider if you were thinking of having another child and your youngest was still breastfeeding?
  - If a friend or relative was considering breastfeeding, what benefit of breastfeeding would you be sure to tell them about?

- **Lifestyle decisions**
  - How do you respond to pressure from family and friends to leave your child before you feel your child is ready for separation?
  - As a parent, you may have found that your views about childrearing differ from those of your parents or in-laws. What has worked for you in handling these disagreements?
  - What is your favorite way to spend time with your baby?
  - How has having a baby changed your life?
  - How can you help everyone feel comfortable when you have guests in your home or when you visit friends who don't share your views on breastfeeding or other aspects of childrearing?

- **Discipline**
  - How are your ideas about discipline different from your partner's?
  - How do you resolve those differences?
  - How have your ideas about effective discipline for children changed since you have become a parent?
  - Life with children is filled with times of joy and times of frustration.
  - How do you handle feelings of anger and frustration toward your child?
  - Parents are often distressed when they see their child become angry.
  - How do you help your child express anger in acceptable ways?

- **Personal growth**
  - How has having a baby changed your marriage?
  - How has being a parent changed you as a person?
  - What have you learned about living with a baby or toddler that you wish you'd known earlier?
  - How has your own childhood shaped the way you respond to your child?
  - How has your baby changed you into a father or mother?

- **Fathering and Mothering**
  - Where can men find the support they need as fathers?
  - How do you react when your child prefers mother's company?
  - What do you enjoy doing with your baby?

- What is the most frustrating aspect of being the parent of a newborn? The most rewarding?
- Parents sometimes have mixed feelings about participating in adult-centered projects and activities that exclude their children. What has been your experience with this?

EMPLOYED BREASTFEEDING MOTHERS MEETING

Another optional meeting the Group might hold in your community is an Employed Breastfeeding Mothers Meeting. These meetings provide specific information and support to employed mothers who want to continue breastfeeding when they return to their jobs. Employed Breastfeeding Mothers Meetings are not intended to replace Series Meetings. Employed mothers benefit from the basic information and ongoing support offered in the four-meeting LLL Series.

An Employed Breastfeeding Mothers Meeting may be the first or only LLL meeting some women attend. Be sure to explain the purpose and services of LLL at this meeting. Many mothers become acquainted with LLL through a special meeting such as this and become long-standing members of the Group.

Choose a Time and Location

Employed mothers benefit from the basic information and ongoing support offered in the four-meeting LLL series.

Choose a meeting time and location that is convenient and appealing to employed women. If women attend during their pregnancy they will be prepared with information and know what to expect both in the normal course of breastfeeding and when returning to the workplace. Groups often hold Employed Breastfeeding Mothers Meetings in a public facility; some make arrangements with places of employment to hold lunch-hour meetings.

Meeting Notices

Develop an Employed Breastfeeding Mothers Meeting notice listing topics you plan to include. You may also want to reassure mothers that their babies are welcome at the meeting, by including on the meeting notice a statement such as "As at all LLL functions, babies in arms and small children who would be unhappy away from their mothers are welcome." Check with your support Leader about review procedures for meeting notices; she can offer suggestions for content or appearance.

After the notice is ready, consider:

- Sending the special meeting notice to employed mothers who have contacted a Leader recently
- Posting the special meeting notice in the community in places that pregnant, employed women frequent (doctors' offices, childbirth classes, maternity shops) as well in places of employment
- Announcing the special meeting at Series Meetings. Encourage women to pass the word on to others who might be interested.

Format

Employed Breastfeeding Mothers Meetings can vary in format from a formal class to a group discussion. If you are planning a one-time meeting, you might prefer the class style to give the mothers as much information as possible in a limited amount of time. If you have the resources to offer an Employed Breastfeeding Mothers Meeting on a regular basis, perhaps once or twice a series, a relaxed informal meeting will better provide long-term support for repeat attendees . Some Leaders have found that employed mothers attending LLL meetings for the first time expect a more formal meeting and have found it helpful to have a structured meeting plan, rather than a few open-ended discussion questions.

Extend LLL hospitality by serving refreshments. Consider offering nutritious snacks with water or fruit juice at the beginning of the meeting. Use the time to talk with each mother and invite her to relax and look over the LLL materials displayed. Some Leaders add a gathering time before the meeting time on the meeting notice. Or, if you prefer, offer refreshments during a meeting break or at the end of the meeting.

Fees and preregistration

For a one-time meeting/class you may want to consider charging a nominal fee to non-LLL members. The fee could be used to cover expenses: handouts, publicity, room charge, refreshments. Charging a fee is optional. If expenses for the meeting are minimal, consider applying the fee to the cost of LLL membership if the mother joins within one year. Some Groups charge a fee that covers the cost of THE WOMANLY ART OF BREASTFEEDING and then give the book to meeting attendees.

People are often tired by the end of a busy workday. Much as they might want to come to a scheduled meeting, when the day actually arrives they may be tempted to stay home. Preregistration and prepayment can strengthen commitment to attend a meeting. Preregistration lets you know how many women to expect.

Handouts, displays, items for sale

Some Groups give an information packet to each attendee, especially for a one-time meeting or class. The cost of information packets can be included in the meeting fee. Contents might include a meeting outline, a meeting evaluation form, a membership flyer, a catalogue, and a selection of pamphlets and tear-off sheets. If you do not provide a packet, you can offer relevant pamphlets and tear-off sheets for sale. Busy employed mothers might appreciate the opportunity to purchase books about breastfeeding and working, nutrition, child development, and parenting.

You may decide not to offer Group Library books for loan at an Employed Breastfeeding Mothers Meeting, especially at a one-time meeting, because it may be difficult for women to return the books. In this case, you can mention the Group Library as an advantage of both LLL membership and attending Series Meetings.

In addition to LLL pamphlets and books, if you have access to a variety of breast pumps, you might want to display them for mothers to examine and ask questions about. You also may want to display posters showing the benefits of breastfeeding and the advantages of LLL membership and have Series Meeting notices and the Leader's business cards available for mothers to take home.

MORE OPPORTUNITIES

Some Leaders have found that employed mothers attending LLL meetings for the first time expect a more structural meeting.

> In addition to LLL pamphlets and books, you might want to display a variety of breast pumps for mothers to examine and ask questions about.

Special considerations

As you plan the meeting, choose a positive approach to help create an inviting atmosphere:

- Greet each mother; remember her name and the name of her baby.
- Communicate enthusiasm and support for the decision to breastfeed.
- Assure mothers that the best way to combine breastfeeding and working is to get breastfeeding off to a good start. Provide information on the basics of breastfeeding.
- Encourage attendance at LLL Series Meetings.
- If mothers are concerned about being separated from their babies, help them explore ways of minimizing the separation. Let them know about alternatives that can help them meet their babies' needs. Assure them that their commitment to breastfeeding and their relationships with their babies are valuable.
- Encourage mothers to use the information and many services LLL has to offer: meetings, books, pamphlets, telephone help, the LLLI Web site.
- Listen to the mothers who come to the meeting and observe their body language. Do they need straightforward information, or do they need to discuss feelings and other issues? Be ready to change your approach, if necessary, to fit the mothers' needs.
- Allow plenty of time to discuss issues important to participants. You can use time efficiently by referring mothers to LLL pamphlets to provide specific details on issues such as milk storage after you have discussed the basic facts.

> Listen to the mothers who come to the meeting and observe their body language. Be ready to change your approach, if necessary, to fit the mothers' needs.

Meeting Focus—Employed Mothers Meetings

If you plan a formal class, LEAVEN May/June/July 1987, pages 37–38, has an extensive meeting outline you may find very helpful. This article is available on the LLLI Web site. If you have not had personal experience with working and breastfeeding, refer to this outline or contact your PL resource Leader for more specific information on combining employment and breastfeeding.

If you offer an Employed Breastfeeding Mothers Meeting as a regular supplement to the LLL Series, consider using questions from the "Making It Work" column in NEW BEGINNINGS (available on the LLLI Web site) or obtaining ideas from articles in your equivalent member publication as conversation starters.

Here are some ideas for meeting focuses.

- **Benefits of breastfeeding**
  - Bonding—only mother can breastfeed
  - Fewer illnesses—benefits mother, baby, and employer, continues even with partial breastfeeding
  - Breastfeeding—a chance to rest
  - Convenience—easy nighttime feedings
  - Happier mother, less absenteeism, means a more productive employee

- **Planning to return to work**
  - Simplifying daily routines at home
  - Finding the right caregiver for baby
  - Planning maternity leave, and your return to work
  - What working hours are best for you
  - Your work wardrobe

- **Getting off to a good start with your baby**
  - Benefits of breastfeeding
  - Establishing breastfeeding
  - Length of maternity leave
  - Finding a caregiver
  - Introducing a bottle

- **Pumping and storing human milk**
  - Selecting a pump, hand expression
  - Transporting and storing milk
  - Finding time and a place to pump at work
  - Finding a "pumping buddy"
  - When and how to start pumping
  - How much milk to leave
  - Introducing the bottle
  - Maintaining your supply

- **Putting it all together, family, employment, and breastfeeding**
  - Sharing family chores, hiring help
  - Planning ahead
  - Your daily schedule (commute time, family time, time to relax)
  - Sleep
  - Simple nutritious meals

MORE OPPORTUNITIES

Possible Title/Focus

Getting Off to a Good Start with Your Baby

Opening Questions

1. What is your biggest concern about combining working and breastfeeding? Note the concerns and make sure they are discussed during the meeting.

2. Today we will be discussing getting off to a good start with your baby. What plans have you made or did you make to get breastfeeding off to a good start?

Listen for, and bring up if not mentioned:
- Try to take a long maternity leave,
- Set aside the early weeks to bond with baby,
- Someone to help with housework/cooking,
- Wait to introduce bottle.

Follow-Up Questions

1. What do you expect from a caregiver?

Listen for, and bring up if not mentioned:
- Time for caregiver to get to know baby is important.
- Caregiver should be receptive to breastfeeding.
- A flexible feeding schedule is helpful.
- Trust your instincts.

EMPLOYED BREASTFEEDING MOTHERS MEETING PLAN

2. How long a maternity leave are you planning to take and why?

Listen for, and bring up if not mentioned:
- The longer the leave, the better.
- Return to work in middle of week.
- Take six to eight weeks to establish milk supply.

2. How did you/do you plan to introduce a bottle? What worked?

Listen for, and bring up if not mentioned:
- Consider using a cup.
- Someone other than mother may want to introduce the bottle.
- Mother may need to be out of house.
- Two weeks before return to work is a good time to start.
- Movement sometimes helps.
- Wrap mother's clothes around bottle.
- Try different nipples.
- Try starting with the baby facing out.
- Have patience!

4. What are the benefits of continuing to breastfeed when you return to work?

Listen for, and bring up if not mentioned:
- A peaceful way to reconnect after a hard day
- Bonding—only mother can breastfeed
- Less illness—benefits mother, baby, and employer, continues even with partial breastfeeding
- Breastfeeding—a chance to rest
- Convenience—easy nighttime feedings
- A happier mother who is rarely absent from work is a more productive employee.

BREASTFEEDING CLASSES

In some communities, parenting and childbirth classes are popular. Some parents prefer a class atmosphere to a support group environment. Some Leaders teach breastfeeding classes as part of a series of childbirth or parenting classes offered by a hospital, clinic, health agency or business. Other Leaders teach independent breastfeeding classes following a regular schedule.

The classes are designed to introduce the basics of breastfeeding to both parents, who usually attend before their baby is born. Consult with your support Leader if you are interested in teaching a breastfeeding class. Breastfeeding Classes are also offered as part of the LLLI Peer Counselor Program. For more information on these classes see the section **Breastfeeding Peer Counselor Program** in this chapter and check the LLLI Web site.

Breastfeeding Meeting/Class for Teens

Pregnant teenagers and teen mothers need basic information, just as all breastfeeding mothers do, but they can benefit from a unique approach. Teenagers often have a strong focus on "self." A Leader may find that Breastfeeding Teen Mothers Meetings meet

A cute baby is a wonderful icebreaker when you are speaking to teens.

the needs of this special group of mothers in the community. All teens, boys and girls, benefit by learning about breastfeeding. Some Leaders are invited to speak to teens in a class at school. In a school, a Leader may address a mixed group of both girls and boys, those who are parents or are soon to be parents as well as those without children.

Special considerations

A Leader needs to keep in mind how teens view breastfeeding.

- Many young people have had little or no contact with breastfeeding babies and mothers.
- Teens are often extremely self-conscious about their bodies.
- Teens may be influenced by societal views that consider breasts to be sexual objects having nothing to do with nurturing a baby.
- Teens may have many misconceptions about the management of breastfeeding and the breastfeeding relationship.

You do not need to sell breastfeeding to teens—most know it is best for babies—just help teens see how breastfeeding can fit into their lives. Because they are teens and believe they can do anything, once they accept the idea of breastfeeding, teen mothers often do very well.

You may want to ask an experienced breastfeeding mother and baby to attend the teen meeting or class. This can be the best way to let teens know that breastfeeding is a normal, natural part of life. A cute baby is a wonderful icebreaker. Teens are often amazed that breastfeeding can be done discreetly, and some may not even notice that a mother is breastfeeding during the meeting.

MORE OPPORTUNITIES

Choose a meeting format and focus

The meeting format varies depending on the audience. A group of teen mothers might prefer a discussion style. In a mixed class of boys and girls in a school, a discussion aid, such as a popular board game or TV game show, modified to focus on breastfeeding, can be helpful. Some Groups bring in home-baked goodies as prizes, giving the winning team first choice. (Check in advance if you plan to do this as some schools have restrictions on food brought in.)

You might begin with a discussion of the advantages of breastfeeding to baby, mother, and father, much as in Series Meeting 1. A meeting for teen breastfeeding mothers or pregnant teens can continue with the basics of breastfeeding when you have established rapport. A class meant to provide an overview of breastfeeding for a mixed group of teens can focus on the benefits of breastfeeding and answers to questions.

Encouraging questions is a good way to be sure that the meeting is meaningful for the teens. Teens may prefer to write their questions ahead of time to avoid embarrassment or discomfort. Prepare one or two questions to help the group warm up. Also, be prepared to answer questions such as these:

- Does breastfeeding hurt?
- How much time does it take?
- How long does a baby breastfeed (age)?
- Can you give mother's milk in a bottle?
- What do you do if your milk leaks?

- Does breastfeeding interfere with having sex?
- Will breastfeeding lead to the baby becoming a homosexual?

Keeping in mind that you are presenting breastfeeding information to teens in a non-LLL group will help you know how to answer these questions. To avoid potentially strong reactions, reveal only what you need to answer the question. Avoid offering information, ideas, or an approach that could shut down communication. Take questions seriously and compliment teens for asking. Remember that humor can be a helpful tool. Answer honestly in a style that suits you; teens appreciate people being themselves and dislike anything that seems phony or condescending.

WRITING FOR LLL PUBLICATIONS

Your personal story about breastfeeding may be just what other breastfeeding mothers would find useful.

Whether or not you think of yourself as a writer, you are most welcome to contribute to a variety of LLL publications.

Group newsletters, Affiliate or Area member publications, and NEW BEGINNINGS inform and inspire LLL members through articles, stories, poems, photographs, drawings, and other information about breastfeeding and parenting that reflect LLL's philosophy and mission. One of your personal experiences as a breastfeeding mother may be just what other breastfeeding mothers would find useful. You might find a basis for a contribution in your personal history written as a Leader Applicant or you may want to describe a more recent experience. You might want to encourage other mothers in your Group to contribute. Through the written word, mothers whom you may never meet can benefit from what you have learned.

Please also consider sharing photographs, together with the written agreement of the mother(s) in the picture, for publication by the Publications Department in your Area and/or by the LLLI Publications Department. Photographs enhance the appeal of written articles and are also very much needed for a variety of publications, even if you do not submit an article.

NEW BEGINNINGS, Affiliate and Area mothers newsletters in many languages have similar guidelines. Contact your support Leader or the editor of the specific publication with any questions about submitting articles. (See **Writer's Guidelines for NEW BEGINNINGS** in Appendix 4.)

Area Leaders' Letters (ALL) provide support for Leaders, giving up-to-date information on breastfeeding and the development of LLL in the Area as well as encouragement for our work as Leaders. Regular contributions come from those with particular responsibilities, such as Area Council members. However, the ALL is a forum where all Leaders can discuss challenges in a friendly, positive way, and offer each other support and ideas. Contributions from all Leaders—both new and experienced—enable this exchange.

You might consider writing about the challenges you face in your work as a Leader and how you've met them or about achievements in day-to-day helping situations or Group work. You might report on a conference session or review books or tapes. You might write an inspirational or humorous article about parenting. Or you might ask your ALL editor for suggestions—she'll be pleased to offer ideas knowing you are willing to help.

Your ALL editor (ALLE) can help you define or develop your topic. Even a short item—such as a meeting or fundraising idea—written quickly by hand during a busy day may serve as a basis for an article.

Whether you welcome editing suggestions or feel uncomfortable with your words being changed, you'll find that any major editing changes are done in close consutation with the author. The next article will go easier…and the one after that, easier still.

LEAVEN, published by LLLI, provides additional support for English-speaking Leaders. Any Leader may submit articles of general Leader interest to the Leaven editor or special column editors. Let your voice be heard!

OPPORTUNITIES IN LLL ADMINISTRATION—AREA, REGION, DIVISION/AFFILIATE

In Chapter 6 **Keeping Up-to-Date,** the LLL support and resource network for Leaders is described. At all levels, volunteer Leaders provide this support. This could be the opportunity you have been looking for to develop your professional skills, contribute in a vital way to the LLLI mission, and work with interesting women without being asked to compromise your belief in family first.

Often Leaders first become involved as part of their Area Council. You might take on a role in the Leader Department, acting as a support Leader for a number of Groups and Leaders in a particular community. In this role, often referred to as District Advisor (DA), District Coordinator (DC), or Area/Assistant Coordinator of Leaders (ACL), Leaders regularly report on their activities to you, and you answer their questions, providing them with support through phone calls, written communication and workshops.

Another role in the Area Council is assisting in Leader accreditation. Often called Coordinator of Leader Accreditation (CLA) or Associate Coordinator of Leader Accreditation (ACLA), these Leaders correspond with Leader Applicants, write articles about Leader Accreditation for Leader newsletters, and present sessions on related topics at workshops or conferences.

The Area Council may also include a Professional Liaison (PL) resource Leader. As a PL Leader, you research specialized medical or legal questions for Group Leaders and help Leaders keep up-to-date on important breastfeeding research by writing articles and presenting information at workshops and conferences.

If you like to organize events, you might enjoy working on a conference committee, or if you prefer speaking, perhaps you would enjoy presenting a session at a workshop or conference. For Leaders who enjoy teaching, training is available to become a Communication Skills or Human Relation Enrichment Instructor/Facilitator, or even a trainer for these Instructors/Facilitators.

There are also many opportunities for Leaders in LLL publications. As well as writing for the various publications (see **Writing for LLL Publications** above), Leaders edit newsletters for Leaders and members, translate books, periodicals, pamphlets, and information sheets into their country's language and even create new pamphlets as needed. Leaders also set up and maintain Web sites.

MORE OPPORTUNITIES

Serving as an LLL administrator could be an opportunity to develop your professional skills, contribute to the LLLI mission, and work with interesting women.

Leaders who are skilled writers, editors, or translators are needed for Area publications jobs, especially in non-English speaking countries where there are usually many urgent needs for material in the national language. If you have good knowledge of English and native level fluency in a language other than English, please consider joining a translation team. (You don't need to live in the country or Area.) You may volunteer through the LLLI Publications Department, through the LEAVEN editor, the International Division Publications Administrator, or directly to the ACL of the relevant Area or Areas.

If you are talented at fundraising or handling money, you might support the Area as a financial coordinator, treasurer, World Walk coordinator, or funding development coordinator.

Training is provided for all of these positions; experience is not necessary. Many Leaders have found work in LLL administration to be a wonderful chance for personal growth in a supportive environment. Your support Leader can let you know what opportunities are currently available.

SPECIAL LLLI COMMITTEES AND WORKING GROUPS

Participating on one of these committees or working groups is a valuable opportunity.

The LLLI Board of Directors accomplishes its work through a variety of committees and working groups. Committee members are recruited by the committee chairmen with the goals and priorities of the Board in mind. Members are drawn from within and outside LLL, subject to stipulations in the Bylaws and the approval of the Chairman of the Board.

Standing committees are formed annually and include: Bylaws, Finance, Audit, Personnel, Program Services, Resource Development, and Action. The chairmen of these committees are appointed by the Chairman of the Board, with the advice and consent of the Board of Directors.

Special committees are commissioned for a specific task by the Chairman of the Board, by the action of the Board, or by a chairman of a standing committee in consultation with the Chairman of the Board. Many of these committees are ongoing, such as the Professional Advisory Board, Planning, and Nominating committees.

LLLI Board Committees and working groups may be announced on LLLINews (see **Online Resources from LLLI** in Chapter 8) or in LEAVEN. Participating on one of these committees or working groups is a valuable opportunity. You are welcome to be in touch with the LLLI Board via the Chairman at any time if you are interested in joining a committee or working group.

ANSWERING THE HOTLLLINE

The HotLLLine is an after-hours service. Mothers in the US who phone 1–800–LALECHE or the LLLI office when it is closed (weekdays from 5 PM to 9 AM Central Time, weekends, and holidays) hear a message asking them to leave their name and address on the answering machine to receive by postal mail the name and telephone number of a local Leader, as well as a copy of the LLLI Catalogue. If a volunteer HotLLLine Leader is available, the message also tells callers that they can reach a Leader for immediate help by calling the number on the recording. This is a nice opportunity for a new Leader to build up her confidence in answering helping calls.

If you are a Leader in the US, you can volunteer for a HotLLLine shift (3 PM to 9 AM weekdays, 9 AM to 3 PM and 3 PM to 9 AM on weekends and holidays). You are expected to be home and available to receive calls during your shift, when you may receive 25 or more calls. During your shift, you will hear only from mothers who call 1–800–LALECHE or the LLLI office and who are willing to pay the cost of a long distance call for immediate help.

You will receive instructions and 20 Leader's Log sheets to record the calls. You will also receive a copy of the International Directory listing Area Coordinators of Leaders, Coordinators of Leader Accreditation, and Affiliate Representatives, so you can refer callers to someone in their own Area or country. After your shift, you send the completed log sheets or the names and addresses of callers to LLLI; mothers receive the LLLI Catalogue and the name and telephone number of a local Leader.

To volunteer for the HotLLLine or for more information, contact the HotLLLine Coordinator at the LLLI office in Schaumburg, Illinois or select "Contact LLLI" on the LLLI Web site.

For information on volunteering to answer the HotLLLine see (available on the LLLI Web site): LEAVEN, Vol. 35 No. 4, August-September 1999, p 5: "The HotLLLine Needs You!"

MORE OPPORTUNITIES

BREASTFEEDING PEER COUNSELOR PROGRAM

The La Leche League International Breastfeeding Peer Counselor Program is a very flexible program designed to give current, accurate breastfeeding information and support to those who, for whatever reason, do not have access to that type of information.

There are three parts to the program:

- LLLI Breastfeeding Peer Counselor Program Administrator Training,
- LLLI Breastfeeding Peer Counselor Training, and
- LLLI Breastfeeding Course.

Each of these components is designed to bring breastfeeding information and support to a wide variety of individuals, health care personnel, agencies, and, of course, to mothers.

The mission of the LLLI Breastfeeding Peer Counselor Program is to reduce infant mortality and morbidity by increasing the rate and duration of breastfeeding among breastfeeding resource-deprived populations. We accomplish that mission by training people who will take the information presented for their own knowledge base, to take back to the women of their communities, and/or for use in administering and supporting the training of Peer Counselors.

Program Administrators are either Leaders or others from the community who are interested in administering a Peer Counselor program, training Peer Counselors, or offering the Breastfeeding Course. They see the value of mother-to-mother support for all parts of the community, have basic breastfeeding knowledge, and are eager to

Peer Counselors have basic breastfeeding knowledge and are eager to share that information with the women of their community in a culturally appropriate and sensitive manner.

share that information with the women of the community in a culturally appropriate and sensitive manner. They take a 30-hour training workshop that gives them background materials, resources, the Peer Counselor Curriculum, and other tools needed to run a successful program. They are then able to use the curriculum to train Peer Counselors or to offer the Breastfeeding Course.

Peer Counselors are usually women who have breastfed a baby for 6 months or so. The most important requirement is that they really understand how important breastfeeding is and have the desire to assist others with successful breastfeeding relationships. They are given training that encompasses all the material in the *Breastfeeding Resource Guide*, plus a communications module and a cultural attitudes module. The training lasts for about 18–20 hours. They are then able to lead support groups, do phone counseling/helping, network with others in the breastfeeding community, and make presentations. Peer Counselors may either volunteer or be paid for their work.

The Breastfeeding Course is the same basic breastfeeding training (18–20 hours) that the Peer Counselor receives, although the communication and cultural modules may be deleted. It is marketed to a different audience; those looking for information only. Giving this course to health care or agency staff helps them meet Steps 2, 3, and 10 in the Baby Friendly Hospital Initiative.

If you are interested in setting up a Breastfeeding Peer Counselor Program, contact the LLLI Breastfeeding Peer Counselor Program Manager at the Schaumburg, Illinois, USA office of LLLI. Check the LLLI Web site for more information.

COOPERATIVE ACTION WITH OTHER ORGANIZATIONS SUPPORTING BREASTFEEDING

La Leche League encounters many opportunities to work with other organizations to help breastfeeding women. The *LLLI Policies and Standing Rules Notebook* contains guidelines for Leaders considering working with other organizations. Some LLL Affiliates have their own Cooperative Action Guidelines. (See **Appendix 1— Action: Cooperative.**)

Perhaps the local LLL Group has been invited to cosponsor a seminar for expectant mothers with another community group or a local hospital. Maybe you've been asked to be part of a local breastfeeding task force or government consortium. You may wonder, "Should LLL be involved in this venture?" "Is it appropriate for me to be involved as an LLL representative?" "Even though this is a good opportunity, am I expected to participate?" The Cooperative Action Guidelines clarify that:

- You may take advantage of the option to participate in cooperative action activities; participation is not required or expected.
- You speak for LLL only on the subject within the scope of LLL expertise— breastfeeding.
- Lists of Leader names, phone numbers, and addresses may be shared with organizations LLL is involved with in cooperative action activities, if such sharing will help to facilitate common goals.
- Follow the Cooperative Action Guidelines any time you are asked to sign or endorse jointly developed written materials on behalf of LLL.
- Neither LLLI nor any of its representatives may accept direct funding from formula manufacturers for any activity.

In most circumstances, you do not need authorization to engage in cooperative action activity. However, every Leader engaged in a cooperative action activity is expected to consult with and report to her appropriate LLL support person before and during her participation. (To learn more about cooperative action or to find answers to specific questions, see the full text of **Cooperative Action—Guidelines for Leaders** in Appendix 1.)

> Working in cooperation with other organizations may be a wonderful opportunity to promote breastfeeding.

WORLD WALK FOR BREASTFEEDING

The World Walk for Breastfeeding is a combination fundraising and promotional event that has been held annually since 1992. Its purposes are to raise money and help draw attention to World Breastfeeding Week. The World Alliance for Breastfeeding Action (WABA) holds World Breastfeeding Week every year from August 1–7. LLLI is a founding member of WABA.

When LLL Groups register for the Walk, they receive a kit with sample promotional products, press releases, insurance forms, a supply of brochures, sponsor forms, and order forms to obtain more supplies, as well as complete information on how to hold a Walk.

Some Groups join with their Chapter or Area to hold a large Walk. This can make the planning easier as well as create a larger gathering, which attracts more media attention. Those participating in the Walk obtain sponsors who pledge to donate a certain amount of money after the walker completes the symbolic Walk. This money is divided between the local Group, Area, Affiliate/Division, and LLLI. It is used to support the organization, fund programs, buy books, and provide continuing education for Leaders at conferences and workshops.

MORE OPPORTUNITIES

Enthusiasm for and participation in the World Walk for Breastfeeding continue to grow. Leaders have held this event in many different countries. In locations where sponsored walks are not common or practical, some Groups, Chapters, Districts or Areas hold an alternative promotional, fundraising event, such as a breastfeeding fair, picnic, or raffle.

Creativity and flexibility enable Groups in a variety of climates and cultures to find ways to join in this show of support for breastfeeding and LLL every year.

For more information, contact your support Leader or your Area or Affiliate/Division Walk Coordinator. Information is also available from the LLLI Public Relations Department World Walk Committee at the Schaumburg, IL office of LLLI and on the LLLI Web site.

LEADER/LACTATION CONSULTANT

The International Board of Lactation Consultant Examiners (IBLCE) is a nonprofit organization established in 1985 to develop and administer professional certification for lactation consultants. It is the only agency recognized by national and international lactation consultant organizations to provide certification for lactation consultants. LLLI and IBLCE are completely separate organizations. A representative from LLLI, selected by the LLLI Board of Directors, representatives from other agencies, and health care professionals serve on the IBLCE Board. When a person has obtained certification from the IBLCE, they are referred to as an International Board Certified Lactation Consultant (IBCLC).

Information about becoming a board certified lactation consultant is available on the LLLI Web site, or you can ask your Professional Liaison Resource Leader. You can also contact the IBLCE via their Web site or write directly to IBLCE at:

International Board of Lactation Consultant Examiners (IBCLE)
7309 Arlington Blvd., Suite 300
Falls Church, VA 22042 USA
(703) 560-7330

Keeping Roles Separate

It is important for a Leader who is also working as a lactation consultant to keep her two roles separate. One is a volunteer commitment and the other is a business. LLLI is a nonprofit organization. To maintain this status, it is important to avoid any possibility of giving the impression that LLL Leaders charge for their services.

> It is important for a Leader who is also working as a lactation consultant to keep her volunteer commitment separate from her business.

LLLI defines the limits and expectations of active Leader status and has established guidelines for Leader/Lactation Consultants. (See Appendix 1, **Leader/Lactation Consultant Guidelines,** for the full text of these guidelines.)

One of the simplest ways to avoid confusion between the two roles is to have two separate phone lines—one for LLL and one for your lactation consultant practice. Another idea is to work as a lactation consultant for an institution such as a hospital or a medical center. When health care providers do volunteer work, they often volunteer in another area of medicine or in a situation completely different from that in which they practice, to avoid confusion between the two roles. It is unethical in the medical community to refer a patient to oneself by saying, "under the auspices of my volunteer work I can't help you, but if you come to my clinic you can be taken care of for such and such a fee."

Perhaps the most complicated situations arise when a Leader has a private lactation consultant practice and is using her home phone for both LLL and her business. If this is your situation, it is appropriate to ask each mother how she found you, and then handle the call in that capacity. Also, it is not appropriate to advertise yourself as a lactation consultant on a phone line that is being given to mothers to call for LLL help.

> To maintain LLL's nonprofit status, it is important to avoid giving the impression that LLL Leaders charge for their services.

When you receive an LLL call you are expected to help the mother to your fullest capacity. This may mean seeing a mother in person or becoming involved in a series of helping calls and follow-ups. LLL Leaders have always been free to visit a mother at home or in the hospital or invite mothers to their own homes as their time and circumstances allow, although it is not part of the basic responsibilities of leadership. If you do not wish to help mothers in this manner, you may refer mothers to a Leader who goes on home/hospital visits, or to another IBCLC. It is not appropriate to offer LLL phone help to a mother and then charge her as a lactation consultant for a visit.

With care and common sense, Leaders, Leader/lactation consultants, and lactation consultants can work together to support breastfeeding mothers and their babies. For more information, contact your support Leader or a Professional Liaison Leader.

Several excellent articles on this topic have appeared in LEAVEN and are available on the LLLI web site:

- LEAVEN, Vol. 26 No. 3, May-June 1990, pp. 39–41: "Guidelines for active Leaders who also work as paid lactation consultants."
- LEAVEN, Vol. 34 No. 4, August-September 1998, pp. 84–85: "Leader/Lactation Consultant: Separating the Two Roles."

- LEAVEN, Vol. 28 No 5, September-October 1992, pp. 75–76: "Leaders and Lactation Consultants."

LLL SERVICE ONLINE

Online communication is an optional activity. It is another tool Leaders can use to help mothers breastfeed. The guidelines on etiquette and empathetic listening that we use in telephone helping and leading meetings apply to email helping, bulletin boards, online chats, etc. Before representing yourself as a Leader in any online activity, it is essential to review the guidelines LLL has established. See **Representing La Leche League Online,** in Chapter 1). When you help mothers online, it is important to keep accurate records and report your activities regularly to your support Leader.

> Before representing yourself as a Leader in any online activity, it is essential to review the guidelines LLL has established.

Some online activities Leaders can engage in are:

- Participating in Leader email lists
- Answering online Help Forms through LLLI or your Affiliate program
- Submitting meeting ideas to the collection on the LLLI Web site
- Working on the LLLI Web site (creating pages, editing/proofreading, writing, translating)
- Working on your Area, country, Affiliate, or Division Web site
- Creating and maintaining a Group Web page (See **Group Web Pages,** in Chapter 4.)
- Leading online LLL meetings or LLL chats
- Serving as a monitor for bulletin boards for mothers on the LLLI Web site, either as a Leader representative or unofficially as a breastfeeding mother.

MORE OPPORTUNITIES

There is more information about online LLL resources in Chapter 6 **Keeping Up-to-Date**. Check with your support Leader and on the LLLI Web site for more information on these opportunities.

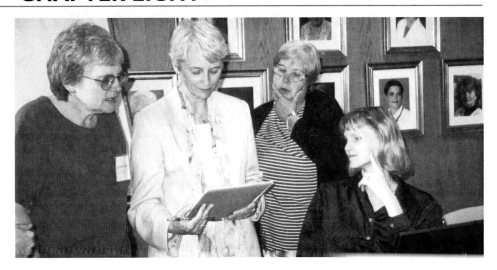

CHAPTER EIGHT

LLLI Services and Programs

LLLI provides a variety of services and programs in order to further its mission: to help mothers worldwide to breastfeed through mother-to-mother support, encouragement, information, and education, and to promote a better understanding of breastfeeding as an important element in the healthy development of the baby and mother. These departments can be contacted at the Schaumburg Illinois USA office of LLLI at:

La Leche League International, Inc.
1400 North Meacham Road
Schaumburg, IL 60173-4808 USA
Phone: 847-519-7730
Fax: 847-519-0035
Email: LLLI@llli.org
Web site: **www.lalecheleague.org**

LLLI SUPPORT DEPARTMENTS

LLLI Education and Member Services Department

The LLLI Education and Member Services Department facilitates:

- LLLI Conferences
- Exhibits
- Continuing Medical and Health Education Programs
- Annual Physicians Seminars
- Lactation Specialist Workshops
- Conference Continuing Education Sessions

A variety of programs and
services help LLLI to
fulfill its mission.

- Enduring Materials.
- Independent Study Modules
- On-Site Classroom Programs
- Medical Associates Program
- Center for Breastfeeding Information
- Research Review Committee
- Lactation Specialist Resources
- Peer Counselor Programs
- 1–800–LALECHE
- HotLLLine
- Professional Breastfeeding Resource Center Memberships
- Memberships

Further information and updates about these programs can be found below, in LEAVEN, in NEW BEGINNINGS, and on the LLLI Web site. **The Peer Counselor Program** and **HotLLLine** are discussed in Chapter 7.

Professional Breastfeeding Resource Center Memberships

Professionals (individuals and organizations) can obtain access to high-quality breastfeeding materials for their clients by joining LLLI as a Professional Breastfeeding Resource Center (BRC) Member. Memberships are available in English and Spanish.

The initial membership package provides the professional with a specialized packet containing LLLI pamphlets and tear-off sheets, one copy each of THE WOMANLY ART OF BREASTFEEDING and BREASTFEEDING PURE AND SIMPLE, and subscriptions to BREASTFEEDING ABSTRACTS and NEW BEGINNINGS. These materials acquaint the professional with LLLI's high quality publications. The membership also entitles the professional to a 15% discount on many items in the LLLI Catalogue.

The Education Department provides ongoing support to the professional with quarterly mailings, including the latest breastfeeding information and new LLLI publications, as well as one hour of consultation with the Manager of the Center for Breastfeeding Information (CBI). BRC members receive a membership card and certificate. Customized renewal memberships are available. Professional Breastfeeding Resource Center Membership brochures are offered in the LLLI Catalogue. Membership is also available on the LLLI Web site.

1-800-LA LECHE

The LLLI Education Department manages a phone line to provide breastfeeding help to mothers. This phone line, 1–800–LALECHE, is toll-free within the USA. Normal long distance charges apply to international calls. LLL Canada also provides a toll-free breastfeeding helpline at 1–800–665–4324. During regular office hours, (Monday-Friday 8 AM–5 PM Central Time) the 1–800–LALECHE number is answered by Leaders who are part of the LLLI staff.

The Leaders answer basic breastfeeding questions, and then refer the caller to her local LLL Leader for follow-up and meeting information. Callers are referred to Leaders listed on the Leader Specialty File when that is appropriate. The mother also receives an LLLI Catalogue.

Leaders who answer 1–800–LALECHE calls are paid staff members. Leaders who live near the Schaumburg, Illinois, USA office of LLLI or within a reasonable call forwarding distance from the office can become operators.

Before and after business hours and on weekends and holidays, a caller to the 1–800–LALECHE number hears a recorded message, allowing her to leave her address to receive an LLLI Catalogue and contact information for a local Leader, as well as giving her the LLLI Web site address. If there is a volunteer Leader scheduled, her name and phone number are included in the message, so callers needing emergency breastfeeding information can place another call to reach her. This after-hours service is called the HotLLLine. For details on volunteering to answer HotLLLine calls see **Answering the HotLLLine** in Chapter 7.

Leader Locator

When a mother calls the LLLI office in Schaumburg, Illinois, the phone message gives her the option of using an automated system to locate a nearby Leader. This system is called the Leader Locator. The caller enters her zip code and the names and numbers of up to three Leaders within 250 miles are given to her. It is important for Leaders to update the information in the LLLI database if they move or have a new phone number in order for the Leader Locator to offer mothers accurate contact information. This service is available 24 hours a day.

Leader Specialty File

Every year, when a Leader in the USA pays her Leader Dues to LLLI she is asked to fill out a form for the Leader Specialty File. This form asks the Leader to check off any specific breastfeeding situations she has specialized knowledge of, either through personal experience or contact with mothers in those situations. This file is available through the 800-Line Leaders as well as the HotLLLine Leaders. It is also available on the LLLI Web site for all Leaders to access.

LLLI SERVICES

Medical Associates Program

The Medical Associates Program is designed for physicians interested in and supportive of breastfeeding. Medical Associates are committed to breastfeeding and to LLLI and its philosophy. Leaders may give a membership brochure to physicians and invite them to join. Medical Associates are usually community physicians in private practice, whereas LLLI Health Advisory Council members are experts in an area of breastfeeding. (See **LLLI Professional Advisory Board,** below.)

Medical Associates are committed to breastfeeding and to LLLI and its philosophy.

The physician who becomes a Medical Associate in the USA receives:

- Certificate suitable for framing
- Medical Associates newsletter, published quarterly
- Subscription to BREASTFEEDING ABSTRACTS
- Subscription to NEW BEGINNINGS
- Subscription to LEAVEN
- 10% discount on many items in the LLLI Catalogue
- Medical Associates Program Directory
- List of LLLI Health Advisory Council members willing to act as consultants to Medical Associates

- Mailings about current events and issues affecting breastfeeding
- Registration discount for LLLI Seminars for Physicians

For more information, contact the Medical Associates Program at the LLLI office or on the LLLI Web site.

Continuing Medical and Health Education Activities

La Leche League International is accredited by the Accreditation Council for Continuing Medical Education (ACCME) to sponsor continuing medical education for physicians. LLLI currently provides Continuing Medical Education (CME) credits through:

- **Annual Seminars for Physicians.** Physician Seminars are offered in the USA for physicians, lactation consultants, and other lactation professionals. LLLI, the American Academy of Pediatrics, and the American College of Obstetricians and Gynecologists cosponsor these workshops. The American Academy of Family Physicians participates as a cooperating organization. (Other Seminars for Physicians are sponsored worldwide by LLL countries or Affiliates.)
- **Lactation Specialist Workshops.** Lactation Specialist Workshops are single-day seminars that are repeated in cities throughout the USA. These workshops provide Continuing Education Recognition Points (CERPS) hours and continuing education credits for lactation consultants, nurses, LLL Leaders and others who work with breastfeeding mothers.
- **LLL Area Health Professional Seminars.** These conferences offer continuing education credits for many fields.
- **Self-study modules.** Self-study modules have been developed using enduring materials criteria and are available through LLLI's catalogue and on the LLLI Web site. These independent study modules offer CME credits and IBCLE CERPs.

La Leche League International is accredited by the Accreditation Council for Continuing Medical Education (ACCME) to sponsor continuing medical education for physicians.

Leaders can help health care providers in their area become more knowledgeable about breastfeeding by giving them brochures for the LLLI Physicians' Seminar, Lactation Specialist Workshops, Area Health Professional Seminars, and LLLI Conferences and encouraging them to attend. Each year, the continuing education programs are announced in LEAVEN about six to nine months in advance, and Leaders are given the opportunity to send for promotional materials. Even though LLLI purchases mailing lists, inserts the brochure in the American Academy of Pediatrics newsletter, and sends out announcements to a large number of health care providers, it has been found that personal contact is the best method of reaching health care providers.

Areas planning to offer CME credits for programs at Area Conferences must pay a fee and obtain appropriate approval of the program. Evaluation and follow-up material must be received at LLLI's Education Department no later than eight weeks after the program. For more details, contact the LLLI Education Department at the Schaumburg, Illinois, USA office of LLLI or through the LLLI Web site. Allow plenty of time so that approval is received before promotional materials need to be printed.

Center for Breastfeeding Information

The Center for Breastfeeding Information (CBI) provides health care providers, researchers, Leaders, breastfeeding counselors, and medical students with a reliable source for breastfeeding information.

For more than 45 years, LLLI has been compiling and updating an extensive collection of professional research articles on breastfeeding. The reference materials at the LLLI office assist Leaders who are helping mothers breastfeed their babies in many ways. The research is also used to reference LLL publications, formulate position statements, provide documentation for LLL breastfeeding management practices, answer challenging breastfeeding questions, and provide material for media releases.

The computerized database contains more than 500 different breastfeeding categories and over 38,000 articles from more than 1,100 professional journals. The collection is updated constantly. The LLLI office also houses a library consisting of 3,000 books and 19,000 professional articles which were donated to La Leche League by Wellstart International.

CBI references are listed by subject, date, author, journal, and title, and can be retrieved in bibliographic lists or on the CBI portion of the LLLI Web site. Copies of complete articles are available for a charge. CBI staff also provides consultations on the material.

Leader requests for information from the CBI are handled through the Professional Liaison (PL) network. Affiliate/Division Professional Liaison staff work directly with the CBI. If necessary, the CBI directs questions to the Professional Advisory Board (PAB).

There is usually no fee involved in researching individual breastfeeding help questions that come through regular PL channels. Leaders who request reference material or background information for individual research needs or personal counseling situations are expected to pay the established fees.

When the CBI is used by professionals and for individual research projects by non-Leaders, fees are determined by research and computer time and by the number of photocopies (with appropriate copyright charges) required to fill the order. Details can be obtained by contacting the CBI at the LLLI office.

Individuals or institutions can purchase a subscription to the CBI that entitles them to BREASTFEEDING ABSTRACTS, LLLI's quarterly update on new research, and prepaid access to CBI services. Please see the CBI brochure (available from the LLLI Web site or the CBI) for current information. In addition, selected bibliographic lists and useful links are provided on the LLLI Web site.

Research review committee

Leader questions about participation in research projects are also passed on to the CBI by the PL support network. The Research Review and Resource Coordinator, with the aid of the CBI Manager, processes research proposals from investigators who seek to enroll LLL members as study subjects. The Research Review and Resource Coordinator then submits the proposals to the Research Review Committee for evaluation. If a research proposal is approved, the Research Review and Resource Coordinator notifies Area Coordinators of Leaders and Professional Liaison Leaders, who assist the researchers in locating members who are willing to participate in the research projects.

Bulletins from the CBI about topics currently in the news are available on the Web site for access by Leaders only.

LLLI SERVICES

For more than 45 years, LLLI has been compiling and updating an extensive collection of professional research articles on breastfeeding

The CBI Manager also assists the Research Review and Resource Coordinator with the development of the Professional Liaison (PL) letter, sent out bimonthly to Affiliate and Division PL administrators, who share it with all other PL Leaders. Bulletins from the CBI about topics currently in the news (hot topics) are available on the Web site for access by Leaders only.

The LLLI Education Department welcomes input from lay and professional sources to help keep its information current. For more information, contact **CBI@llli.org** or phone the LLLI office.

Funding Development Department

The Funding Development Department has primary responsibility for raising funds in support of the programs and services of LLLI. These programs and services in turn support LLL's mission.

Like most nonprofit organizations, LLLI relies heavily on philanthropic support to fulfill its mission. Contributions from individuals, corporations, foundations, and through special events such as the World Walk for Breastfeeding are an investment in the future of LLLI. The Center for Breastfeeding Information (CBI), the Breastfeeding Peer Counselor Program, the Education Department, and the Leader Accreditation Department, along with 1–800–LA LECHE, are examples of core programs whose sustainability would not be possible without continued generous philanthropic support.

> Contributions from individuals, corporations, foundations, and through special events such as the World Walk for Breastfeeding are an investment in the future of LLLI.

To learn more about funding development, and how you may become involved as a donor and/or fundraising volunteer, contact the Director of Funding Development and Advancement at the LLLI Office or via the LLLI Web site.

External Relations and Advocacy Department

The External Relations and Advocacy Department coordinates LLLI's consultative status with the United Nations Children's Fund (UNICEF), formal working relations with the World Health Organization (WHO), and registration with the United States Agency for International Development (USAID). The External Relations and Advocacy Department also facilitates LLLI activities with the World Alliance for Breastfeeding Action (WABA), which include the distribution of the annual World Breastfeeding Week (WBW) Action Folder in the USA, Canada, and English-speaking Caribbean as well as activities related to the Global Initiative for Mother Support (GIMS). In addition, the department oversees LLLI's membership in the Child Survival Collaborations and Resources Group (CORE). The department collaborates with Area, Division, and Affiliate administrators on projects, grants, and cooperative efforts with international nongovernmental agencies. It also coordinates global cooperative action, develops international position papers for conferences and forums and maintains the Advocacy pages on the LLLI Web site. Currently, there are nine LLL Leaders around the world who volunteer their time to assist the External Relations and Advocacy Department in its activities with international agencies and nongovernmental organizations.

For more information, contact the External Relations and Advocacy Department at the LLLI Office in Schaumburg, Illinois, USA.

Public Relations Department

The LLLI Public Relations Department is responsible for providing information about the organization to the rest of the world. It does this in a variety of ways from assisting in overseeing the LLLI Web site content to sending the media news releases about important events and new breastfeeding information, and supplying facts and arranging interviews with LLL representatives when reporters, authors, producers, or speakers ask for information about breastfeeding or La Leche League.

The Public Relations Department is also active whenever widespread media attention is focused on an inaccurate or slanted view of breastfeeding. The Public Relations Department responds to media reports that portray LLL or our volunteers inaccurately. It also challenges advertising that uses our name or logo without permission.

When these incidents occur, the Public Relations Department tracks down the source of the information, and using research from the Center for Breastfeeding Information or other credible sources, works to correct the misinformation. On occasion, it writes letters to editors or producers or, in the case of a widespread story, issues media releases to correct the misinformation or counteract the unfavorable publicity. Area and Affiliate/Division administrators receive appropriate information via LLLINews, an official LLL email announcement list, to address the concerns of mothers who may be calling with questions. To obtain statements and media releases issued by the Public Relations Department, contact your support Leader or the Public Relations Department at the LLLI office or go to the LLLI Web site.

It is important for the Public Relations Department to be kept informed about media coverage on breastfeeding and La Leche League. You can help by sending copies or URL links of articles about breastfeeding, along with complete information about the source of the article, to the Public Relations Department. If the information appears on radio or television, obtain the name of the show, time and date of broadcast, and complete address of the station or network where it was broadcast. It is not always possible or appropriate to respond officially to every media item regarding breastfeeding.

Certain television shows, radio programs, or print media may portray breastfeeding humorously. Although these can be annoying, LLLI has limited resources and responds only to portrayals of breastfeeding that can be viewed as damaging. Consider writing yourself; in many cases, letters from individuals are far more effective than those written on behalf of an organization.

> When these incidents occur, the Public Relations Department tracks down the source of the information and works to correct the misinformation.

LLLI SERVICES

Publications Department

The Publications Department distributes more than two million publications each year, providing current, accurate, referenced information on all aspects of breastfeeding through books, pamphlets, and periodicals published for a variety of audiences. Books published by LLLI cover topics related to breastfeeding and parenting. They are frequently translated into languages other than English. Our two major books are THE WOMANLY ART OF BREASTFEEDING, now in its sixth revision, and THE BREASTFEEDING ANSWER BOOK, now in its third revision.

Concise information on specific topics is published in both pamphlet and tear-off sheet formats. Tear-off sheets offer basic information in an inexpensive and easy-to-use form. Leaders often use this format in new mothers' packets. Pamphlets offer more in-depth information on a specific topic for the breastfeeding mother who requires more background, and are useful for mailing to mothers who call for information. Pamphlets and tear-off sheets are often translated into languages other than English or used as a starting point for adaptation in other languages.

NEW BEGINNINGS, the LLLI member magazine, features personal stories about breastfeeding mothers and babies. Question-and-answer columns offer suggestions from readers in response to classic situations. Technical articles provide information on subjects of interest to breastfeeding mothers. LEAVEN, the LLLI magazine for Leaders, includes articles on a variety of topics specific to helping breastfeeding mothers and managing a La Leche League Group. (See **Writing for LLL Publications**, pages 190-191 for how to contribute to these publications.)

BREASTFEEDING ABSTRACTS is an eight-page quarterly publication for health care providers and others interested in clinical applications of new knowledge in the field of lactation. Each issue includes an informative article along with abstracts of recent breastfeeding research. Professional books of interest are sometimes reviewed in its pages. LLLI also publishes an annual summary of facts about breastfeeding with brief descriptions of relevant and credible research articles on breastfeeding and mothering.

Book Evaluation Committee

The primary responsibility of the LLLI Book Evaluation Committee (BEC) is the annual publication of the *LLLI Bibliography* (No. 174-13). This is prepared in conjunction with the LLLI Publications Department. The BEC Chairman and the LLLI Staff Liaison for the BEC are listed in the LLLI Personnel Directory (No. 405-13). A Leader can recommend recently published books for the LLLI Bibliography by contacting the LLLI BEC Chairman. (See **Appendix 1, Book Evaluation Committee.**)

> Book Evaluation Guidelines are used to determine whether a book is appropriate for inclusion in the LLLI Bibliography

Book Evaluation Guidelines

Book Evaluation Guidelines help evaluators determine whether a book is appropriate for inclusion in the *LLLI Bibliography*. Books that conflict significantly with LLLI philosophy or promote a cause that detracts from LLL's focus on mothering through breastfeeding will not be approved. However, a book that presents the beliefs or experiences of an author may be approved even when these beliefs and experiences go beyond LLL's purpose, philosophy, and mission if they do not conflict significantly with LLLI philosophy. (See **Appendix 1, Book Evaluation Guidelines.**)

Summary statements are included with each entry in the LLLI Bibliography. The LLLI Bibliography is available on the LLLI Web site and through the LLLI Catalogue. Significant differences between a book's content and LLLI philosophy will be noted in the summary. (See **Appendix 1, Bibliography, LLLI.**)

Appeals and review

If you have a question about a book's inclusion in the Group Library or in the LLLI Bibliography, you can direct the question to your support Leader or in writing to the LLLI BEC Chairman. Your request should include your specific concerns.

A Leader who wishes to register her disagreement with the results of an evaluation by the LLLI BEC can appeal the decision. If enough Leaders initiate appeals, a review of the book's evaluation will be made. If the issue in question was not addressed in the original evaluations, the BEC Chairman will send a copy of the LLLI Book Evaluation Guidelines and a current evaluation form to the concerned Leader. The Leader may reevaluate the book in question according to the guidelines and return copies of the completed form to the BEC Chairman and the LLLI Staff Liaison.

If ten or more Leaders from a broad geographical area pursue an appeal, an additional review will be undertaken by a committee including the BEC Chairman, LLLI Staff Liaison, LLLI Publications Director, a representative from the Leader Accreditation Department, a representative from the Leader Department, and a representative from the Professional Liaison Department, when appropriate. This committee will consider the current concerns and previous evaluations before making a recommendation to the LLLI Executive Director.

Based on this recommendation, the LLLI Executive Director or her designate will determine the status of the book in question. The LLLI Board of Directors retains final authority to approve or not approve a publication for the LLLI Bibliography. (See **Appendix 1, Book Evaluation Guidelines.**)

Alumnae Association

The LLLI Alumnae Association is the vehicle through which La Leche League members and Leaders continue a lifelong affiliation with LLLI. Membership in the Alumnae Association can provide a natural transition for members and retiring Leaders who want to maintain their LLL connection, as well as a place for active Leaders and members to connect with other active and retired Leaders and members.

Through its coordinator and volunteer Alumnae Council, the Alumnae Association strives to:

LLLI SERVICES

Membership in the Alumnae Association can provide a natural transition for members and retiring Leaders who want to maintain their LLL connection.

- Ensure the existence of LLL for present and future generations of mothers, children, and grandchildren,
- Provide support and encourage learning among Leaders,
- Promote the mission and philosophy of LLLI in the community and workplace,
- Locate and be attentive to the needs of retired Leaders worldwide,.
- Serve as a resource to Areas, Affiliates, Divisions, and LLLI for planning, support, and program development,
- Oversee special projects for LLLI,
- Recognize the accomplishments of former Leaders and members, and,
- Support LLLI financially.

The Alumnae Association offers:

- CONTINUUM, a newsletter with articles on personal growth, changing family relationships, women's health issues, current breastfeeding research, book reviews, and news about LLLI and Alumnae activities,
- Social events and sessions and activities at Area, National, Affiliate, Division, and LLLI Conferences,
- A variety of trips, as varied as a Caribbean cruise and Grand Canyon hikes,
- Special projects, such as a retiring Leader survey, and,
- Extra benefits, such as a 10% discount on most items from the LLLI Catalogue, registration discount for LLLI Conferences, and optional term life insurance.

For more information, contact the LLLI Alumnae Association Coordinator at the LLLI office or via the LLLI Web site. Contact your support Leader for information on local alumnae associations.

LLLI Professional Advisory Board

Much of the credibility of La Leche League International comes from the fact that a board of prestigious professional advisors supports the organization.

> The Professional Advisory Board is composed of men and women recognized for their expertise in and support for breastfeeding and related fields

The LLLI Professional Advisory Board is appointed by the LLLI Board of Directors and made up of three active Councils: Health, Legal, and Management. Each is composed of men and women recognized for their expertise in and support for breast-feeding and related fields. These men and women act as advocates for LLLI, consult on complex breastfeeding-related issues, evaluate new or conflicting research, review LLLI publications, speak at conferences and seminars, and advise LLLI on legal, financial, and other business management issues. Health Advisory Council members ensurethat La Leche League recommendations and positions are based on research and sound medical advice.

Members of the Advisory Councils may reply to specific questions channeled through appropriate LLL sources such as the Professional Liaison network. They are not available to reply to specific questions from individual Leaders. (See **Support for the Leader Dealing with Medically or Legally Related Issues,** in Chapter 6.)

Online Resources from LLLI

LLLI's Online Communications staff provides a variety of resources on the Internet to Leaders, members, and the general public. The LLLI Web site at **http://www.lalecheleague.org** meets a wide range of needs. Via the Web site, Leaders, breastfeeding mothers, professionals who work with breastfeeding mothers, and others interested in breast-feeding can:

- Find answers to common breastfeeding questions through the extensive collection of Frequently Asked Questions (FAQ) files;
- Learn how to help LLL—by becoming a member, Leader, or Peer Counselor or by making a financial donation;
- Read inspiring and informative articles from NEW BEGINNINGS, LEAVEN, and BREASTFEEDING ABSTRACTS;
- Locate breastfeeding books and products, as well as Group supplies, in the online LLLI Catalogue;
- Read LLLI's press releases since 1995;
- Find an LLL Group or Leader in their vicinity or find one for a friend;
- Ask an accredited LLL Leader a breastfeeding question by means of the "Help Form" programs sponsored by LLLI and many Affiliates;
- Attend an online LLL meeting;
- Discover enriching activities to participate in, such as the World Walk for Breastfeeding, LLLI Conferences, and local Area, Regional, National, and Affiliate/Division Conferences;
- Search the Center for Breastfeeding Information database, which has thousands of breastfeeding references, and browse the collection of selected bibliographies;

- Learn about the LLLI Alumnae Association; or
- learn how they can join LLL or contribute to its mission.

New features and services are continually being added!

The OnLLLine Chronicle: News from La Leche League International is a service from the Online Communications Department. This free online newsletter, available to anyone who wants to subscribe, includes:

- Breastfeeding news
- What's new on the LLLI Web site—there's something new almost every day!
- Upcoming workshops, conferences, and seminars
- New LLLI publications—hot off the press!
- LLLI advocacy and outreach activities
- News releases from LLLI
- Featured quotes and breastfeeding briefs from NEW BEGINNINGS, one of our FAQs, or another LLL publication
- Announcements

The OnLLLine Chronicle is distributed via email to all subscribers around the middle of each month. Directions for subscribing and an archive of past issues are available on the LLLI Web site.

Online breastfeeding help and support can be helpful to women who are unable to attend meetings or do not have a Group near them. The mother who feels uneasy about attending a meeting alone or who has questions about LLL may find sampling our organization through our online services to be a good way to learn more about us. After becoming comfortable with LLL Leaders and members via online chats or email, mothers often make the decision to attend a Group meeting. Online LLL meetings and chats are also wonderful options for mothers who are in isolated areas, homebound, or otherwise unable to attend a local meeting. (See **LLL Services Online** in Chapter 7.)

While English is generally regarded as the language of the Internet, LLLI continues to move rapidly to add other languages to our Internet resources for parents, members, and Leaders, as are many Areas and Affiliates on their own Web sites. The original material and translations on the Web sites are all provided by volunteers, as is much of the design and maintenance of the LLLI Web site, as well as management of other LLL Internet activities. Paid LLLI staff provide direction and many other materials and services.

> The mother who feels uneasy about attending a meeting alone may find sampling our organization through our online services to be a good way to learn more about us.

LLLI SERVICES

APPENDIX

The forms, policies, and guidelines included in the Appendix may be copied by Leaders for LLL use.

LLLI POLICIES AND GUIDELINES

The Policies and Guidelines included in Appendix One are those that are referred to in THE LEADER'S HANDBOOK. The complete and current LLLI Policies and Standing Rules Notebook is available on the LLLI Web site (**http://lalecheleague.org**) on the Leader password protected pages. To obtain the password, please contact your support Leader.

ACTION: COOPERATIVE

LLLI and all its representatives have the option to take advantage of opportunities to cooperate with others. Cooperative action is limited to LLL's scope of expertise—breastfeeding. *(Apr 94)*

Policies and Standing Rules: Appendix 10—Cooperative Action—Guidelines for Leaders: Mixing Causes Statement

Helping mothers worldwide to breastfeed, so that they can learn mothering through breastfeeding, is the main focus of the work of La Leche League as defined by the LLLI Mission Statement and Bylaws, ARTICLE II. PURPOSE. The main focus of LLLI does not prevent interaction with other organizations whose purposes are compatible with the LLLI mission. LLLI and all its representatives have the option of taking advantage of opportunities to cooperate with others who support, promote and protect breastfeeding in accordance with established guidelines. The La Leche League Group is not to be used as a forum for a Leader's non-LLL interests or to do the work of organizations other than LLL. Leaders may not use their Leader status for commercial gain derived from non-LLL activity or to promote their personal non-LLL interests.

Questions for Leaders to consider prior to agreeing to cooperative action activity

A Leader is expected to discuss these questions with her LLL support person before agreeing to any cooperative action. The PL Program should also be consulted for anything involving health care providers and legal issues.

Should LLLI be involved in this venture?

1. *What are the goals of the proposed Cooperative Action?*
   Are they specific? Measurable? Achievable? Compatible with LLL?

2. *Who are all the parties involved?*
   Are their missions and purposes compatible with LLL?

3. *How will LLL benefit from involvement in this venture?*
   What are the benefits to mothers and babies? The local LLL Group? LLLI? Does it help LLL to achieve its mission?

4. *Will LLL be compensated either directly or indirectly?*
   Will my participation result in expense to my Group or Area in terms of either money or resources?
   Will LLL be offered payment or an honorarium for my participation?
   Will LLL materials be used/purchased? As LLL's representative, will my expenses be paid?
   (Note: Compensation is not a requirement of LLL participation. However, costs and potential income need to be considered.)

Should I be involved in this venture as LLL's representative?

1. *What specifically am I being asked to do?*
   Attend meetings, generate ideas, write, speak, organize activities, give one-on-one help? What is the required time commitment?

2. *Am I the best qualified Leader available?*
   Do I have the experience, abilities, qualifications, expertise needed for my participation? Am I aware of and willing to access LLL resources available to me that would assist me with this work?

3. *Do I have enough time and energy to fulfill my primary Leader responsibilities and to participate fully in this cooperative venture?*
   Does it merit Leader time and energy being channeled away from regular LLL work?
   Will my LLL Group suffer if I become involved?

To decline participation in cooperative action

At no time is an LLL Leader required to participate in cooperative action even if it is determined that her participation would be beneficial to LLL.

If you decide to decline participation, be honest and courteous, taking care to protect LLLI's image and promote our mission and purpose. Discuss your approach with your LLL support person. If appropriate, use a graceful statement that leaves the door open for possible future involvement, such as, "after consultation with other Leaders, I have decided to decline your offer at this time." You do not need to offer a justification for your decision, particularly if it is personal (e.g., lack of time). If you are declining because you feel that LLL participation is inappropriate, you may want to cite LLL policies in a non-confrontational style.

If you decline participation with a letter, discuss it with your LLL support person prior to sending it and provide her with a copy of the final letter for her files.

Guidelines for Leaders Involved in Cooperative Action Activities as LLL Representatives

Consultation/reporting requirements

Under most circumstances, authorization is not required for a Leader to engage in Cooperative Action activity. However, every Leader engaged in a Cooperative Action activity is expected to establish a consult/report relationship with her appropriate LLL support person before and during her participation. Specific reporting guidelines are determined by each Division or Affiliate. LLLI retains the final authority over all Cooperative Action activity including the right to terminate any activity that is not in compliance with written guidelines.

These are typical consulting/reporting relationships:

Local level: A Leader contacts DA, who reports to the ACL.
Area level: Contact ACL who reports to the appropriate Regional personnel, DD, or Affiliate Head.
National level: Contact DD/Affiliate Head, and/or ED.

Cooperative Action Report

When a Leader accepts the responsibility of representing LLL in a Cooperative Action activity, she needs to file a written Cooperative Action Report with her LLL support person that includes the following information:

- The name of the organization(s) seeking LLL cooperation with pertinent information about the activity. Include the organization's name, address, phone/fax number, and contact person.
- The name(s) and positions of LLL personnel participating.
- Proposed goals, plans and timeline for the joint project(s).
- Reason(s) LLL/LLLI was asked to participate.
- Methods to be used in publicizing what the organization is doing to promote breastfeeding and related subjects.
- Way(s) in which LLL/LLLI will benefit through participation.
- Costs/Compensation to LLL/LLLI, if any.

Acknowledgment of LLL participation

In any written listing of the participants that includes credentials, "LLL Leader" needs to appear beside the name of LLL representatives.

Limitations of cooperation

LLL expertise

An LLL Leader representing LLL/LLLI on a board, panel, task force, committee, or other similar group is authorized to speak for LLL only on subjects within the scope of LLLI expertise which includes providing mother-to-mother support for breastfeeding and helping mothers worldwide to breastfeed so that they can learn mothering through breastfeeding.

LLLI POLICIES

Signing a Document on Behalf of LLLI

Special caution should be used when a proposal requires a Leader to sign anything intended for publication or distribution to the public. Any LLL representative who signs a document on behalf of LLLI must have it reviewed by the ACL or her designate (for example, Outreach Coordinator) and, if legal or health care issues are involved, by the APL. A Leader should be aware that she is not obliged to sign anything, even after having participated in groundwork, unless that part dealing with breastfeeding is accurate according to LLLI resources. A mandatory disclaimer must be prominently included in the document to the effect: "La Leche League International agrees with the breastfeeding information contained in (…). All other information is outside LLL's scope of expertise." The Leader is to send a copy of any such document to her LLL support person.

Breastfeeding promotion projects funded by formula manufacturers

Neither LLLI nor any of its representatives may accept direct funding from formula manufacturers for any activity.

Sharing Leader lists

Lists of Leader names, phone numbers, addresses may be shared with organizations LLL is involved with in Cooperative Action Activities if such sharing will help to facilitate common goals.

When Leader lists are shared, the Leaders involved are to be notified.

Leaders will have the opportunity to have their names excluded from such lists. These requests should be noted in Area Leader Directories, which are to be updated annually.

Requests for sharing Leader lists are to be reviewed by the appropriate LLL administrator (within Area—ACL, Division—DD, Affiliate—Affiliate Head, LLLI—ED). Permission for use of lists will be withdrawn if the proposed activity is found to be incompatible with LLLI's mission, purpose, or policies.

LLL endorsement of jointly developed materials

Materials and/or projects that are jointly developed through cooperation with other organizations may be endorsed either by LLLI or one of its units (Group, Area, country). The wording of the endorsement should reflect the level of LLL involvement and responsibility for the project: "LLL of (Group, Area, country) endorses...", "Co-sponsored by LLL of ...", "in cooperation with LLL of..."

Jointly developed materials for which endorsement is sought are to be reviewed through normal LLL review processes by the LLL administrator at the level that the materials will be used (within Area—ACL, Division—DD, Affiliate—Affiliate Head, LLLI—ED). Final copies of any such materials/project descriptions are to be sent to LLL administrators and kept on file for a minimum of five years.

Upon favorable review of written materials, the Leader will be authorized to include the statement, "La Leche League International agrees with the breastfeeding information contained in (...). All other information is outside LLL's scope of expertise."

In no instance will any materials supported by companies which manufacture or distribute infant formula receive LLLI endorsement.

(*Feb 92; rev May 89, Oct 90, Oct 91; completely replaced Feb 95; rev Feb 98*) Cross reference: Action: Cooperative Sponsorship, Endorsement, Authorization, or Approval by LLLI

ACTION BY LEADERS

Leaders may act as interested private citizens or as LLL Leaders to promote breastfeeding to public officials, heads of state, and other recognized government groups at any time. Such advocacy is especially appropriate when action is pending anywhere that may affect breastfeeding.

Under the Lobbying Disclosure Act of 1995, the United States Internal Revenue Service does not count the activities of volunteers as lobbying. Therefore, advocacy by volunteer Leaders does not affect the nonprofit status of LLLI in the USA.

Outside the USA, Leaders are advised to determine whether advocating breastfeeding to government groups will affect the legal status of LLL in that country. (*Jun 94; rev Jun 94, Feb 98*)

BIBLIOGRAPHY, LLLI

The *LLLI Bibliography* is a list of books, published in print, audio or video format, or on digital media, found to be supportive of LLLI's mission, purpose, and philosophy and helpful to parents. The books published by LLLI most fully reflect LLLI philosophy and are the only books recommended by LLLI. Additional books included in the list are approved by the LLLI Book Evaluation Committee according to the LLLI Book Evaluation Guidelines; inclusion on the list does not imply LLLI's endorsement of that book. (*effective October 31, 1997; recorded Feb 98*)

BIBLIOGRAPHIES, LLL

In order to reflect local language and culture, Areas and Affiliates may establish field bibliographies of books evaluated according to the LLLI Book Evaluation Guidelines. These field bibliographies are considered as additions to the *LLLI Bibliography*. Areas and Affiliates that choose to establish a field bibliography assume responsibility for communicating their current list to the Chairman of the LLLI Book Evaluation Committee and the LLLI Director of Publications each time their field bibliography is updated.

The entire group of lists, consisting of the LLLI and all the LLL field bibliographies, compose the LLL Bibliographies. (*effective October 31, 1997; recorded Feb 98*)

BOOK EVALUATION COMMITTEE

The LLLI Executive Director shall establish an LLLI Book Evaluation Committee (BEC) composed of LLL Leaders to determine which books are included in the *LLLI Bibliography* according to the LLLI Book Evaluation Guidelines. The LLLI Executive Director shall designate an LLLI staff liaison to facilitate the work of this committee.

The Book Evaluation Committee shall prepare a summary paragraph for each entry in the *LLLI Bibliography*. Qualifying statements or disclaimers regarding the evaluation of a book for the *LLLI Bibliography* are included in this summary.

The procedures of this committee shall include an opportunity for Leaders to appeal the committee's decisions. The LLLI Board of Directors retains final authority to approve and to remove books for the *LLLI Bibliography*. (*effective October 31, 1997; recorded Feb 98*)

BOOK EVALUATION GUIDELINES

Books included in the LLL Bibliographies shall be evaluated according to the Book Evaluation: Principal Criteria. (*effective October 31, 1997; recorded Feb 98*)

Policies and Standing Rules: Appendix 36—Book Evaluation Guidelines: Principal Criteria

The purpose of the evaluation process is to select books

- supportive of LLLI's mission, purpose, and philosophy;
- helpful to parents;
- within the parameters of the principal criteria listed below.

Content (subject matter)

Books dealing directly with breastfeeding and/or relationships impacting breastfeeding are generally of greatest potential interest to LLL members and will be given priority for review and possible inclusion in the *LLLI Bibliography*.

Professional books substantially dealing with breastfeeding are usually of interest primarily for LLLI Catalogue sales and for Leader reference. Leaders may share these with Group members as appropriate.

Books that include information beyond LLLI's mission, purpose, and philosophy (e.g., preschool options, vaccination, teaching children how to handle money, etc.) may be acceptable if:

1. the author maintains an objective stance in describing a variety of perspectives, and
2. does not promote an idea that is inconsistent with LLLI's mission, purpose, and philosophy.

Books focusing on topics that may go beyond the concerns of the mother currently breastfeeding (e.g., school age/teenage/adult children, education, caring for elderly parents, marriage enrichment, grieving) may be included in the *LLLI Bibliography* when the topic is of potential interest to LLL members and the author's approach is congruent with LLL philosophy.

Children's books and tapes may be included in the *LLLI Bibliography* if they have illustrations of breastfeeding, encourage loving family relationships, or promote family-centered activities.

Books that primarily and specifically advocate a religious philosophy are not acceptable for the *LLLI Bibliography*. However, a book containing accurate, worthwhile information on breastfeeding or other topics related to LLLI's mission, purpose, and philosophy wherein the author's personal faith is an integral part of the presentation may be recommended for approval if the religious philosophy does not overshadow the topic(s) for which the book is being evaluated.

Tone

LLLI's goal is to provide materials that aid readers in making informed decisions. Books that present a balanced and informative case for the advantages of a particular attitude or practice are preferred. Books that persuade primarily by highlighting the pitfalls of the "opposition" should be avoided.

LLLI POLICIES

Breastfeeding Advocacy A limited exception to the tone of a book is the one written with the intent of provoking a strong reader response and motivating the reader to action. The most important aspect of evaluating this kind of book is to determine whether the information presented is current, accurate, and fair, and whether the author limits discussion and criticism to the issues. Such books will be listed in the *LLLI Bibliography* under "Breastfeeding Advocacy" and will be subject to regular evaluation as protocols and issues can date quickly.

Criticism As LLLI grows in size and reputation the opportunities and the inclination for others to criticize increases, too. A less than positive view toward some aspect of LLLI does not preclude recommending a book for approval. (*effective October 31, 1997; recorded Feb 98*)

Policies and Standing Rules: Appendix 37 – Book Evaluation: Appeals and Review

In the event of disagreement with the Book Evaluation Committee's decision to approve, not approve, or remove a book from the *LLLI Bibliography*, any Leader may pursue an appeal.

All concerns about a book should be directed in writing to the Chairman of the Book Evaluation Committee and the BEC's LLLI staff liaison, as soon as possible after notification to Leaders of the results of the book's evaluation.

If the issue in question was not addressed in the original evaluations, the BEC Chairman will send a copy of LLLI's Book Evaluation Guidelines and a current evaluation form to the concerned Leader. This Leader may reevaluate the book in question according to the Guidelines and return this completed form to the BEC Chairman with a copy to the LLLI staff liaison as a matter of record.

If ten or more Leaders from a broad geographical area pursue an appeal, an additional review will be undertaken within 90 days by a review committee including:

- BEC Chairman,
- LLLI staff liaison for the BEC,
- LLLI Director of Publications,

- a representative from the Leader Accreditation Department,
- a representative from the Leader Department,
- a representative from the Professional Liaison Program, when appropriate.

This committee will consider the current concerns, review any files on this book, and produce a brief, one-page recommendation to LLLI's Executive Director.

Based on these recommendations, the LLLI Executive Director or her designate, with input as needed from other LLLI resources, will determine the status of the book in question. The LLLI Executive Director may delegate the responsibility of making a final decision to any staff or administrator she feels is most qualified to make a decision.

The LLLI Executive Director will provide a periodic report to the Program Services Committee of the LLLI Board of Directors on Leader appeals of Book Evaluation Committee decisions.

The LLLI Board of Directors retains final authority to approve or not approve a publication for the *LLLI Bibliography*. (*effective October 31, 1997; recorded Feb 98*)

COPYRIGHTED MATERIAL, LLLI

LLLI copyrighted materials may not be duplicated by anyone without the permission of the LLLI Executive Director. (*May 78*)

DEFINITION OF ACTIVE LEADER

An active LLL Leader pursues the La Leche League mission through basic Leader responsibilities as defined in the Policies and Standing Rules Notebook and/or other service to LLL. An active Leader's fees are current, she keeps up to date with Leader education, and she communicates regularly with the organization. (*Oct 91, Mar 01*)

DIRECTORIES, LA LECHE LEAGUE

La Leche League Directories shall not be used for non-League activities. (*Jun 84; rev Nov 85*)

DONATIONS OF MONEY, GOODS AND SERVICES: ACCEPTANCE BY LLLI

LLLI may accept money, goods, and services from individuals, groups, organizations, and other sources that are compatible with the goals and policies of LLLI as long as they do not put an undue strain on LLLI staff resources and do include an overhead sum, which may be negotiated for restricted gifts and grants. (*Feb 82*)

GRIEVANCE PROCEDURE FOR LEADERS AND GRIEVANCE COMMISSION

The Grievance Commission is established to carry out the Grievance Procedure for Leaders, which provides an avenue for Leader complaints not resolved through the usual communication channels of LLL. (*Jul 99*)

Policies and Standing Rules: Appendix 40—LLLI Grievance Procedure for Leaders and Grievance Commission
Grievance Procedure Purpose

The La Leche League International Grievance Procedure provides an avenue for Leaders who feel their complaints have not been resolved through the usual and appropriate LLL channels. The Grievance Procedure is conducted by the Grievance Commission, established by and responsible to the LLLI Board of Directors.

The Grievance Procedure confers no contractual or other legally enforceable rights on any Leader.

Scope of procedure

The Grievance Procedure is available to Leaders.

A Leader may file a grievance with the Coordinator for the Grievance Commission within one year of her last attempt to resolve the grievance through the usual and appropriate channels of communication.

The Grievance Procedure is intended to address issues arising from implementation of LLLI policy.

The Grievance Procedure is not intended to address disagreements with LLLI policies in general. To register dissent with an LLLI policy, Leaders write directly to the LLLI Board of Directors.

In circumstances that do not fall within the scope of this procedure, an individual may request access to the Grievance Procedure, which may be granted by the Board of Directors.

General principles and procedures

The Board of Directors is responsible for informing Leaders about the Grievance Procedure.

General expenses to implement the Grievance Procedure shall be designated in the budget for the Board of Directors. Lack of available funding may affect the implementation of the procedure.

The Coordinator for the Grievance Commission is responsible to the Board of Directors for implementing the Grievance Procedure according to these general principles and procedures.

1. Grievances are submitted to the Coordinator of the Grievance Commission. All submissions must be in writing: by post, fax, or electronic mail (email). A grievance that makes formal use of this procedure should be explicitly labeled with a reference to the LLLI Grievance Procedure in order to be distinguished from a letter of complaint traversing the usual channels of administration and communication.

2. Together the Coordinator and grievant will review the situation and what steps have been taken within the usual and appropriate LLL channels. The Coordinator may facilitate the grievant in accessing any usual and appropriate LLL communication channels not yet utilized.

3. Upon receipt of the grievance the Grievance Coordinator notifies all parties identified in the grievance. The Grievance Coordinator sends a list of Grievance Commission members to all parties involved. Each party involved informs the Coordinator whether there are any members of the Grievance Commission with whom they are unwilling to work. The Coordinator designates one member of the Grievance Commission to serve as facilitator and notifies all parties. The Coordinator may serve as a facilitator.

4. The parties to the grievance and the facilitator work together to determine a plan for proceeding, including time frames and regular assessments of progress. Steps include, but are not limited to:
   i) Requesting information from, consulting, and collaborating with the Board of Directors, LLLI staff, and any administrators who might be able to assist in grievance resolution;
   ii) Providing relevant information about pertinent LLLI guidelines, policies, and resources available;
   iii) Laying out the facts and coming to agreement on any facts in dispute;
   iv) Determining what policies of LLLI are applicable;
   v) Determining if appropriate procedures were followed.

5. The facilitator helps the parties develop and agree on a course of action.

6. The facilitator outlines the implementation process for agreement by the parties to the grievance.   **LLLI POLICIES**

7. At the completion of the process, the facilitator who processed the grievance and the Coordinator of the Grievance Commission submit a report to the Chairman of the Board of Directors of LLLI. This report may point out issues in procedure or policy that are believed to warrant reconsideration or further study by the Board of Directors; the report may suggest actions to the Board of Directors.
   - Any files in the hands of an administrative body of LLL must be turned over to the facilitator in a timely fashion at the request of the facilitator, who makes information in any files accessible to all parties to the grievance, while recognizing the confidentiality of anyone not party to the grievance.
   - Face-to-face meetings including parties to the grievance and the facilitator may be held if agreed upon by all parties to the grievance and the facilitator, and if the expenses of such meetings are shared equally by all parties to the grievance.
   - During the operation of the grievance procedure, the facilitator may consult with other members of the Grievance Commission, with the exclusion of Commissioners whom parties to the grievance identified as those with whom they are unwilling to work.
   - Accurate written records are kept at all stages of the Grievance Procedure by the facilitators and reviewed by the Coordinator or her designate. The status is shared with all parties to the grievance at least every two months.
   - The Grievance Commission reserves the right to terminate the procedure if, after its best efforts, it determines that agreement cannot be reached, or when financial resources are not available for further pursuit.

Grievance Commission

The Grievance Commission is herein established by and responsible to the Board of Directors of La Leche League International to implement the LLLI Grievance Procedure to:

- review grievances from Leaders that have not been resolved by the usual administrative support structure of LLLI for the purpose of resolving such grievances to the mutual satisfaction of all parties to the grievance;
- communicate any suggested actions to the Board of Directors after such review.

Appointments and membership

The Board of Directors appoints a Coordinator for the Grievance Commission for a two year term at the Annual Session, with the term continuing until the Annual Session two years later. Individual members of the Grievance Commission and the LLLI Board of Directors are responsible for submitting recommendations for the Coordinator of the Grievance Commission to the Chairman of the Board thirty days in advance of the Annual Session.

Members of the Grievance Commission are nominated by the Coordinator for the Grievance Commission and are appointed to serve on the Grievance Commission upon approval by a majority of the Board of Directors of LLLI. Nominees must be recommended by at least two Leaders, members of the Board of Directors of LLLI, or other Grievance Commission members. Membership of the Grievance Commission should strive to reflect the diversity of La Leche League in terms of geography, culture, language, and range of experience as a Leader, with additional consideration for those with expertise that might assist the work of the Grievance Commission.

The Grievance Commission consists of a minimum of six members in addition to the Coordinator of the Grievance Commission.

The minimum term for Grievance Commission members shall be three years, after which time each member's term shall be renewable annually upon recommendation by the Coordinator of the Grievance Commission and approval by a majority of the Board of Directors.

Members of the Grievance Commission:

- are knowledgeable about LLL policies, procedures, and resources;
- listen and respond in an objective and caring way with regard to issues, people, or departments involved;
- address people and issues without pre-judgment, anticipation, or tendency to direct outcomes;
- think independently, critically, and clearly;
- identify issues and present them clearly, concisely, and dispassionately, both in person and in writing;
- practice strict confidentiality;
- exercise efficiency in meeting time schedules; and
- collaborate with Commission members for constructive outcomes.

Duties

The Grievance Commission shall carry out the LLLI Grievance Procedure, including but not limited to:

- receiving complaints;
- respecting administrative decisions that accurately reflect the intent of LLLI policy made by the Board of Directors;
- providing confidential, sensitive, empathic listening;
- making every effort to offer a fair hearing to all parties involved;
- approaching all parties to a grievance flexibly and creatively, taking into account logistic, language, and cultural factors;
- making every effort to facilitate the resolution of grievances;
- consulting and collaborating directly with volunteer and paid staff in La Leche League if directed to do so by the Board of Directors of LLLI;
- reporting to the LLLI Board of Directors regularly, with a minimum of one report 45 days in advance of each meeting of the Board of Directors.
- submitting an annual budget for implementation of the Grievance Procedure to the LLLI Board of Directors and Executive Director as part of the financial planning process of LLLI. (Jul 99; rev Feb 02)

GROUP SERIES MEETINGS

The order of Series Meetings shall be:

- Advantage of Breastfeeding to Mother and Baby
- Baby Arrives: The Family of the Breastfed Baby
- The Art of Breastfeeding and Overcoming Difficulties
- Nutrition and Weaning

The wording of these titles may be varied although the emphasis should remain the same. (*Nov 82; rev Feb 88*)

GROUP LIBRARIES

As part of La Leche League's service to mothers, each LLL Group should endeavor to provide a lending library composed of publications selected from the LLL Bibliographies.

The Basic Group Library will include, to the extent possible, four basic books:

1. The most recent edition of The Womanly Art of Breastfeeding in the appropriate language,
2. A nutrition-oriented text such as Whole Foods For The Whole Family or an alternative book of similar nature appropriate in the relevant country,
3. A book that presents an overview of childbirth,
4. A book on parenting that supports LLLI's concept of loving guidance.

Areas and Affiliates may specify guidelines for choosing the three basic books on nutrition, childbirth, and loving guidance from the LLL Bibliographies. Priorities for selecting additional books will be according to the Group's needs.

Summaries for each entry are included in the LLL Bibliographies to assist Leaders in selecting additional books for Group Libraries. A copy of the summary should also be affixed to the corresponding book as a new book is added to the Group Library. These summary paragraphs include all disclaimers specified by the Book Evaluation Committee and should be the only disclaimers used. (*effective October 31, 1997; recorded Feb 98*).

HOME BIRTH: MEDICAL SUPERVISION

While LLLI supports alert participation by the mother in childbirth, the organization does not recommend or encourage a home birth without medical supervision.

In any discussion of non-supervised home birth at LLL meetings the Leader will clearly state LLLI's concern about the risks involved and guide the discussion toward other topics. LLLI policy on home birth should be made clear during the Leader application process. (*Feb 78; rev Oct 86*)

INSURANCE, LIABILITY

Liability Insurance shall be carried for the Board of Directors, Officers, and Leaders. (*LLLI Bylaws, Article X. Feb 81*)

LEADER ACCREDITATION

LLL Leaders are accredited by LLLI and are recognized as LLL Leaders worldwide. (*Nov 82*)

"Applying for Leadership" is adopted as LLLI policy and included in the LLLI Policy and Standing Rules Notebook as an Appendix.

"Applying for Leadership" includes:

- LLLI Prerequisites to Applying for Leadership
- LLLI Criteria for Leader Accreditation
- LLLI Prerequisites to Applying for Leadership—Guidelines for Leaders

(*Jun 85; rev Nov 85; completely replaced Feb 98; rev Oct 98*)

LLLI POLICIES

Appendix 18—Applying for Leadership—LLLI Prerequisites to Applying for Leadership

Personal breastfeeding experience

Mother has breastfed her baby for at least nine months when she applies for leadership. Baby was nourished with mother's milk until there was a nutritional need for other foods (i.e., about the middle of the first year for the healthy, full term baby). If baby has weaned, the baby was nursed for about a year and the transition from breastfeeding respected the baby's needs.

Note: Special consideration may be given to a woman whose personal breastfeeding experience is outside the realm of a normal course of breastfeeding.

Mothering experience

Mother values nursing at her breast as the optimal way to nourish, nurture, and comfort her baby. She recognizes, understands, and responds to baby's need for her presence as well as for her milk. She manages any separation from baby with sensitivity and respect for the baby's needs.

Organizational experience
- Is a member of LLL.
- Supports LLLI purpose and philosophy.
- Has attended at least one series of meetings (where available) and has demonstrated a commitment to LLL.
- Owns and is familiar with the contents of the most recent edition of The Womanly Art of Breastfeeding (if available in her language) as a primary resource for LLL Leaders.
- Has a recommendation from an LLL Leader.

Personal traits

- Has sufficient command of language to complete the application and preparation for accreditation and to fulfill the responsibilities of LLL leadership.
- Has an accepting and respectful attitude toward others.
- Exhibits warmth and empathy toward others.
- Demonstrates or is willing to develop effective communication skills.

LLLI Criteria for Leader Accreditation.

To be accredited as an LLL Leader, a woman will meet the following criteria:

- She has met the LLLI Prerequisites to Applying for Leadership (as listed above).
- She has nursed her baby for about a year.
- She has demonstrated understanding of LLLI philosophy.
- She has conveyed her knowledge of basic breastfeeding management, outlined in Breastfeeding Management Skills Criteria.
- She has demonstrated leadership skills and attitudes, outlined in Leadership Skills Criteria.
- She has completed the LLL Leader accreditation process.
- She has signed the LLL Leader Statement of Commitment.

La Leche League is a worldwide, educational, nonsectarian, non-discriminatory service organization.

Breastfeeding Management Skills Criteria

Upon completion of her application, the newly accredited Leader will be able to demonstrate knowledge of **basic** breastfeeding management and problem solving techniques, **basic** lactation physiology of the mother and baby, and of the **normal course of breastfeeding** as described in the most recent edition of THE WOMANLY ART OF BREASTFEEDING, which will be owned by the newly accredited Leader, **if it is available in her language.**

The newly accredited Leader will have completed the LLLI *Breastfeeding Resource Guide*, if available in her language, or its counterpart. If the LLLI *Breastfeeding Resource Guide* or its LAD-approved counterpart is not available in her language, she will have identified appropriate resources in her language, as available and as she is able, in the following categories of breastfeeding management. The categories include but are not limited to:

- LLL resources available to Leaders
- Mother-to-mother helping techniques
- Structure and function of the breast
- Management of breastfeeding
- Positioning techniques
- Infant anatomy, sucking mechanisms, and breastfeeding behavior
- Infant reflexes
- Potential problems (e.g., nipple or breast problems, slow or low weight gain, thrush, allergies)
- Role of maternal and infant nutrition
- Solid foods
- Weaning
- Premature infants
- Jaundice
- Hand-expression and pumping
- Working and breastfeeding

The *Breastfeeding Resource Guide*, if available in an Applicant's language, or its LAD-approved counterpart will be completed by the Leader Applicant as part of her application in the way that the Applicant, Leader, and LAD representative determine is best suited to her individual situation (e.g., completed alone by the Applicant using resources available to her, completed at an Applicant workshop, or completed in parts in collaboration with another Leader or LAD representative).

A newly accredited Leader will be able to demonstrate knowledge of how to use LLL information and resources, if available and as she is able. Ownership of THE BREASTFEEDING ANSWER BOOK is strongly recommended, if available in her language. Other recommended (but not required) resources where available include, but are not limited to: LLL Professional Liaison Programs, LEADER'S HANDBOOK, LEAVEN (or another LLL Leader publication in her language), NEW BEGINNINGS (or another LLL member publication), the LLLI Web Site (including links from the LLLI Web Site), breastfeeding resources available to her on the Internet, and other resources in her language.

Leadership skills criteria

Upon completion of her application, a Leader Applicant will have demonstrated awareness and understanding of the leadership skills necessary to assume the responsibilities of leadership. The Applicant, with the help of the contact Leader (where available), will have completed a checklist of topics to discuss in preparation for leadership, if one is available in her language.

Upon completion of her application, the Leader Applicant will have demonstrated that she:

- Understands the importance of acceptance and respect for individual choices regarding breastfeeding and parenting.
- Can communicate effectively in providing mother-to-mother help.
- Is familiar with LLL resources and can gather, organize, and retrieve pertinent information.
- Understands and agrees to work within LLL guidelines for consulting, documenting, and reporting.
- Understands and agrees to work within LLLI policies as presented in the LLLI Bylaws, Policies and Standing Rules Notebook, The Leader's Handbook, and other LLLI publications.

These skills and attitudes are covered in THE LEADER'S HANDBOOK and are learned through reading, personal experience, attendance at Series meetings, LLL conferences and workshops, and discussion with sponsoring Leader(s) and LAD representative(s). These skills and attitudes are demonstrated in the Personal History, during Series meetings and during completion of the "Preview of Questions Mothers Ask."

LLLI Prerequisites for Leadership—Guidelines for Leaders

Introduction

1) La Leche League International (LLLI) accredits Leaders to carry out its purpose and mission. Leaders are a diverse group of women representing a broad spectrum of cultures, bound together by a common philosophy and a mother-to-mother approach to providing breastfeeding help.

2) The credibility and authority of LLLI are due, in major part, to the fact that all LLL Leaders are experienced breastfeeding mothers. LLL wants to attract prospective Leaders who have or are willing to develop the knowledge, experience, and skills needed to help mothers breastfeed and gain a better understanding of mothering through breastfeeding. Collectively LLL Leaders provide a variety of real life examples of mothering through breastfeeding and ways that challenges to breastfeeding can be overcome. The LLLI Prerequisites to Applying for Leadership are written in broad terms recognizing that mothers in a variety of circumstances can and do embrace LLLI philosophy and put it into practice.

3) These guidelines are designed to help a Leader and interested mother discuss the prerequisites and together evaluate whether or not the mother is ready to apply for leadership. A Leader's close contact with mothers and potential Applicants, along with her knowledge, observations, and use of LLL resources, places her in a unique position to help a mother decide whether or not to apply.

LLLI POLICIES

4) In preparation for discussing leadership with a mother, it is a Leader's responsibility to be familiar with the LLLI Application Packet (No. 485) or the LLL Affiliate Application Packet (which both include information about current LLLI policies related to leadership accreditation) as well as with THE WOMANLY ART OF BREASTFEEDING and THE LEADER'S HANDBOOK. A Leader can consult a LAD representative with any questions or concerns prior to or at any time during an application.

5) Before a woman can apply to become an LLL Leader, she needs the support of at least one active Leader (who could be a LAD representative). After consultation with co-Leaders, the Leader writes a recommendation affirming that the mother meets the LLLI Prerequisites to Applying for Leadership and that she will help the mother prepare for leadership. After a mother begins her application, she works with one or more Leaders and LAD representatives to fulfill the remaining LLLI Criteria for Leader Accreditation.

Personal Breastfeeding and Mothering Experience Prerequisites

6) In order to meet the Personal Breastfeeding and Mothering Experience Prerequisites, a mother has experienced mothering through breastfeeding in a way that includes being available and responsive to her baby's needs. This experience, combined with what she learns from other mothers and from LLL resources, provides her with a strong base for helping mothers.

7) The Personal Breastfeeding and Mothering Experience Prerequisites are interrelated and to be considered as a whole, without overemphasizing individual phrases or sentences. A Leader can use LLLI philosophy statements, policy statements, and these guidelines to stimulate discussions with the interested mother as they examine together how the mother's experiences reflect her understanding of mothering through breastfeeding as presented in THE WOMANLY ART OF BREASTFEEDING.

8) Leaders discuss and clarify LLLI philosophy statements with potential Applicants using resources such as THE LEADER'S HANDBOOK and questions similar to these:
- What is your understanding of each concept statement? Are any concepts unclear to you? Do you have reservations about any of the concepts?
- How do you see your experiences reflecting the concepts?
- How could your experiences and understanding of each concept help you fulfill the role of a Leader?

9) A mother may have experienced situations, usually short term, in which substitutes for human milk and/or nursing at mother's breast were determined to be or were accepted as necessary. The Leader and mother, in their discussion of the Personal Breastfeeding Experience Prerequisite, consider the mother's understanding of her baby's needs and LLLI philosophy and how this understanding is revealed in her subsequent experience of mothering through breastfeeding.

10) The "special consideration" note applies only to the Personal Breastfeeding Experience Prerequisite. It has relevance in unusual situations that can challenge a mother's ability to breastfeed, such as a physical limitation of mother or baby. When a mother's breastfeeding experience differs from that described by the prerequisite and might warrant this special consideration, the Leader should consult with a LAD representative.

11) A mother who makes every effort to meet her baby's needs for nurturing and nourishment at her breast and who has demonstrated awareness of and responsiveness to her baby's need for her presence can fulfill the Mothering Experience Prerequisite. A mother can sometimes combine commitments that take her away from her baby with an experience of mothering through breastfeeding that is consistent with LLLI philosophy. A mother who experiences extensive, ongoing separation from her baby is unlikely to fulfill the Mothering Experience Prerequisite.

12) When considering the Mothering Experience Prerequisite with a mother who has experienced separation from her baby, Leaders can use the following as the basis for dialogue and insight:
- How the mother demonstrates that she recognizes and understands the baby's intense need for her presence and how she responds to meet this need;
- Any impact of separation on mothering through breastfeeding;
- The arrangements the mother makes/has made to lessen separation between mother and baby, and/or to minimize disruption of breastfeeding;
- The mother's presentation and explanation of LLLI philosophy in light of her experience;
- How the mother thinks she would help other mothers experiencing situations similar to her own.

13) After discussions using the guidelines provided above, if a Leader recognizes that a mother is incorporating LLLI philosophy into her life, that mother very likely meets the Personal Breastfeeding and Mothering Experience Prerequisites. If a Leader is unsure about whether the mother's experiences thus far fit within the prerequisites, she can consult with a LAD representative.

Organizational experience prerequisite

14) The Organizational Experience Prerequisite establishes that a mother knows enough about LLL and the role and time commitments of an LLL Leader to make an informed decision about leadership. It also provides the Leader with an opportunity to get to know the mother well enough to write a recommendation.

Personal traits prerequisite

15) The Personal Traits Prerequisite helps a Leader identify mothers who have a foundation for developing effective leadership skills. Effective leadership relies on a woman's attitude and approach toward mothers who seek help as well as the way she presents herself and communicates with others. As a mother moves from seeking information and support for herself to offering these to other mothers, a Leader can note the mother's current attitudes and skills, as well as her willingness to learn and interest in learning. During the application, an Applicant will have the opportunity to build on the foundation of her personal traits and further develop the skills she would need to help mothers as an LLL Leader.

16) Leader Applicants need adequate language skills to be able to complete the application. This includes having or acquiring adequate knowledge about breastfeeding and the communication skills needed to be a Leader. If there are challenges to accessing LLL information due to low literacy, language barriers, or disabilities, Leaders, Applicants, and LAD representatives work together to facilitate access to or develop necessary resources.

Conclusion

17) The Leader's observations and opinions are important as she talks with a mother about LLL leadership, both before and during an application. If the Leader is satisfied that a mother fulfills the Prerequisites, she can encourage the mother to apply for leadership.

When the Leader writes her recommendation, she bases her comments on the prerequisites and these guidelines, her interactions with the mother and their discussions about LLL leadership, her recognition that the mother is incorporating LLLI philosophy into her life, and her perception of the mother's willingness to learn.

18) If, at any point before or during the application, a Leader has doubts about whether a mother fulfills the prerequisites or can meet the criteria for leadership, it is the Leader's responsibility to consult with a LAD representative. If a Leader determines that a mother does not meet the prerequisites, it is her responsibility to inform the mother of the reasons for the decision and to inform her of the appeals process outlined in the Application Packet.

LEADER ACCREDITATION APPEALS

A brief description of the appeals process will appear in the Leader Application Packet. *(Feb 98)*

Appendix 38 —LLLI Leader Accreditation Appeals Policies and Process

Before each Board meeting, LAD Directors will prepare a report on accreditation appeals for the LLLI Executive Director and Board of Directors. The LLLI Executive Director, in consultation with the LLLI Board of Directors and LAD Directors, will develop an appropriate format for the Appeals Report from LAD Directors to the LLLI Executive Director and LLLI Board of Directors. *(Feb 98)*

Policies and Standing Rules: Appendix 38——LLLI Leader Accreditation Appeals Policies and Process

Introduction

A Leader Applicant or mother interested in applying for LLL leadership may disagree with a decision regarding her application made by a local LLL Leader or the Leader Accreditation Department (LAD) representative. In order to afford her an opportunity to make her questions known and addressed, LLLI offers a Leader Accreditation Appeals Process for the following situations:

1. The local LLL Leader or LAD representative determines that an Applicant or interested mother does not meet the LLLI Prerequisites to Applying for Leadership.

2. An Applicant is asked by a LAD representative to withdraw her application at any time after the application has begun.

The appeals process shall focus on dialogue that fosters respect, understanding, and collaboration. Dialogue will be used to facilitate an outcome with increased under-

standing and resolutions that include everyone involved in the appeals process.

LLLI POLICIES

Definitions

Within the scope of this policy, an **interested mother** is a mother who has expressed an interest in becoming a Leader but whose application has not been allowed to proceed.

Applicant refers to a mother whose application for leadership has been accepted.

LLL Leader is someone who has been accredited by LLLI as an LLL Leader.

LAD representative refers to members of the LLLI Leader Accreditation Department, hereafter referred to as LAD (e.g., ACLAs, CLAs, RALAs, ADRALAs, Affiliate LAD Administrators, or Director of the LAD).

LLLI LAD administrative body refers to the international group of LAD administrators who are responsible for coordinating the work of accreditation in recognized LLL entities. (This includes implementing policies and procedures in the training of LAD personnel and work with Applicants and Leaders.) This group is coordinated by the LAD Director and currently it includes: one representative from each Affiliate, one from each US Division, and one from each International Division Region.

Stage 1

Interested mother is not recommended for leadership application.

A. When a decision not to recommend an interested mother is made by an LLL Leader, she explains her decision to the interested mother and informs her of her right to correspond directly with a LAD representative who provides her with complete information about the appeals process.

B. If the interested mother wishes to appeal, she corresponds with the appropriate LAD representative (with a copy to the LLL Leader), explaining why she feels that she meets the LLLI Prerequisites to Applying for Leadership or should be recommended for leadership, or providing new information which may affect her potential application. The Leader may at any time reverse her prior decision and notify the LAD representative.

C. The LAD representative writes the interested mother with her recommendation or decision after consulting, if necessary, with the interested mother, the Leader, and LAD support staff.

D. If the initial decision not to recommend an interested mother is reversed, her application may be initiated.

E. If the initial decision is upheld, and the interested mother is not satisfied with the response, she may exercise the option under Stage 2.

Stage 2

Initial Leader decision not to recommend an interested mother is upheld by the LAD representative and the mother wishes to appeal to the LAD representative at the next administrative level.

The initial decision to halt an application was made by a first level LAD representative in consultation with LAD support staff, and an Applicant or interested mother wishes to appeal to the LAD representative at the next administrative level, with or without support of the Leader.

A. The Applicant or interested mother continues her appeal to the next level LAD representative. She may respond to the issues involved in the previous LAD representative's decision and explain why she still feels that she meets the LLLI Prerequisites to Applying for Leadership or should otherwise be recommended for leadership. The LAD representative making the previous decision may reverse her decision and 1) recommend the interested mother for leadership application, or 2) communicate to LAD support staff her reasons for wanting to continue a halted application.

B. The next level LAD representative writes the interested mother with her recommendation or decision after consulting, if necessary, with the interested mother, the Leader, and LAD support staff.

C. If the previous decision is reversed, the application will be initiated or continue.

D. If the decision is upheld, the Applicant or interested mother may exercise the option under Stage 3, if she is not satisfied with the decision. The local LLL Leader may choose to support the Applicant or interested mother in her appeal, or the Applicant or interested mother may pursue an appeal on her own.

Stage 3

Applicant or interested mother appeals to LLLI LAD Director.

A. The Applicant or interested mother writes the LAD Director to continue her appeal. She may respond to the issues involved in the LAD representative's decision and explain why she still feels that she meets the LLLI Prerequisites to Applying for Leadership, should be recommended for leadership application, or should continue her application. The LAD representative making the previous decision may reverse her decision and 1) recommend the interested mother for leadership application, or 2) communicate to LAD support staff her reasons for wanting to continue a halted application.

B. At her discretion, the LAD Director may consult with members of the LLLI LAD administrative body who have not been directly involved in the decision being appealed.

C. The LAD Director sends her decision with rationale in writing to the Applicant or interested mother (with a copy to the Leader and all LAD representatives who have been involved in the appeal).

D. If the previous decision is reversed, the application is initiated or continued.

E. If the decision is upheld, the Applicant or interested mother may exercise
the option under Stage 4. The local LLL Leader may choose to support the Applicant or interested mother in her appeal, or the Applicant or interested mother may pursue an appeal on her own.

Stage 4

Applicant or interested mother appeals to the LLLI Leader Accreditation Review Committee.

A. The Applicant or interested mother informs the LAD Director that she wishes to appeal to the LLLI Leader Accreditation Review Committee. She may respond to the issues involved in the LAD Director's decision and explain why she still feels that she meets the LLLI Prerequisites to Applying for Leadership, should be recommended for leadership application, or should continue her application.

B. If the LAD Director does not wish to reverse her decision, she forwards the file in a timely manner to the LLLI Leader Accreditation Review Committee.

C. Within a reasonable amount of time, the LLLI Leader Accreditation Review Committee reaches a final decision and communicates that decision in writing to the Applicant or interested mother (copying the Leader and all LAD representatives who have been involved in the appeal). The decision of the LLLI Leader Accreditation Review Committee will be reported to the Chairman of the LLLI Board, LLLI Executive Director, and the LAD Director.

D. The LLLI Leader Accreditation Review Committee decision is final.

General LLLI Leader Accreditation Appeals Policies

1. When receiving the Leader Application Packet, all interested mothers will be informed of the existence of an appeals process and given the name of the appropriate LAD representative to contact for complete information.

2. In order to access the appeals process, a mother must contact a LAD representative.

3. An Applicant or interested mother or LLL Leader who wishes to appeal a decision that halts or prevents an application should do so within 60 days of receiving the written notice of a decision. If there are extenuating circumstances that caused a delay of longer than 60 days, the person receiving the appeal should take these into consideration.

4. All Applicants or interested mothers will be notified in writing of appeals decisions within a reasonable amount of time. Responses will outline rationale for decisions and LLLI or LAD resources upon which the decision is based. Later reviewers will comment in writing on these citations if they decide to reverse a decision.

5. At any point in the appeals process, LAD representatives may consult with other LAD support people and with administrators outside the LAD, if it will help with conflict resolution and/or objectivity. If other LAD or other LLLI administrators are brought into the dialogue, their opinions will be documented in the file.

6. The appeals process shall focus on dialogue that fosters communication and respect by working together to increase understanding of the LLLI Prerequisites to Applying for Leadership and the LLLI Criteria for Leader Accreditation.

7. All communications used in an appeals process must be documented, including email, telephone calls, video or audiotapes, or in-person meetings. Copies of appeals files will be kept by the last LAD representative involved in the appeals process, and the LLLI Leader Accreditation Review Committee if the appeal reached that level. *(Feb 98; rev Feb 99)*

LLLI POLICIES

LEADER ACCREDITATION APPEALS: AFFILIATES

When implementing their appeals process, it is expected that Affiliates will incorporate the following:

1. All Applicants and interested mothers will be informed of the existence of an appeals process.
2. Applicants and interested mothers will be notified in writing of decisions on their appeals.
3. LAD representatives will consult with other LAD support staff as appropriate and if necessary to help with conflict resolution.
4. The LLLI LAD Director will be informed of appeals decisions reached within Affiliates.
5. If all prior stages in the Affiliate appeals process are exhausted, Applicants and interested mothers may make a final appeal to the LLLI Leader Accreditation Review Committee as outlined in "LLLI Leader Accreditation Appeals Policies and Process," Appendix 38. *(Feb 98)*

LEADER ACCREDITATION: APPLICATION FEE

A Leader Application fee will be charged. *(Nov 80; rev Nov 85)*

LEADER ACCREDITATION: REMOVAL

A Leader's accreditation may be removed for philosophy discrepancy, discrediting LLL, and/or behavior that continually causes conflict or interferes with her effectiveness as a Leader. Before removal of a Leader's accreditation is considered, that Leader must be informed of the Grievance Procedure. *(May 82; rev Feb 83, Jul 99)*

LEADER: BASIC RESPONSIBILITIES

A La Leche League Leader:

- Helps mothers one-to-one, by telephone or in person, keeping accurate records of these helping situations.
- Plans and leads monthly Series meetings.
- Supervises the management of the Group, including membership, finances, Group workers, Group Library, and materials for sale; informs the Area Coordinator of Leaders (usually through the District Advisor/Coordinator) about her LLL activities through written monthly reports.
- Keeps up-to-date on all important breastfeeding information, taking advantage of LLL's opportunities for continuing education through publications, meetings, correspondence, and the network of resource Leaders.
- Takes an active role in helping other mothers find out about leadership and helps them prepare to become LLL Leaders. *(Feb 98)*

LEADER ELIGIBILITY

An applicant shall not be considered ineligible for leadership on the basis of any of the following factors: race; creed; color; physical disability; marital status; financial or social position; political or social views. Since an LLL Leader is a mother who has breastfed a baby, a man cannot become an LLL Leader. *(Jan 75)*

LEADER/LACTATION CONSULTANT: GUIDELINES

The Leader who maintains a dual role as a Leader/Lactation Consultant will observe guidelines for Leader/Lactation Consultants. *(Oct 89)*

Policies and Standing Rules: Appendix 21——Guidelines for Leader/Lactation Consultants

1. An active Leader/Lactation Consultant cannot make referrals to herself for pay.

2. An active Leader/Lactation Consultant cannot advertise herself as a Lactation Consultant on LLL phone recordings or at LLL Group meetings.

3. The Leader discount on purchasing materials from LLLI is intended to produce revenue for the local Group or Area. The Leader/Lactation Consultant is expected to return such profits to LLLI, her Group, or Area. However, she may purchase materials at a commercial bulk rate and retain the profit as any business may do.

4. A Leader/Lactation Consultant using LLLI materials and resources to help a paying client is expected to reimburse LLLI for the cost of those materials or resources, or to make a donation to LLLI, her Group, or her Area.

5. Leader/Lactation Consultants may advertise in written LLL materials or exhibit at LLL functions to the same extent as other individuals and organizations thst promote breastfeeding and offer breastfeeding information and support. Free exchange of information promotes cooperation and harmony and benefits everyone in the long run. Exclusion promotes lack of cooperation. *(Oct 89)*

   Cross reference: Leaders/Lactation Consultant: Guidelines

LLL LOGO AND LLL NAME PROTECTION

The October 1992 revision of the "Policy for Use of the LLL Logo and Name, La Leche League" shall be added to the PSR and replace any existing statements therein. *(Oct 92)*

Policies and Standing Rules: Appendix 26—LLL Logo and Name Protection

The LLL logo is the registered trademark of La Leche League International. The name La Leche League is also a registered trademark of the organization.

Protection of the logo and name

Registration of the logo through the United States Patent and Trademark office protects the use of the logo. The name La Leche League is also registered and protected.

Use of the logo within LLL
For official LLL business

LLL Groups, Chapters, Districts, Areas, Divisions, and Affiliates may use the LLL logo and name La Leche League for official business on stationery, forms, publications, notices, etc., as described in the "Guidelines for Correct Presentation of the Logo and Name" which is included in this policy.

When an item is sold:

A La Leche League representative or member may use the LLL logo or name La Leche League on an item which is sold if 1) the item is approved by the Executive Director or her designate and 2) a royalty of 5% of the retail selling price is paid to LLLI for the use of the logo. See the policy "Procedures for Approval of Items Sold." Sales of these items must benefit an LLL Group, Chapter, District, Area, Division, Affiliate, or LLLI.

Procedure for approval:

Within La Leche League, approval is required for the use of the LLL logo or name: 1) when the logo and/or name appears on an item to be sold 2) when the logo and/or name is incorporated into a design for the first time. Approval is granted by the Executive Director or her designate.

If the logo or name is used alone, no approval is necessary. Use the "Guidelines for Correct Presentation of the Logo and Name" which follows.

Use of the logo outside LLL
How to obtain permission to use the LLL Logo:

Other organizations, businesses, or publications may use the logo only with the express, written permission of the LLLI Executive Director. Requests will be considered on an individual basis and all terms of the agreement including royalties will be determined by the Executive Director.

Infringement:

If the logo, name, or a confusingly similar mark is used by another organization, business, or publication, LLLI will inform the infringer in writing of the infringement and request that he cease using the LLL logo or name. Further action will be taken as needed.

Guidelines for correct presentation of the LLL logo and name
The logo must be an exact reproduction of the design shown to the left. Camera-ready artwork and electronic files of the logo are available from LLLI on the Leader Order Form, No. 175, 176, 177.

The line around the oval is part of the logo design. The light and dark areas of the logo design can be reversed. There are no color restrictions for the logo or name. There are no typestyle restrictions for the name La Leche League.

LLLI POLICIES

The logo and name can be incorporated into a design (such as a state or country map) if the entire logo and/or name are kept intact. If incorporated in a design, the placement of the Registration Mark ® for the logo is the same as if the logo stood alone. The Registration Mark which is shown as a circle around a capital "R," is placed at the lower right hand area of the logo, outside the oval and next to the mother's hand. No Registration Mark is required with the name La Leche League when it is used by anyone within the organization.

The Registration Mark must be used when the logo is applied to printed matter. However, on an item like jewelry it can be omitted.

The entire design must be in good taste. It can be submitted to LLLI c/o the Public Relations Department, if there is a question as to whether the design is appropriate and correct. In all cases, the judgment of the Executive Director is final.

If either the logo or name is used inappropriately, the person will be notified through the proper established channels. *(Oct 92; rev Feb 99)* *Cross references: Logo, LLL Logo and LLL Name Protection.*

MAILING LISTS

At the discretion of the LLLI Publications Director, sale of LLLI mailing lists shall be permitted hereafter. Names of individuals wishing to be excluded from these lists shall not be included in any sale. *(Oct 84; rev Feb 92)*

MISSION STATEMENT

Our Mission is to help mothers worldwide to breastfeed through mother-to-mother support, encouragement, information, and education, and to promote a better understanding of breastfeeding as an important element in the healthy development of the baby and mother. *(May 89; rev Apr 93)*

PHILOSOPHY, LA LECHE LEAGUE INTERNATIONAL
Appendix 1 (date unrecorded)

Policies and Standing Rules: Appendix 1—La Leche League International's Philosophy

LLLI believes that breastfeeding with its many important physical and psychological advantages is best for baby and mother and is the ideal way to initiate good parent-child relationships. The loving help and support of the father enables the mother to focus on mothering so that together the parents develop close family relationships which strengthen the family and thus the whole fabric of society.

LLLI further believes that mothering through breastfeeding deepens a mother's understanding and acceptance of the responsibilities and rewards of her special role in the family. As a woman grows in mothering she grows as a human being and every other role she may fill in her lifetime is enriched by the insights and humanity she brings to it from her experiences as a mother.

The purpose of LLLI is distinct. The purpose as stated in the Bylaws does not prevent interaction with other organizations with compatible purposes but La Leche League will carefully guard against allying itself with another cause, however worthwhile that cause might be.

The basic philosophy of LLLI as expressed in THE WOMANLY ART OF BREASTFEEDING is summarized in the following concepts:

- Mothering through breastfeeding is the most natural and effective way of understanding and satisfying the needs of the baby.
- Mother and baby need to be together early and often to establish a satisfying relationship and an adequate milk supply.
- In the early years, the baby has an intense need to be with his mother which is as basic as his need for food.
- Breast milk is the superior infant food.
- For the healthy, full-term baby, breast milk is the only food necessary until the baby shows signs of needing solids, about the middle of the first year after birth.
- Ideally the breastfeeding relationship will continue until the baby outgrows the need.
- Alert and active participation by the mother in childbirth is a help in getting breastfeeding off to a good start.
- Breastfeeding is enhanced and the nursing couple sustained by the loving support, help, and companionship of the baby's father. A father's unique relationship with his baby is an important element in the child's development from early infancy.
- Good nutrition means eating a well-balanced and varied diet of foods in as close to their natural state as possible.
- From infancy on, children need loving guidance which reflects acceptance of their capabilities and sensitivity to their feelings. *(rev Feb 98)*

POLICY STATEMENTS: CONCEPTS

Policy statements corresponding to concepts summarizing the basic philosophy of LLLI are grouped in Appendix 17—Concept Policy Statements.

Mothering through Breastfeeding *(Apr 94)*; Mother and Baby Together Early and Often *(Apr 94)*; Mother/Baby Relationship *(Feb 85)*; Breast Milk As Superior Infant Food *(Apr 94)*; Starting Solids *(Apr 93)*; Weaning *(Oct 92)*; Father's Role *(Feb 92)*; Nutrition *(Feb 84)*; Loving Guidance *(Oct 86)*.

Policies and Standing Rules: Appendix 17—Concept Policy Statements

Mothering through Breastfeeding

Breastfeeding provides a complete way of meeting a baby's primary needs, which include touch, acceptance, and warmth, as well as food. Every time a mother puts her baby to breast she uniquely and naturally satisfies this whole complex of needs. The intimate interaction between mother and baby, which deepens as the breastfeeding relationship continues, serves as the framework for increasing the mother's capacity to understand her baby as it enhances the baby's responsiveness to mother's cues. The "mothering hormone," prolactin, which is produced in response to the baby's suckling, further encourages the mother's sensitivity to her baby.

While it is certainly possible to satisfy a baby's primary needs in the absence of breastfeeding, there is no other act which so beautifully and automatically grants all of these needs at the same time. *(Apr 94)*

Mother and baby together early and often

The terms "early and often" are used rather than an arbitrary time limit for establishing a milk supply and breastfeeding relationship. Special circumstances can impose separation in the early weeks after birth, presenting challenges to the mother and baby. With an understanding of how "early and often" prevents difficulties, every effort can be made to keep mothers and babies together and nursing from birth. *(Apr 94)*

Mother/baby relationship

In considering a mother for leadership, the focus shall be on the mother's breastfeeding experience, on her awareness of her baby's need for her presence, her continuing flexible availability to her baby, and her willingness to support the philosophy of LLLI. *(Feb 85)*

Breast milk as superior infant food

Breast milk is a complete infant food containing all the nutrients in ideal proportion for optimal human growth. The growing infant's changing needs are matched by appropriate changes in the composition of his mother's milk, Breast milk provides more than nutrition. Beginning as colostrum, breast milk works with the infant's developing immune system to provide protection against a wide array of illnesses, a benefit which extends beyond infancy. Breast milk is easily digested and eliminated and also reduces the infant's exposure to allergens and allergic illnesses. Furthermore, the psychological benefits of breastfeeding are invaluable: frequent opportunities for touching, holding and eye contact serve as important stimuli for the infant's development. Unique and unduplicated, breast milk is the superior infant food for babies at all economic levels around the world. *(Apr 94)*

Starting solids

For the full-term healthy infant, breast milk alone provides optimal nutrition for growth and development during the early months of life. When a mother considers starting other food and drink, the focus shall be on the mother's awareness of her baby's specific nutritional needs and signs of readiness, rather than upon the baby's age or outside factors.

Physiological and behavioral signs of readiness for other foods and drink include, but are not limited to:

- The baby's appetite increases and does not subside after several days of intensive nursing.
- The baby is able to sit up unsupported, facilitating eating and swallowing.
- The baby not only reaches for and tastes food, but also swallows it.
- The baby can digest other foods and drink, as evidenced by the appearance of the baby's stool.
- The baby's teeth are appearing. (Apr 93)

Weaning

Natural weaning is the gradual end of the breastfeeding relationship between a responsive mother and her growing child. As the child matures, his changing physical and emotional needs are increasingly satisfied through means other than breastfeeding. Although the child usually initiates natural weaning, the mother continues to take an active role by determining in each situation whether nursing or some other approach will best meet her child's needs. A mother demonstrates her commitment to natural weaning through her sensitivity to her child's individual needs and readiness; her flexibility in responding to the unpredictable course of natural weaning and her understanding of and trust in the fundamental stages of a child's development. *(Oct 92)*

Father's role

In considering a mother for leadership, the focus shall be on her understanding of the father's role, not as a mother substitute, but as a unique figure in the baby's life. Recognizing that mothers' circumstances vary and that they may have little control over a father's presence, involvement, or philosophy, the emphasis should be on her ability and willingness to help others appreciate a father's contribution to the breastfeeding relationship. *(Feb 92)*

Nutrition

LLLI POLICIES

Nutrition information and recommendations in THE WOMANLY ART OF BREASTFEEDING shall be considered the essence of our approach to the subject of nutrition and recommendations in WHOLE FOODS FOR THE WHOLE FAMILY shall be considered examples of the application of this approach. *(Feb 84)*

Loving guidance

The goal of the policy on Loving Guidance, i.e., helping a child grow to be a loving, caring, self-disciplined adult, is ideally reached by an emphasis on discipline/teaching methods and attitudes that foster learning while maintaining self-esteem. This process reflects awareness of, sensitivity to, and respect for developmental needs, capabilities, and individuality. In considering a mother for leadership, the focus will be on the entirety of her relationship with her child and her willingness to support the philosophy and goal of loving guidance by example and word. Harsh or restrictive physical or verbal methods, or a lack of parental attention, concern, or intervention are inconsistent with the philosophy and goals of the Loving Guidance policy. Yet, we understand and accept isolated lapses from our ideals as we continually strive to grow in our understanding of Loving Guidance. *(Oct 86)*

SELLING ITEMS WITH LLL'S NAME OR LOGO

The Executive Director is vested with the right to approve all items offered for sale under the auspices of LLL. A percentage of the retail price of items sold bearing the League's name, logo, or other emblem shall accrue to LLLI. *(Feb 87)*

APPENDIX 2—GROUP FINANCIAL INFORMATION

Income Record

Month _____ Year _____

Group Name _____ **Treasurer** _____

Date	Received From	Total Amount	Membership Dues	Womanly Art	Books	Other Sales	Sales Tax	Donations	Other Income	Savings Transfer

Expense Record

Month _____ Year _____

Group Name _____ **Treasurer** _____

Date	Paid to	Total Amount	Dues— LLLI	Dues— Area	Dues— Group	Pamphlets	Womanly Art	Books for Resale	Books for Library	Other Sales Items	Meeting Supplies	Postage and Phone	Other Expenses	Savings Account

Financial Report Form

GROUP NAME _____ **Date of Report** _____

Group Treasurer _____

Leader (s) _____

Report covers period from _____ **to** _____

Beginning Balance

Income		Expenses	
Membership Dues		Membership Dues (LLLI)	
Womanly Art		Membership Dues (Area)	
Other Books		LLLI Group Dues	
Other Sales		Womanly Arts	
Donations		Pamphlets	
Other Income		Library Books	
Interest		Books for Resale	
World Walk		Other Sale Items	
Sales Tax		Meeting Supplies	
Fundraisers		Postage & Telephone	
Miscellaneous		World Walk	
(specify):		Sales Tax	
		Miscellaneous (specify):	
Total Income		**Total Expenses**	
Transfers from Savings		Transfers from Savings	

Closing Balance (total income less total expenses)

Supplementary Financial Information

Savings Account

Beginning Balance	$ _____
Transfers to Savings	_____
Interest	_____
Transfers from Savings	_____
Closing Balance	_____

Unpaid Bills

To	Amount	Date

Inventory

Item	No. on Hand
Womanly Art	
Other books for resale	
Other items for resale	

Group Assets   Value

Library Books	
Videos/Slides	
Miscellaneous	

LA LECHE LEAGUE OF YOUR AREA
2004-2005 ANNUAL GROUP FINANCIAL REPORT

This report covers the annual reporting period from APRIL 1, 2004 to MARCH 31, 2005.

GROUP NAME: _____   GROUP EIN _____

LISTED LEADER Name and Address _____

TREASURER'S Name and Address _____
TREASURER'S Phone Number _____

COUNTY OF GROUP _____   TOTAL SALES TAX RATE _____

1. BEGINNING BALANCE (closing balance from previous report "Total of all accounts")   _____

INCOME
2. MEMBERSHIPS   _____
3. WOMANLY ART OF BREASTFEEDING   _____
4. OTHER BOOKS/ITEMS FROM LLLI   _____
5. DONATIONS   _____
6. FUNDRAISING   _____
7. MISCELLANEOUS   _____
8. SALES TAX   _____
9. TOTAL INCOME   _____

10. TOTAL INCOME + BALANCE (Line 1 + Line 9 = Line 10)   _____

EXPENSES
11. LLLI GROUP AFFILIATION DUES & LEADER DUES
       (list each Leader on back of page)   _____
12. LLL IOWA/USWD ASSESSMENT @ $20/LEADER/
       LEADER RESERVE/AWOR LEADER
       (list each Leader on back of page)   _____
13. LLLI MEMBERSHIP PORTION @ $17.00/MEMBER   _____
14. LLL AREA/DIVISION MEMBERSHIP PORTION @ $5.50/MEMBER   _____
15. PHONE EXPENSES, GROUP SUPPLIES, LIBRARY ADDITIONS   _____
16. WOMANLY ART OF BREASTFEEDING   _____
17. OTHER BOOKS/ITEMS FROM LLLI   _____
18. LEADER EDUCATION (ACF, DW, HRE, ETC.)   _____
19. FUNDRAISING   _____
20. 20% FUNDRAISING INCOME TO AREA   _____
21. MISCELLANEOUS (if more than $35, please itemize)   _____
22. SALES TAX   _____
23. TOTAL EXPENSES   _____

24. TOTAL INCOME - EXPENSES = NEW BALANCE   _____

PLEASE FILL IN WITH FIGURES AS OF 3/31
       BALANCE IN: CHECKING ACCT.   _____
                            SAVINGS ACCT.   _____
                            CASH ON HAND   _____
TOTAL (This TOTAL should equal year's balance)   _____

INFORMATION ON GROUP FUNDRAISERS: On the back, please share information on each Group fundraiser, including the type of fundraiser, how much money was raised, and whether it was a worthwhile fundraiser for the amount of work involved. This form is required to be completed and returned to Laura Leader, Area Financial Coordinator, 2345 W 6th St., Anytown, Your Area 50613 by June 1, 2005. Keep one copy for your files.

Ordering from LLLI Using a Group Account
Note: Leaders who order from Affiliate/Area Order Departments may follow different procedures.

1. Orders can be placed by mail, telephone, fax, or email.

   Mail: LLLI Order Department
   P.O. Box 4079
   Schaumburg Illinois 60168-4079 USA
   Phone: 847-519-9585 Order Department
   847-519-7730 main switchboard
   Fax: 847-519-0035
   Email: **orderdepartment@llli.org**
   Web: **www.lalecheleague.org**

   ❑ Do not include a credit card number on email orders because this address is not secure. Items to be ordered can be emailed; credit card number can then be given during a quick call to the Order Department.
   ❑ Credit card orders can be placed using the Web address because this is secure. Click on LLLI Catalogue.

2. **Use a current order form; check the date on the copy you are using.** The *Leader Order Form* (No. 400-20 from LLLI) is updated at least twice a year. Using a current form assures current prices and availability.

3. **Use a Group Account Number.** A new Group is automatically issued a Group Account Number by LLLI. An order received without a Group Account Number, a credit card number, or full payment will be returned unprocessed. The Group Account Number must be written on remitted checks as well.

4. **The Listed Leader is responsible for Group orders.** No matter who compiles it, every order must be signed by the Listed Leader who is responsible to LLLI for all orders placed by her Group. The Listed Leader's name and address should appear in the "bill to" section of the order form. The Listed Leader receives all correspondence from LLLI regarding the Group Account.

5. **Designate where the order should be shipped.** Even though the Listed Leader is responsible for all Group orders, an order can be shipped to another Group member. The "ship to" name and address on the order form can be changed with each order.

6. **Prepay the order when possible.** Whenever feasible, the Group Treasurer should fully or partially prepay orders. It is important to write the Group Account Number on both the check and order form even if the order is prepaid. The remittance copy of the Invoice that the Listed Leader receives will show any balance due. This balance should be paid within 30 days.

7. **Check the package contents when the order arrives.** Remove the Invoice or Shipping List from the pocket on the outside of the box and check the order against it. Your order may be shipped in more than one box.

8. **If the Ship to and Bill to names are different, a Shipping List will be enclosed with the package and the Invoice will be mailed to the Listed Leader.** On the Shipping List all items will be listed as "Back Ordered" because the Shipping List is printed before the order is marked as shipped in the computer system. If an item is actually back ordered, this will be indicated on the Invoice.

FINANCES/ORDERING

9. **Give the Invoice to the Group Treasurer.** The Invoice should be kept on file and checked against the Group check register and expense record sheet. Payment should be sent to LLLI (within 30 days) with any balance due. Include the Group Account Number and Invoice Number with payment. Additional orders will not be processed if the Group Account shows a balance due for more than 60 days.

10. **A monthly statement will be sent to the Listed Leader from LLLI** if money is owed or there is a credit on your Group Account. It may cover several invoices if the Group has ordered several times during the month or if invoices have not been paid over a period of several months.

11. **Keep accurate records when making partial payments to LLLI.** Payments are credited against the earliest outstanding invoice.

12. **Each Group has a $200 (US) credit limit with LLLI.** Any new order plus the account balance due must not exceed $200 including shipping and handling charges. In order to access this $200 credit available to LLL Groups, your Group and Leader Dues must be current and no balances can be outstanding on your Group Account for more than 60 days.

13. **LLLI depends on timely payments.** LLLI relies on its Groups to keep their accounts current to ensure continuing financial stability. If each of the more than 3,000 LLL Groups owed only $25 (US) to LLLI, there would be $75,000 outstanding. If a Group is having difficulty paying bills, its Leaders should reevaluate how funds are being used. The Area is responsible for monitoring Group financial stability. The Area Finance Coordinator will be notified if a Group's Account is not kept current.

Sample Inventory Record

INVENTORY RECORD			Year	2003	
Item	Number in Stock	Sold	Purchased	Balance on Hand	Date
Womanly Art	6	2	0	4	Oct 31
Whole Foods	3	1	0	2	Oct 31
Motherwise	3	3	10	10	Oct 31
LLL Mugs	5	1	0	4	Oct 31
Baby slings	2	0	0	2	Oct 31
Womanly Art	4	3	10	11	Nov 30
Whole Foods	2	1	0	1	Nov 30
Motherwise	10	2	0	8	Nov 30
LLL Mugs	4	0	0	4	Nov 30
Baby slings	2	1	0	1	Nov 30

Sample Letters Encouraging Membership

To a mother who indicated interest in LLL Membership on the sign-in sheet:

Dear _____,

Thank you for attending our recent La Leche League meeting. We hope you enjoyed the meeting and had your questions answered.

On the sign-in sheet you indicated that you are interested in LLL membership. Our Group relies on membership for a large part of our operating budget. Your membership also ensures support for breastfeeding mothers worldwide. Membership in the USA is $36 per year.

Some tangible benefits for you are a subscription to New Beginnings [or equivalent member publication] and 10% off books and other items in the *LLLI Catalogue* in addition to the local benefits of phone help, support group meetings, and our lending library.

I have enclosed a self-addressed stamped, envelope for your convenience. Please make your check payable to LLL of _____. Thank you in advance for your membership. We hope to see you at our next meeting.

To a mother who has attended two meetings and has not yet become a member:

Dear _____,

We hope you enjoyed attending our recent La Leche League meeting. It was nice to see you again.

We encourage mothers who attend our meetings to become members of LLL. Not only do you benefit from membership but your payment also helps LLL continue for mothers throughout the world.

Membership in the USA is $36 a year. You receive a subscription to New Beginnings [or equivalent member publication] and 10% discount on books and other items from the *LLLI Catalogue* as well as the local benefits of support group meetings, phone help, and our lending library.

Sometimes mothers get busy looking through the Group Library or talking with mothers and don't have time to seek out ___, our Treasurer, before they leave the meeting. For your convenience I have enclosed a self-addressed, stamped envelope. Please make your check payable to LLL of ___.

Thank you in advance for your membership. We hope to see you at our next meeting.

Sample Letters Encouraging Membership

To a new member along with her Membership Card:

Dear _____,

Thank you for joining La Leche League of ___. Enclosed is your membership card. This card entitles you to 10% discount on books and other items from the *LLLI Catalogue*. You will be receiving your first issue of NEW BEGINNINGS [or equivalent member publication] soon. Thank you again for supporting LLL in our community and throughout the world.

To a mother whose membership is due for renewal:

Dear _____,

Your membership in La Leche League will expire (month and year) . We hope that you enjoy LLL meetings and NEW BEGINNINGS [or equivalent member publication] and will renew your membership for the next year. Your membership also helps ensure that breastfeeding support will be available for mothers in the future.

You may also receive a reminder to renew from La Leche League International. Please consider renewing through our Group. When you renew through our Group some of the money helps us add to our library and purchase supplies. We rely on memberships for a large part of our budget.

Membership for the next year is $36. Please make your check payable to LLL of ___. I have enclosed a self-addressed, stamped envelope for your convenience. If you have any questions, please call me.

Again, thank you for your support of LLL of ___.

6 Ways to Encourage and Promote Membership*

- Create a membership atmosphere - Inform people about membership - Invite and encourage membership
- Make it easy to become a member - Appreciate members - Maintain contact

1 Create a membership atmosphere

- Think about what attracted you to membership and provide the same elements at Group meetings and over the telephone.

- Arrange seating for comfort and easy hearing and seeing. Be sure mothers are greeted and given assistance if they need it. Set out the Group Library where it is inviting. Use nametags.

- Expect people to want to be members. Use introduction time to give information about how.

- Be enthusiastic, sincere, and honest. There are many reasons to suggest membership and no reasons to apologize.

- Make Series Meetings fun, with fresh approaches to topics.

- Recognize that some things we are accustomed to are new to others, for instance, nursing toddlers, mothers leaving and returning with their babies and toddlers, children in the room during the meeting. During introductions and whenever else it seems relevant, explain briefly and invite questions.

- Promote the Group Library: highlight the variety of topics; refer to books on the Series Meeting topic and relevant to the interests and concerns of the women present.

- Encourage participation during the meeting. Show appreciation for specific contributions to the discussion.

- Talk about membership during the meeting, when people are immersed in what LLL offers.

- Spark interest in NEW BEGINNINGS or your local members' publication by quoting from it during the meeting.

- Remember mothers' and babies' names.

- Throughout the meeting, listen to and respect all viewpoints; introduce LLL information and philosophy as another (not as "the") way, for people's consideration.

- Build a feeling of belonging: send cards to mothers when they give birth and create an opportunity at the meeting for them to talk about the birth or early nursing.

- At the end of the meeting, encourage people to come back and to bring a friend.

- Group jobs and Evaluation/Enrichment meetings build strong ties to the Group and LLL. Mention the jobs that need to be done and invite meeting participants to volunteer for them.

- After the meeting, send a note to or call first-time attendees. Refer to something each said or did that added to the meeting and invite her to attend the next one. Encourage her to call you if she has any questions or concerns. Call again a few days before the next meeting.

- At Evaluation Meetings, talk about first impressions and the Group's purpose. Encourage Group workers to maintain the respectful atmosphere, avoid mixing causes, keep the discussion on track, listen to new mothers, and not hold side conversations.

2 Inform people about membership

- Give a pamphlet or borchure about membership to newcomers.

- Mention that LLL is a charitable organization and that Leaders, too, pay dues.

- Mention that the money saved (by not having to purchase formula and related equipment, for instance) can more than cover the cost of La Leche League membership.

- Refer to the benefits of membership during the meeting and other conversations.

3 Invite and encourage membership

- During introductions, say how long you have been a member of LLL.

- Write a "Welcome to LLL" letter for your New Mother Packets; include information about membership and an invitation to become a member.

- Make coupons to give to each participant at a meeting, offering a discount on a purchase or renewal to a member who brings a new member to the Group.

- Offer a discount on the purchase of THE WOMANLY ART OF BREASTFEEDING with each membership.

- Include a column entitled "Do you wish to become a member or renew your membership?" on the attendance sign-in sheet. This informs people of the expectation and seeing concrete evidence of other's interest can encourage people to show theirs as well. The Group Treasurer follows up—during refreshment time or soon after the meeting.

- As a theme for a membership drive, draw a picture of your town or use an LLL logo; write members' names on appropriately shaped stickers (or paper cut-outs) and try to "reach around" or "surround" the area by a certain date.

- Briefly discuss your membership advantages poster (perhaps add a comparison list of what can—and can't—be bought for the same amount) and have a "special": in addition to the

---

* Depending on where you live, member could be subscriber, supporter, or contributor.

benefits listed on the poster, women who purchase memberships at the meeting will receive a small gift (something inexpensive the Leader buys and wraps prior to the meeting).

- Create a new member packet that includes the membership card, 12 logo stickers, added discount coupons for purchase of specific LLLI-published books (if your Group can afford this).

- Introduce the Treasurer at the beginning and the end of the meeting. Ask her to talk about membership toward the end, so people will know who she is and feel more comfortable about approaching her.

4 Make it easy to become a member

- Send follow-up letters to women who attend for the first time. Include a welcome note, information on the benefits— to the member and to LLL—of membership, and specific information on how to become a member.

- Follow up telephone helping calls with an envelope containing information about LLL and membership.

- Hold a fundraising event in which people can earn a membership or renewal. The profits (beyond participants' memberships) would go into a membership scholarship fund.

- Offer membership scholarships for those who cannot afford the cost. Suggest women pay what they can afford and complete the memberships from the fund.

- Offer installment plans for memberships.

5 Appreciate members

- Thank people who are members and mention specific ways memberships have helped the Group and LLL.

- Make a chart to show where membership money goes. Along with the chart of where membership dollars go, display your Group's yearly budget at meetings so people will see how their money is spent (and needed) locally.

- When you purchase a new Library book, highlight it at the meeting and announce that it was purchased with membership funds from the last few months. Thank the people whose memberships made the purchase possible.

- Have a thank-you tea or potluck for members.

- Work toward 100% membership; announce when the Group achieves it; give yourselves a round of applause. (You could also celebrate during snack time.)

- Remember that you are valuable to the women you help and that memberships help bring the valuable resource of LLL Leaders and Group to your community, area, country, and world. Remind Group members and participants that they are valuable to each other and that their memberships help to ensure the same resource—of LLL Leader and other mothers—to their community, country, and the world.

- Display your Group affiliation certificate at meetings and talk about how memberships make the Group and larger organization viable (and available).

6 Maintain contact

- Call to remind members—including those who no longer attend meetings—about a month before their memberships expire and ask for their continuing support.

- Create the Group job of "Membership Coordinator" to keep track of members, prepare and distribute member packets, remind people about renewals, etc.

- Invite members—including those who no longer attend meetings—to picnics and other social gatherings. (Remember to also "invite" them to Area Conferences.)

- If you have a Group newsletter, in addition to making it available at meetings, send it to members who no longer attend.

Note: We have not credited ideas to specific people or publications. Most have been tried and modified by so many people it would be difficult to find out where they originated. So, if one of these ideas is "yours," Thank you!

These ideas—gleaned from a variety of Area Leader publications as well as from LEAVEN—were developed by La Leche League Leaders and Groups. Try the ones that are attractive to you. Add to them. Send your ideas to your Area Editor or LEAVEN.

"The financial support of mothers who came before us ensured that La Leche League is here for us today. I invite you to join La Leche League today so we can be here for others in the future."

"Think of membership as an inexpensive monthly outing with your baby in a friendly environment where you find helpful information, have access to a library of great books about parenting and breastfeeding, and enjoy nutritious snacks."

Processing Membership Dues

Note: Outside the USA procedures are different.
Check with the District Advisor/Coordinator, Area Treasurer, or Area Coordinator of Leaders.

1. Give the mother a receipt. Her LLLI Membership Card will be mailed to her along with a welcome letter.

2. Send LLLI an LLLI Circulation Department NEW BEGINNINGS Card (No. 172-13 from LLLI) for each member along with a check for the LLLI portion of the membership. Type or print the information; it is very important that the name and address are legible.

   Blank 3 x 5 inch file cards can be used as long as they are completed with the same information as the LLLI card. Paper may be used if cards are not available. Be sure to type or print.

   Indicate on each card whether the membership is new or renewed. If a mother was a member at any time, treat it as renewed. If a renewing member has moved, send both of her addresses clearly marked "old" and "new," including postal codes for both. If the mother has moved more than once since she was last a member, send the last address that appeared in LLLI's files if possible.

   When a mother's address changes, it is also important for her to notify LLLI directly so she continues to receive NEW BEGINNINGS.

3. A card must be sent for each member but money can be combined in one check. Write __ members @ __ and the members' names on the memo line of the check.

   Write separate checks for memberships and invoices since these are handled by separate LLLI departments.

4. Enter the membership in three places in the Group's records: on the income record sheet, in the check register (for the deposit or the check to LLLI), and on the expense record sheet.

5. Send in the Area portion of memberships monthly or by the series as required by the Area. If memberships are sent only every four months, the money should be earmarked for that purpose.

   Make appropriate entries in the check register and on the expense record sheet.

6. Send memberships in promptly! Remember, new members are waiting to receive their NEW BEGINNINGS or equivalent member publication.

MEMBERSHIP

Please Print

Name – Last   First   Husband's

Address

City   State/Province

Zip/Postal Code   Country

Phone #

Are there any changes to your name and address simce your last tenewal? If so please print correction below:

NEW_____ RENEW_____

172-13

LLLI Membership Categories

Type of Membership	Breakdown of Fees					Benefits						
	Fee	LLLI	Division	Area	Group	Membership Card	New Beginnings	Leaven	Continuum	LLLI Catalogue (Optional)	Term Life Insurance (Optional)	Reduced LLLI Conference Registration
Regular	$36	$22	$2.25	$3.25	$8.50	X	X			10%	X	X
2 Year	$65	$39	$4.25	$6.00	$15.75	X	X			10%	X	X
3 Year	$95	$57.50	$6.25	$8.75	$22.50	X	X			10%	X	X
Family	$52	$26	$5.50	$5.50	$15.00	X	X			10%	X	X
Active Leader	$30					X	X	X		15%	X	X
Leader Reserve	$34					X	X	X		15%	X	X
Leader Family	$44					X	X	X		15%	X	X
Sustaining	$115	$65	$5	$10	$35	X	X			10%	X	X
Alumnae	$25	$25				X	X		X	10%	X	X

Repeater's Survey Card

1. **I'm interested in helping the Group in some way (i.e. hostess, librarian, treasurer, etc.).**   ☐ yes   ☐ no

2. **I'd like to learn more about LLL.**   ☐ yes   ☐ no

3. **The idea of becoming an LLL Leader interests me.**   ☐ yes   ☐ no

4. **I have these ideas for improving the Group/Series meetings:**

_____

_____

_____

183-13

Last Name _____ First _____ Phone No. _____

Address _____

City _____ State/Province _____ Zip/Postal Code _____

Child's Name	Birth Date	Nursed?

Hospital _____ Due Date _____

Dues Paid _____ Today's Date _____ No. 185-13

LA LECHE LEAGUE MEETINGS

	TOPIC	DATE
I.	Advantages of Breastfeeding to Mother and Baby	_____
II.	Baby Arrives; the Family and the Breastfed Baby	_____
III.	Art of Breastfeeding and Overcoming Difficulties	_____
IV.	Nutrition and Weaning	_____

Time: At the home of:

Address:

Group Leader(s):   Phone:

These informal meetings are open to all women interested in breastfeeding. Babies are always welcome. Call your La Leche Leader at any time, for breastfeeding help or to purchase a copy of THE WOMANLY ART OF BREASTFEEDING. Loan copies of this book are also available.

1255-13

Breastfeeding...
It Makes A Difference

The American Academy of Pediatrics declared human milk to be the preferred food for all newborns. It recommended babies be exclusively breastfed for at least six months and that breastfeeding be continued for a minimum of 12 months or longer.

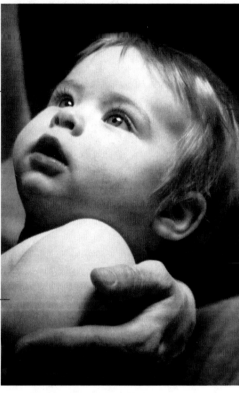

Mothers who breastfeed are healthier

Human milk gives infants the most complete nutrition possible and provides the optimal mix of nutrients and antibodies necessary to thrive.

Breastfeeding saves money

No packaging; less pollution

Breastfed babies have fewer, less serious illnesses and allergies

Exclusive breastfeeding naturally spaces pregnancies

Join LLLI and provide your child with the very best start in life.

To become a member, contact your local Group Leader or LLLI.
Local Group Leader:

LA LECHE LEAGUE
INTERNATIONAL
1400 North Meacham Road • Schaumburg,
IL 60173.4840 USA • 847.519.7730 •
fax 847.519.0035 • 1.800.LA.LECHE
www.lalecheleague.org • lllhq@llli.org

418-13

MEMBERSHIP

INTERESTED IN
BREASTFEEDING?

La Leche League offers breastfeeding support and information through:

• Monthly meetings

• Telephone help from experienced Leaders

• Lending library and books for sale

• More than 40 years experience helping thousands of mothers

• Special couples and toddlers' meetings

• New Beginnings, a bimonthly journal for parents

Give us a call!

ARLINGTON HEIGHTS		PALATINE/ROLLING MEADOWS		MOUNT PROSPECT CENTRAL	
3rd Tues at 7:30 pm		3rd Tues at 7:30 pm		3rd Wed. at 7:30 pm	
Claire	555-1234	Jennifer	555-1234	Diana	555-1112
Denise	555-2345	Monica	555-2345	Fergy	555-2111
Ruby	555-3456	Linda	555-3456	*Elizabeth	555-7408
*Vanessa	555-4567	*Paula	555-4567		

MOUNT PROSPECT/WHEELING		MOUNT PROSPECT WEST	
3rd Tues at 7:30 pm		2nd Thur at 9:30 am	
Joy	555-1234	Marsha	555-1234
Tootie	555-2345	Jan	555-2345
*Natalie	555-3456	Cindy	555-3456
Blair	555-6789		

*Breast pumps and other breastfeeding aids are avaliable directly from these LLL Group Leaders
FOR GROUPS IN OTHER AREAS, CALL LLLI AT 1-800-LA-LECHE.

Sample Joint Meeting Notice

L A L E C H E L E A G U E
I N T E R N A T I O N A L
Breastfeeding Information & Support

Planning to Breastfeed?

Monthly Meetings Discuss:
✔ Advantages of Breastfeeding
✔ Childbirth and the new baby at home
✔ The art of breastfeeding and overcoming difficulties
✔ Nutrition and weaning

For breastfeeding and/or meeting information call:

www.lalecheleague.org

171-13

LA LECHE LEAGUE
BREASTFEEDING INFORMATION & SUPPORT

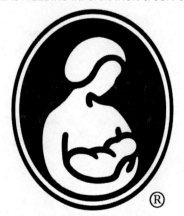

®

MONTHLY MEETINGS DISCUSS:
• advantages of breastfeeding
• childbirth and the new baby at home
• the art of breastfeeding and
  avoiding difficulties
• nutrition and weaning
Pregnant women, mothers, & babies welcome

For BREASTFEEDING
and/or MEETING
INFORMATION CALL:
Allison
555-4675

Sample Posters

BREASTFEEDING?
Or considering it?
Breastfeeding is:

Free
Environmentally Sound
Convenient
Healthiest for mother and baby

La Leche League offers:

• Lending library with books on breastfeeding,
  childbirth, parenting and nutrition
• Mother-to-mother support
• Leaders accredited by La Leche League International
• Latest breastfeeding information
• 24-hour telephone help

La Leche League of Bloomsburg

meets the first Thursday of each month at 7:30 pm
Call a Leader for directions.

Meeting Schedule

Jan 8 The Benefits of Human Milk
Feb 5 Fathers & Siblings of the Breastfed Baby
Mar 5 Breastfeeding: Questions Mothers Ask
Apr 2 Thoughts on Weaning

La Leche League Leaders are available to answer breastfeeding questions.
For more information call:
Lisa 555-3456
Luann 555-3467
Nancy 555-1234

Sample Forms and Guidelines

LEADER'S LOG

Name   Date

Address   Time

Phone

Question/Problem

Doctor has said

Infant Name

                    (Age)   (Weight)

Other Family Members

LEADER'S RESPONSE

Suggestions

LLL/Information sent

Referred by/Referred to

Follow up   Leader's Name

No. 94

Ed. Note: *In some situations a Leader may be required to use a specific format. Check with your District Advisor/Coordinator or Area Coordinator of Leaders.*

La Leche League
ANNOUNCES

its series of monthly meetings for Breastfeeding Mothers

I. Advantages of Breastfeeding to Mother and Baby

Date_____   Time_____

II. Baby Arrives; the Family and the Breastfed Baby

Date_____   Time_____

III. The Art of Breastfeeding and Avoiding Difficulties

Date_____   Time_____

IV. Nutrition and Weaning

Date_____   Time_____

THE WOMANLY ART OF BREASTFEEDING, now in its sixth edition (1997), has become a classic. Its practical, down-to-earth, and warmly supportive approach has made it a favorite of mothers who rely on its sound medical backing and up-to-date research into all aspects of the breastfeeding relationship. Available in bookstores or through local LLLGroups.

Breastfeeding is a simple and natural process, but you may need support and information on the correct positioning of the baby at the breast, working and breastfeeding, avoiding problems, and overcoming any difficulties that may occur.

Knowing other women who have breastfed their babies can be helpful and reassuring. Having accurate, up-to-date information is also important.

Attending La Leche League meetings can help you learn about breastfeeding from other nursing mothers. At these monthly meetings, mothers share not only their questions and concerns but also the benefits and joys of breastfeeding. Being in touch with La Leche League can give you the network of support you need.

Membership in La Leche League is just $36 per year. Members receive a bimonthly journal called NEW BEGINNINGS, filled with warm personal stories from breastfeeding parents along with up-to-date research, book reviews, and much more. To find out about other benefits of membership, call the La Leche League Leader listed below.

If you have questions, call the following La Leche League Leader(s):

_____

Meeting Location _____

Your Hostess is _____ phone number _____

Babies are always welcome at La Leche League meetings.
This will be the only notice sent for this series. Please mark your calendar.

La Leche League International
1400 N. Meacham Road
Schaumburg, IL 60173-4808 USA
www.lalecheleague.org

Leader Change of Address/Status Form—USA

If you move or change your status, follow the steps below to be sure that all areas of LLL are notified.

1) Complete form and mail it to Customer Service Department: PO Box 4079, Schaumburg IL 60168-4079 USA.
2) Send a copy of form to your Area Secretary (AS). If moving to a new area notify the new ACS or ACL.
3) If this involves a change in Group information, complete a Group Change Form (DCF) with your DA and/or AS.
(You may attach a label from LEAVEN or NEW BEGINNINGS or copy name, address, and codes exactly below.)

Current Information on File at LLLI

Name_____ New LLLI Leader ID No._____

Address_____City_____State_____Zip Code_____

Telephone Number (include area code)_____ New Group ID Account No._____

Were you Listed Leader of this Group?_____ Email Address_____
(*If yes, please fill in box at the bottom of the page*)

New Information for LLLI Records (Please Print)

Change of Name, Address, Phone, or Zip Code   **Effective**
Date_____

Name_____ New LLLI Leader ID No._____

Address_____City_____State_____Zip Code_____

Telephone Number (include area code)_____ New Group ID Account No._____

Email Address_____

Language

Fluent in language other than English (specify speaking, reading, and writing)
1._____
2._____

Change of Leader Status

If you change your status after you have paid your dues this year, you will continue to receive LEAVEN and NEW BEGINNINGS until the end of the year. We will change your status code in the computer and the following year your billing will reflect your new status. When you are no longer active on a regular basis your choices are: (Check below)

_____**LEADER RESERVE**—This category is for the Leader who is no longer regularly active but is expected to take on an occasional assignment if called upon by her ACL or DC. She can receive NEW BEGINNINGS and LEAVEN.

_____**RETIRED LEADER**—We don't like to lose a single Leader, but when the time comes, we want you to know that mothers everywhere appreciate the fact that you were there. We are grateful to you. You will receive a complimentary one-year subscription to CONTINUUM.

_____**ALUMNAE MEMBER**—After your one year complimentary CONTINUUM subscription expires, become and Alumnae member. The retired Leader who still wants the contact and support of other LLL people can join the Alumnae Association. An Alumnae member receives Alumnae News, and a 10% discount on orders. A one-year membership is $25.

_____**REACTIVATE**—You need to contact your ACL to reactivate as a Leader, and include a payment of Leader dues.

Other Change:_____

Change in Group Listed Leader

BE SURE TO SEND IN GROUP DIRECTORY CHANGE FORM TO YOUR AREA SECRETARY
TO OFFICIALLY CHANGE LISTED LEADER FOR THIS GROUP

Will you continue to be Listed Leader?   ☐ Yes   ☐ No

If no, who is the new Listed Leader? Name_____

Address_____City/State/Zip_____

Phone_____Email_____

Signature_____Date_____

USA COA/2

La Leche League of _____ Meeting Sign-In Sheet

Date _____   Meeting _____   Hostess _____

Name	Address	Phone number	Children's names & ages/ Due date	Willing to bring refreshments?	Willing to host a 4-meeting series?	Membership paid through (mo./yr.)?

TOTALS: New mothers _____   Members _____   Repeaters _____   Leaders _____   Applicants _____   Babies _____   Toddlers _____   Children _____

Medical Questionnaire

When a mother asks for LLL information about a medical situation, check all LLLI resources, including the BREASTFEEDING ANSWER BOOK, THE WOMANLY ART OF BREASTFEEDING, NEW BEGINNINGS, LEAVEN, LLLI pamphlets, and the LLLI Web site. If these do not furnish enough information, mail, phone, fax, or email the following information to your local Professional Liaison Leader. See your Area Directory for her name and check with local support people for procedures in your community.

Submitted by:

Leader's Name	Address	City/State (Province)	Zip (Postal Code)	Date

Forwarded to:

APL/AAPL	PL Resource Person	Center for Breastfeeding Information
Date	Date	Date
Signed	Signed	Signed

Question/Problem: Please include all relevant facts (use additional pages if necessary)

What has the mother done already?

Infant: Age, birth weight; present weight; nursing (how often?); solids started (when?); vitamins, supplementary feedings; pacifier; sleeps through the night or long period of time; general health; illness; symptoms of problem (how long, etc.)

Information Leader has offered:

Mother: Age, general health, birth experience; stress; diet; vitamins; herbs; medications; menstrual periods; illness; symptoms of problem (how long, how often.)

Health care provider has suggested:

LLL Resource Person suggests:

Once this form is completed, it is top priority to reply promptly, or refer the question to the appropriate resource person.

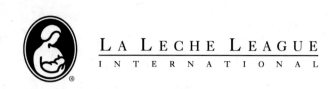

LA LECHE LEAGUE INTERNATIONAL | STYLESHEET

A stylesheet is a set of house rules intended to ensure consistency of format, spelling, capitalization, abbreviation, word usage, and other technicalities peculiar to an organization or publisher. Consistent style helps LLL publications to appear professional and credible.

Grammar and usage questions not covered by this stylesheet use a standard guide such as *The Chicago Manual of Style* (University of Chicago Press), *Gregg Reference Manual* (Macmillan/ McGraw Hill), *A Dictionary of Modern English Usage* by HW Fowler (Oxford University Press), or *The Canadian Style: A Guide to Writing and Editing* (Department of the Secretary of the State).

CAPITALIZATION, ABBREVIATION, AND USAGE

Abbreviations may confuse readers. Use them at your discretion. Job titles and names of departments vary around the world, so those abbreviations are not shown here. Spell out all titles and departments on first reference in an article. Capitalize the following words and phrases as shown. Do not abbreviate unless indicated in parenthesis.

Affiliate
Area
Board of Directors
Center for Breastfeeding Information (CBI)
Chapter
Couples Meeting
District
Division
Enrichment Meeting
Evaluation Meeting
Founder
Founders' Advisory Council (FAC)
Group

Health Advisory Council (HAC)
Help Form(s)
Internet
La Leche League (LLL)
La Leche League International (LLLI)
Leader, co-Leader
Leader Applicant
Legal Advisory Council (LAC)
Legal Associate
Library (e.g., Group Library)
Listed Leader
LLLOnline
Management Advisory Council (MAC)

Medical Associate
Meeting 1, 2, 3, 4
Planning/Evaluation Meeting
Region
Series Meeting
Toddler Meeting
Treasury (e.g., Area Treasury)
URL
Web site
World Wide Web

Do not capitalize **email, leadership, member, membership, mother,** or **newsletter.** Capitalize "conference" or "workshop" only when referring to a specific conference or workshop that is the subject of the article.

ADDRESS, PHONE, FAX, EMAIL

Spell out state/province in text if publication circulates outside of your country; no commas before and after postal code. Two-letter postal abbreviations may be used in block style; no punctuation is necessary.

Byline: Lisa Leader, Town, State/Province, Country

Text: Lisa Leader, 45 Anniversary Road, Town, State/Province 55555 Country. Phone/fax: 555-555-5555, LisaL@lll.org (email).

Block: Lisa Leader
40 Anniversary Road
Town State/Province 55555
Country
phone: 555-555-5555
fax: 555-555-0000
mailto:LisaL@mailprovider.org

PLURALS AND POSSESSIVES

LEADER'S HANDBOOK
Area Leaders' Letter
When an administrative position is abbreviated (for example, ACL, for Area Coordinator of Leaders) :
ACLs (more than one ACL)
ACL's (belonging to the ACL)
ACLs' (belonging to more than one ACL)

NUMBERS

USE: Meeting 1, 2, 3, 4
USE: Publication No. 5

One through ten: spell out in text
11 and up: use number

If a sentence begins with a number, spell it out or rewrite the sentence. Months by name, not number (Ex: 5/7 means 5th day of July to some, 7th day of May to others)

COMPOUND WORDS OR SEPARATE WORDS?

Compound words:
breastfeeding
cosleeping
fundraising
postpartum

Separate words:
breast milk (human milk or mother's milk preferred)
health care provider or health care professional

PREFERRED WORDING

USE: La Leche League or LLL
AVOID: League used as a noun or adjective

USE: an LLL Series Meeting (pronounced el-el-el)
AVOID: a LLL Meeting

USE: La Leche League
AVOID: the La Leche League ("La" means "the")

USE: Group worker, member, attendee
AVOID: LM, League or LLL Mother/Mom, Group Mother/Mom

USE: Leader Applicant, Applicant
AVOID: LA

USE: preparation for leadership, application, application period or time
AVOID: application process, applicancy

USE: La Leche League International Conference, LLLI Conference
AVOID: International Conference, Orlando Conference

USE: Founder, co-Founder
AVOID: Founding Mother

USE: Chairman
AVOID: Chairwoman, Chair

USE: mother(s), child(ren)
AVOID: mom(s), kid(s)

USE: email, email list
AVOID: chat loop, email loop, listserv, or listproc

When describing personal experiences, use personal pronouns for milk and babies wherever possible:

USE: my milk, her milk, my baby, her baby, his baby, our baby
AVOID: baby (without "a," or "the")

PUBLICATIONS

Capitalize all letters of books and periodicals published by LLLI. Caps and small caps may be used. THE WOMANLY ART OF BREASTFEEDING may be referred to as THE WOMANLY ART on second reference. No other shortened forms or abbreviations of other titles should be used.

ex: BREASTFEEDING ABSTRACTS
     THE BREASTFEEDING ANSWER BOOK
     THE FUSSY BABY
     THE LEADER'S HANDBOOK
     LEAVEN
     NEW BEGINNINGS
     WHOLE FOODS FOR THE WHOLE FAMILY
     WHOLE FOODS FROM THE WHOLE WORLD
     THE WOMANLY ART OF BREASTFEEDING

Italicize or underline
     Books not published by LLLI
     Pamphlets, brochures, tear-off sheets, etc.
     Names of Area Leaders' Letters

Enclose in quotations
     Conference session titles
     Titles of articles
     Names of Area memos and bulletins

References

Books: Author(s) last name, Initial. Title [caps if LLLI], edition. City, State: Publisher, year; pages.

> Sears, W. and Sears, M. *The Baby Book*. Boston: Little Brown, 1993; 2-17.

> THE WOMANLY ART OF BREASTFEEDING. Schaumburg, IL: LLLI, 1997; 55-56.

Articles from periodicals: Author(s) last name, Initial [use "et al." if more than three]. Article title [lower case after first word unless proper noun]. Periodical title [italicize or underline, caps for LLLI] date; volume(issue)[omit volume and issue for LLLI]: pages.

> Mortensen, E.L., Michaelsen, K.F., Sanders, S.A., et al. The association between duration of breastfeeding and adult intelli-

gence. *JAMA* 2002; 287(15):2365-71.

> Land, C. Autism and the breastfeeding family. LEAVEN Feb/Mar 2002; 10-11.

LLLI pamphlet: Author(s) last name, Initial [if applicable]. Pamphlet title [italicize or underline]. LLLI, date. Publication No. ___.

> Gotsch, G. *Pacifiers: Yes or No?*. LLLI, April 2002. Publication No. 324-17.

> *Breastfeeding Makes a Difference*. LLLI, June 2002. Publication No. 1196-17.

INTERNET REFERENCES:

Standards for including references to Web sites are still changing, so these guidelines will evolve depending on need for clarity and accuracy. Web sites may be shown as sources to help readers find more information. Show both home page and mailing address of the organization whenever possible, so readers without Internet access may also find information. Avoid listing Web sites that have a high potential for mixing causes.

www.lalecheleague.org
La Leche League International
1400 N. Meacham Rd.
Schaumburg IL 60173-4808 USA

Avoid using Web sites as references for factual information, since Web sites may change frequently. Find a printed source for factual information or consider omitting the passage from the article.

USAGE:

A Web site is a collection of pages under one domain name (such as lalecheleague.org). "LLLI Web site" refers to all the pages on the site, or the concept of having a Web site. "LLLI Web page" refers to a single page within the Web site. Ex. "Look for our Group's Web page on the LLLI Web site."

New Beginnings Writers' Guidelines

The purpose of New Beginnings is to inform and inspire LLL members worldwide through articles, stories, poems, and other information about breastfeeding and parenting that reflect LLL's philosophy and mission.

What we're looking for

Narrative features—Mothers' stories, Focus on Fathers, Growing Families

- The primary purpose is to tell a personal story.
- Use a first person perspective, and a conversational tone.
- Leave the reader with hope.
- Strike a balance between describing details and sharing feelings.
- Photos of your child and/or family add to the appeal of these stories. (We will do our best to return photos after use; however, they are occasionally lost, so it is best not to send the only copy of a favorite photo. Please identify everyone in the photo. Digital images must be at least 300 dpi and must be in jpg or gif format.)

Mothers' stories

- Focus is on breastfeeding and/or mothering issues.
- Stories usually concern children under the age of about one year, but may vary depending on the underlying theme of the story.

Focus on Fathers

- Presents a celebration of the father's unique role in the life of his breast-fed baby.

Growing Families

- Shows how LLL philosophy can be applied as children grow older.

Informative features—feature articles, Information Please, Eating Wisely

- The primary purpose is to develop an idea or discuss a topic.
- Usually there is a third person perspective; personal examples may add interest or help illustrate a point.
- A more formal tone is used. Include references (use books from Group Libraries where possible).
- Balance general statements and claims with supporting evidence and examples.

Feature articles

These are written with the first-time mother in mind and reflect LLL philosophy. References are helpful, because they provide a way for mothers to find out more about a topic that interests them. References to books available from LLLI or in LLL Group Libraries are preferred.

Information Please

Provides current, referenced information about the benefits of human milk and other topics related to breastfeeding.

Eating Wisely

Thoughtful, creative stories are designed to increase the readers' understanding about nutrition and provide practical information about feeding families.

Toddler Tips, Staying Home Instead, and Making It Work

These question-and-answer columns pose real or hypothetical situations about different aspects of mothering and breastfeeding. Our readers send a variety of responses, which helps us to mimic the atmosphere at LLL meetings (both online and in person), where a mother can ask a question and gather ideas from others in similar situations. Leaders are encouraged to contribute to these columns.

Things to avoid

- Broad generalizations (example: "No mother would . . ." or "All women feel . . ." Very few things are true or false for every mother.)
- Brand names (except where it would add to the sense of the story)
- Mixing causes
- Describing in detail experiences that go beyond the general topic of mothering through breastfeeding (example: circumcision, vaccinations, home schooling, alternative medicine, home birth, vegan/kosher/non-dairy diets)
- Criticizing health care professionals

Length

Write what needs to be said—no more, no less. A column inch is about 40 words. One-page articles or columns are 800–900 words. Lead articles may be 2000–3000 words.

Submitting articles or stories

All submissions will be acknowledged. Submissions that are accepted for publication become the property of LLLI and will be edited for clarity, grammatical usage, and adherence to LLLI publishing guidelines. Authors whose submissions are published will receive two complimentary copies of the issue in which their work appears. Submissions may be held for a time before publication. We are unable to return unused submissions.

Send submissions to:
LLLI Attn: NEW BEGINNINGS Editor
1400 N. Meacham Rd.
Schaumburg, IL 60173
EditorNB@llli.org
Please remember to include your mailing address when sending submissions via email.

FORMS

Date Received: _____
Date Answered: _____

La Leche League
Monthly Activity Report

_____
Group Name

Meeting   1 2 3 4 *or* Special Meeting: _____

_____   _____
Date and Time of Meeting   Location of Meeting

_____   _____
Meeting led by   Completed by

Attendance:
_____ # of Leaders
_____ # of Leader Applicants
_____ # of moms at first meeting
_____ # repeaters (*not Leader Applicants*)
_____ # visitors: (*nurse, midwife, baby-sitter,*
              grandmother, other _____)
Other Leaders Attending:

_____ **Total adults at meeting**
_____ Total # of babies, children, & toddlers
_____ # of pregnant moms

Group:
          ❏ Is Doing Well   ❏ Needs Help

Library Additions:

Group Activity:
_____ Memberships collected
          New _____ Renewals _____
_____ WABs sold
_____ Other items sold: _____

Financial Activity:
Bank Balance: $_____
Expenses pending: $_____
Donations from Leaders: $_____
          (*cash value of stamps, phone calls, etc.*)
Quarterly tax & membership report to Area filed:
          ❏ Apr   ❏ Jul   ❏ Oct   ❏ Jan

          Phone Helping Calls:
_____ # of Leaders answering calls this month
_____ via phone
_____ via e-mail/fax
_____ personal (*home/hospital visit; casual contact*
              at church/store/community meeting, etc.)
_____ **Total number of helping calls this month**

My thoughts about the meeting:

Generally, the meeting was   ❏ terrific   ❏ just fine   ❏ so-so   ❏ not too good   5/00 em

SAMPLE MEDIA RELEASES

Many Groups submit short articles like these to the newspaper in their community to announce their meeting each month. An interesting fact about breastfeeding and/or La Leche League can be mentioned along with meeting information and Leaders' phone numbers. Be sure to include a name and phone number at the top of each news release so an editor can contact you if there are further questions.

Meeting 1

La Leche League to Meet

ANYTOWN—Planning to breast-feed? Then you'll want the information and encouragement that La Leche League provides. Leaders are experienced breastfeeding mothers, accredited by La Leche League International. Whether you're pregnant or already nursing, LLL has something for you—tips and techniques shared by mothers who have enjoyed a successful breastfeeding relationship.

Services available include monthly informational meetings, lending library and 24-hour phone help for breastfeeding problems or questions. All mothers and their babies are welcome.

A new series of meetings is starting on (date) at (time). For directions to the meeting or more information, please call (Leaders' first names and phone numbers).

Meeting 2

La Leche Meeting Set

ANYTOWN—Breastfeeding is the most convenient way to feed a baby. It saves time and energy for a busy mother. Discussion at the next meeting of La Leche League of ____ will cover this and other topics, such as getting breast-feeding off to a good start, how often and how long a baby nurses, the father's role and returning to work when nursing.

If there's a new baby in your life or you are expecting, you are encouraged to bring your questions and concerns to the meeting on (date) at (time).

Other LLL services include a lending library and 24-hour telephone help. For directions to the meeting or help with a breastfeeding concern call (Leaders' first names and phone numbers).

Meeting 3

Mother-to-Mother

ANYTOWN—Mother-to-mother support is the heart of La Leche League. No book on breastfeeding can equal talking to experienced nursing mothers and seeing their happy babies. At La Leche League Meetings mothers find a continuing source of information, inspiration and support.

La Leche League Leaders guide discussion at the meetings and answer questions from the group or individually. The next meeting, "The Art of Breastfeeding and Avoiding Difficulties" will be held (date) at (time) in (public place).

For directions to the meeting or more information, please call (Leaders' first names and phone numbers).

Meeting 1

LLL Begins New Series

Colostrum is the first milk produced by a new mother. Not only is it specifically suited to a newborn's nutritional needs but it protects baby against infection with its immunoglobulins, leukocytes and anti-inflammatory factors not available in artificial feeding products. As a result of this free "health insurance," breastfed babies enjoy good health, see their doctors less often and allow their parents to miss less work.

Learn more about the advantages of breastfeeding for baby and the whole family, borrow books on breastfeeding and parenting and meet other mothers and mothers-to-be at a new series of four monthly meetings

La Leche League of ____ meets (date) at (time). Babies are welcome at our meetings. Call (Leaders' first names and phone numbers) for more information or directions.

Meeting 4

La Leche League

ANYTOWN—Studies have confirmed that breastfeeding offers mothers protection against breast cancer and that the risk decreases as the duration of breastfeeding increases.

Continued breastfeeding, weaning and nutrition are topics for discussion at the La Leche League meeting held (date) at (time). LLL Leaders are available to answer questions during the discussion or one-to-one after the meeting. For directions to the meeting or more information, please call (Leaders' first names and phone numbers).

Meeting 2

Breastfeeding

ANYTOWN—Are you looking for information about how to start breastfeeding? Do you have questions about how often or how long babies nurse? Do you have concerns about spoiling your baby, managing household tasks with a new baby or helping the baby's father feel comfortable in his role? Are you thinking about returning to work and wonder if it's still possible to nurse?

Learn more about these issues and the breastfeeding family at a meeting of La Leche League of ____ on (date) at (time). The program will be "There's a New Baby in Your Life." All mothers and mothers-to-be are welcome. Babies are welcome, too!

For directions to the meeting or more information, please call (Leaders' first names and phone numbers).

Meeting 3

Avoiding Breastfeeding Difficulties

ANYTOWN—Many breast-feeding problems—low milk supply, soreness, baby fussiness——can be avoided if a mother is well informed about breastfeeding. La Leche League provides information, encouragement and support.

Mothers and mothers-to-be who would like to learn more about the normal course of breastfeeding are invited to the LLL of _____ meeting held (date) at (time).

Babies are welcome at our meetings. Call (Leaders' first names and phone numbers) for more information or directions.

Meeting 4

La Leche League to Meet

ANYTOWN—La Leche League believes breastfeeding gives babies the best possible start in life. LLL also emphasizes continued wholesome nutrition for the whole family, encouraging a balanced diet of foods in as close their natural state as possible.

"Breastfeeding and Beyond" will be the topic at the next LLL of _____ meeting on (date) at (time). Mothers and expectant mothers are invited to attend this discussion on nutrition and weaning. Babies are welcome too. For directions to the meeting or more information, please call (Leaders' first names and phone numbers).

General

La Leche League

ANYTOWN—La Leche League meetings emphasize the joys of breastfeeding while they inform and encourage mothers who wish to nurse their babies. LLL offers mother-to-mother help in a series of four meetings based on the book THE WOMANLY ART OF BREASTFEEDING, published by La Leche League International.

Discussions at meetings include the latest medical research as well as mothers' personal experiences. LLL services include a lending library and 24-hour phone help for breastfeeding problems and questions.

LLL of _____ meets (date) at (time). Mothers with their nursing babies and mothers-to-be are welcome. For directions to the meeting or more information, please call (Leaders' first names and phone numbers).

Employed Mothers Meeting

Working and Breastfeeding

A breastfeeding mother planning to return to work or be away from her baby for any length of time needs to know the "when" "where" and "how" of pumping and storing breast milk. These and other topics of interest to employed breastfeeding mothers will be addressed at a special "Breastfeeding and Working" meeting presented by LLL of _____.

LLL Leaders will provide information and handouts to interested mothers and mothers-to-be. The meeting will be held (date) at (time) in (public place). For directions to the meeting or more information, please call (Leaders' first names and phone numbers).

General

Breastfeeding

ANYTOWN—Whether you breastfeed your baby six days, six weeks or six months, you'll find La Leche League meetings supportive and informative.

LLL of _____ will meet on (date) at (time). Mothers with their nursing babies and mothers-to-be are welcome. For directions to the meeting or more information, please call (Leaders' first names and phone numbers).

General

Breastfeeding Saves Money

Save up to $30 a week! Sound too good to be true? Breastfeeding instead of purchasing an artificial feeding product for your baby can save a family money.

Expectant and new mothers can learn more about breastfeeding at the La Leche League of _____ meeting on (date) at (time). Meeting discussion will include the latest medical research as well as mother's personal experiences. Attend and meet other mothers who are new parents like yourself. Leaders accredited by La Leche League International lead the discussion and are available to answer individual questions.

For directions to the meeting or more information, please call (Leaders' first names and phone numbers).

RADIO ANNOUNCEMENTS

The radio is another way to increase the awareness of LLL in the community. One main idea with supporting points is presented in each announcement. Short sentences are easy to read and comprehend on the air. Include a name and phone number at the top of each radio announcement so someone can contact you if there are further questions.

Economic Advantages

Mother's milk is the best food for babies. And giving your baby the best saves you money too.

- Mother's milk is free and available around the clock.
- Mothers don't need to eat more to make plenty of milk for their babies. A normal balanced diet is all you need.
- Breastfeeding promotes infant health because mother's milk contains natural immunities. You save money on doctor visits and expensive medicines.

If you'd like information or need help nursing your baby, call La Leche ("lay-chay") League at (phone number).

Employed Mothers

Many women wonder if they can continue nursing their babies when they return to work. The answer is "yes"! Research shows that it's easier to combine working and breastfeeding when you take these three steps:

- Take the longest maternity leave you can. Your milk supply will be better established, and you'll feel more confident in your nursing and mothering.
- Try to work shorter hours at first. This will make all aspects of mothering easier.
- If you'll have to miss a feeding, try to plan for collecting your milk at work. This helps you keep up your milk supply.

Mothers who combine breastfeeding and working say that it's convenient and worthwhile. For more information, call La Leche ("lay-chay") League at (phone number).

General Breastfeeding

Mother knows best—did you know that mother's milk is the superior infant food?

- It contains the right nutrients, in the right amounts. And the milk changes as the baby grows, adapting to the baby's needs.
- Milk supply adjusts to the baby's need. In general, the more a mother nurses her baby, the more milk she has.
- Mother's milk is always fresh, warm and ready to serve. Breastfeeding is safe and convenient.

La Leche ("lay-chay") League is available to help women who are interested in breastfeeding. Call (phone number).

Immunities in Human Milk

Mother's milk is the superior infant food. Breastfeeding benefits infant health.

- Babies cannot become allergic to their own mother's milk.
- Mother's milk contains natural immunities, so babies have fewer illnesses.
- When a baby does get sick, mother's milk is good medicine. Doctors have remarked how quickly breastfed babies recover.

MEDIA RELEASES

Women who are interested in breastfeeding can call La Leche ("lay-chay") League at (phone number).

GLOSSARY OF LLLI ABBREVIATIONS

AIPC—Agreement of International Principles of Cooperation

ACC—Area Communications Coordinator

ACL—Area Coordinator of Leaders

ACLA—Associate Coordinator of Leader Accreditation

ACE—Area Coordinator of Events

ACS—Area Conference Supervisor

AFC—Area Financial Coordinator

ALL—Area Leaders' Letter

ALLE—Area Leaders' Letter Editor

APL—Area Professional Liaison

BEC—Book Evaluation Committee

BEG—Book Evaluation Guidelines

CBI—Center for Breastfeeding Information

CE—Continuing Education

CEU—Continuing Education Unit

CERP—Continuing Education Recognition Point

CME—Continuing Medical Education

CLA—Coordinator of Leader Accreditation

CSD—Communication Skills Department

CSI/CSF—Communication Skills Instructor/ Communication Skills Facilitator

DA—District Advisor

DC—District Coordinator

EUS—Eastern United States Division

ED—Executive Director

FAC—Founders' Advisory Council

HAC—Health Advisory Council

ID—International Division

LLL—La Leche League

LLLI—La Leche League International

LAC—Legal Advisory Council

LAD—Leader Accreditation Department

MAC—Management Advisory Council

MA—Medical Associate

PAB—Professional Advisory Board

PC—Peer Counselor

PCPA—Peer Counselor Program Administrator

PSR—Policies and Standing Rules Notebook

PL—Professional Liaison

OPLR—Online Professional Liaison Resource

USWD—United States Western Division

Index